Breast Cancer 3
Advances in Research and Treatment

Current Topics

Breast Cancer
Advances in Research and Treatment

Edited by **WILLIAM L. McGUIRE, M.D.**

Volume 1 • **CURRENT APPROACHES TO THERAPY**

Volume 2 • **EXPERIMENTAL BIOLOGY**

Volume 3 • **CURRENT TOPICS**

A Continuation Order Plan is available for this series. A continuation order will bring delivery of each new volume immediately upon publication. Volumes are billed only upon actual shipment. For further information please contact the publisher.

Breast Cancer 3
Advances in Research and Treatment

Current Topics

Edited by
William L. McGuire, M. D.

University of Texas Health Science Center
San Antonio, Texas

Springer Science+Business Media, LLC

Library of Congress Cataloging in Publication Data

Main entry under title:

Breast cancer.

Includes bibliographical references and index.
Vol. 1 has special title.
1. Breast—Cancer. [DNLM: 1. Breast neoplasms. 2. Breast neoplasms—Therapy.
WP870 B8245]
RC280.B8B673   616'.9'94'49   77-23505
ISBN 978-1-4899-2665-4 (v. 3)

ISBN 978-1-4899-2665-4   ISBN 978-1-4899-2663-0 (eBook)
DOI 10.1007/978-1-4899-2663-0

© Springer Science+Business Media New York 1979
Originally published by Plenum Press, New York in 1979
Softcover reprint of the hardcover 1st edition 1979

Contributors

J. Bailar, III, National Cancer Institute, National Institutes of Health, Bethesda, Maryland 20014

Gary C. Chamness, Department of Medicine, University of Texas Health Science Center, San Antonio, Texas 78284

Richard B. Everson, National Cancer Institute, National Institutes of Health, Bethesda, Maryland 20014

Pietro M. Gullino, Laboratory of Pathophysiology, National Cancer Institute, National Institutes of Health, Bethesda, Maryland 20014

Untae Kim, Department of Pathology, Roswell Park Memorial Institute, New York State Department of Health, Buffalo, New York 14263

Marvin A. Kirschner, New Jersey Medical School, Newark Beth Israel Medical Center, Newark, New Jersey 07112

Marc E. Lippman, National Cancer Institute, National Institutes of Health, Bethesda, Maryland 20014

William L. McGuire, Department of Medicine, University of Texas Health Science Center, San Antonio, Texas 78284

James A. Rillema, Department of Physiology, Wayne State University School of Medicine, Detroit, Michigan 48201

Eugeniusz Samojlik, Department of Medicine, Division of Endocrinology, and The Specialized Cancer Center, The Milton S. Hershey Medical Center, The Pennsylvania State University, Hershey, Pennsylvania 17033

Richard J. Santen, Department of Medicine, Division of Endocrinology, and The Specialized Cancer Center, The Milton S. Hershey Medical Center, The Pennsylvania State University, Hershey, Pennsylvania 17033

Preface

Breast cancer continues to be a major problem. In Volume 1 of this series we dealt exclusively with topics concerned with therapy. In Volume 2 we explored various aspects of experimental biology which are critical to our developing better methods of diagnosis and treatment. In the present volume, we turn to a series of individual topics of considerable interest, including systemic methods for hormonal ablation, screening for early cancer, male breast cancer, and more.

The first chapter addresses the question of why some breast tumors metastasize and others do not. Based on elegant animal tumor models, Kim believes that metastasizing tumor cells are the undesirable by-product of the host immune surveillance mechanism. Unstable membrane structures lead to shedding of membrane constituents, abnormal locomotive properties, and evasion of the host defense system. Factors which alter membrane structure will therefore have to be considered in our approach to the management of early breast cancer.

With the advent of adjuvant chemotherapy and its demonstrated success in certain patient subsets, it is logical to design adjuvant therapies which also include an endocrine manipulation. Surgical adrenalectomy has long been used in the advanced disease setting but there is considerable reluctance to use major ablative surgery in the adjuvant setting because of the associated morbidity. Santen and Samojlik offer a rational alternative, medical adrenalectomy. In this chapter they review the physiologic basis for adrenalectomy and various non-surgical approaches that have been used to achieve adrenal steroid suppression. They present a thorough pharmacological approach for optimally combining aminoglutethimide and hydrocortisone to block estrogen precursor production. It would appear from the clinical correlations that medical adrenalectomy may be equivalent to surgical adrenalectomy.

It is fashionable and important to understand how tumors *grow*, but the biochemical events leading to and surrounding tumor *regression* have not been sufficiently emphasized. Gullino brings us up to date with regard to regression of hormone-dependent mammary tumors. He is able to make four generalizations from considerable data. (1) The collapse of cell populations occurs in the absence of obviously toxic stimuli. (2) When physiological death occurs it is not simply the result of a sudden removal of vital supplies; tumors regress in an organized manner. (3) RNA and protein synthesis occur very early in involution. (4) Mobilization of phagocytes and lysosomal activity appear more often to be a secondary event following conditions that invite lysosomal attack, rather than a primary cause of regression. These insights should provide fresh clues for more effective therapy design.

Turning to intracellular mediators of mammary tumor cell growth and function, the chapter by Rillema reviews the role of cyclic nucleotides, binding proteins, and kinases, as well as prostaglandins and polyamines. Since an antagonist has been identified for each of these possible mediators, clinical application should soon follow. For example, there is now a resurgence of interest in the use of methyl GAG to block polyamine synthesis in patients with a variety of malignancies.

Now that all agree that estrogen receptor determinations should be obtained on all breast cancer patients. the inevitable question is—who, how, and where? Chamness and McGuire focus on "how" and discuss the background of receptor assays, proceeding to critically examine virtually all of the published methods. The special problems of assaying progesterone, androgen, and glucocorticoid receptors, as well as estrogen receptors, are presented. This chapter should serve as a valuable reference for those concerned with choosing one assay technique over another.

For decades, investigators have been trying to identify a particular hormonal environment that would promote the development of breast cancer. Many hypotheses have been put forth based on urinary excretions of various steroids in women at various risks of developing breast cancer. Kirschner critically examines these data, beginning with both endogenous and exogenous estrogens, the androgens and their metabolites, progesterone, prolactin, and thyroid and pituitary hormones. He forces us to conclude that, as yet, no clear-cut pattern of abnormal hormone production or abnormal hormone milieu has been found in women at increased risk for breast cancer. This is certainly disappointing. Nevertheless, an immense amount of epidemiological data exists associating hormones and breast cancer; clearly, we must sharpen our thinking and hypotheses, because therein may be an answer to preventing the disease.

In the past year, there has been hardly anything to match the controversy surrounding mammographic screening for early breast cancer. Because of the sharp differences of opinion regarding the risk versus benefit of routine screening, the National Cancer Institute and the American Cancer Society have issued guidelines for the proper use of mammographic screening. Bailar has been one of the visible figures in calling attention to the risks and in the present chapter provides an overview of the data leading to the present guidelines. It is likely that as more data on benefit accrue from the breast cancer demonstration projects, and as improved technology results in lower doses of radiation being delivered, the guidelines may change yet again.

We tend to ignore the male in most discussions of breast cancer in view of the relatively low incidence of the problem. In this volume, however, Everson and Lippman provide us with a complete account of the disease in males, from etiology to diagnosis and treatment. In addition, new data is provided regarding steroid receptor status. The latter should be important since the endocrine approach to treatments is analogous to that of the female with breast cancer.

In summary, Volume 3 of this series covers a wide range of topics, all of which we hope will provide stimulating reading for basic biologists as well as clinicians caring for breast cancer patients.

William L. McGuire, M.D.

May, 1979

Contents

3. Medical Adrenalectomy for Treatment of Metastatic Breast Carcinoma

Richard J. Santen and Eugeniusz Samojlik

4. Actions and Metabolism of Intracellular Mediators in Neoplastic Mammary Cells

James A. Rillema

5. **Methods for Analyzing Steroid Receptors in Human Breast Cancer**

   Gary C. Chamness and William L. McGuire

6. The Role of Hormones in the Development of Human Breast Cancer

Marvin A. Kirschner

7. Risks and Benefits of Mammography

J. Bailar, III

8. Male Breast Cancer

Richard B. Everson and Marc E. Lippman

Factors Influencing Metastasis of Breast Cancer

UNTAE KIM

1. Introduction

Metastasis is the most critical attribute of all human cancers, particularly for those of nonvital, surface organs such as the breast. In general, patients undergoing removal of small breast tumors, prior to the development of axillary lymph node metastases, have a better cure or long-term survival rate than those with large tumors or axillary involvement. The ten-year survival rate of women with small breast cancers treated with standard extirpative surgery has been reported to be more than 80%, dropping to about 50% when one to three axillary lymph nodes are involved, and to 25% when more than three nodes are positive.[1,2] Consequently, greater efforts are being directed toward the early detection of breast cancer by various means. However, even some small tumors may have already spread to the regional lymph nodes by the time they are clinically detected, and, in other instances, the cancer may recur and disseminate widely after an extended period of dormancy. The annual mortality rate of breast cancer patients, reported as 39%, has not changed over the past 40 years.[3] This lack of improvement in the survival rate can be attributed mainly to our deficient understanding of the biology of metastasis, and, more directly, to the insufficient

UNTAE KIM • Department of Pathology, Roswell Park Memorial Institute, New York State Department of Health, Buffalo, New York 14263.

knowledge of its mechanisms. Therefore, a critical analysis of factors influencing metastasis of breast cancer may be a useful and timely task.

2. Pathogenesis of Metastasizing Mammary Cancer

Unlike human cancer, most animal solid tumors, including mammary tumors, grow expansively at the site of origin without infiltrating the surrounding tissues or metastasizing to distant organs, even when they become very large. These fundamental differences in the biological characteristics of human and animal tumors may lie in their respective pathogeneses. Most laboratory investigators tend to favor fast-growing animal tumor models which have been induced with potent chemical, viral, or physical carcinogens, and select those with a short latency period. Such tumors are usually highly immunogenic,[4] due probably to the lack of sufficient time to undergo host immunoselective processes. In contrast, human cancers, except for some of those caused as the sequelae of occupational or industrial hazards, usually occur late in life, and their longer latency period may be attributable to a more subtle exposure to oncogens, developing through various immunological and endocrinological selective forces generated by the host and leading to less immunogenic tumors. These assumptions were tested in laboratory animals by subjecting them to various immunological stimulations and inhibitions during the carcinogenic period. The procedure was successful in yielding many spontaneously metastasizing mammary tumors in female rats with biological, biochemical, and immunological characteristics resembling those of human breast cancer.[5,6]

2.1. Induction of Spontaneously Metastasizing Mammary Tumors

It is well established that all carcinogens have an immunosuppressive effect on laboratory animals,[7] and that further immunological intervention, such as neonatal thymectomy, enhances tumorigenesis in certain strains of rodents.[8-12] The effect of neonatal splenectomy on the development of the host immune surveillance mechanism, however, is not clear.[13-15] Furthermore, neither thymectomy nor splenectomy in adult animals seems to cause any clinically recognizable immunodepression, although adult thymectomy has been reported to produce diminished *in vitro* blastogenic response to phytohemagglutinin (PHA) and concanavalin A (con A) by the host spleen cells.[16] Squartini[17] reported that either neonatal thymectomy or splenectomy in the high-mammary-tumor strain of virgin BALB/cf(C3H) mice caused decreased mammary tumor incidence and delayed the tumor onset, but when both ablations were combined the incidence increased back to the level of normal mice. In RIII mice, on the other hand, neither procedure alone had any appreciable effect on the tumor incidence, but it decreased markedly when the ablations were combined. In force-bred female BALB/cfRIII mice, thymectomy delayed tumor onset, but it had no effect on the overall tumor incidence. It has also been reported that some of the sarcomas induced in neonatally thymectomized mice were rejected by intact syngeneic mice upon transplantation, suggesting a possible antigenic modification in these tumor cells.[12] Thus, it is reasonable to postulate that the absence of thymus and/or spleen in chemical carcinogen-fed female rats affects not only the tumor incidence, but also the biological properties of the induced tumors. An experiment to this effect was carried out in conjunction with specific and nonspecific immunological stimulations during the tumor development to promote immunoselection of certain tumor cell clones.

2.1.1. Chemical Mammary Tumorigenesis

Four groups of ten highly inbred, young-adult W/Fu female rats each were fed 200 mg of 3-methylcholanthrene. A week prior to the feeding, the first group was thymectomized, the second splenectomized, the third thymectomized and splenectomized, and the fourth left intact. The surgical immunosuppression caused a 20, 31, and 45% increase, respectively, of mammary tumor incidence over the control group in an 18-month period. In a parallel experiment, the incidence in general was decreased by 30–40% when such animals were immunostimulated with injections of sheep red blood cells and dinitrophenol sulfonate-conjugated bovine gamma globulin prior to the development of tumors.

A total of 213 primary mammary adenocarcinomas were induced in the first experiment, with each rat producing more than one tumor and occasionally as many as six. Among these tumors, 13 (6.1%) regressed spontaneously before they reached 5 mm in average diameter, and, in rats where a surgical excision of an early-appearing, putatively more antigenic tumor was done in order to evoke host immune response against similarly antigenic latent tumor cells, 16 additional primary mammary tumors, some as large as 12 mm in diameter, regressed completely. Of the 184 progressively growing primary tumors, 93 were transplanted into normal syngeneic female rats when they reached an average diameter of about 15 mm, of which three were rejected. Twenty-nine of the 90 successfully transplanted tumors (32.2%) metastasized spontaneously in the secondary host, 15 of them originating from the surgically immunosuppressed groups in which an early-appearing tumor had been excised. Thus, four types of immunologically distinct tumors induced in this experiment can be identified: (1) containing antigen incompatible with the autochthonous hosts, although small numbers of these tumor cells may escape or "sneak through"[18]; (2) growing well in autochthonous hosts, but rejected by normal syngeneic hosts upon transplantation; (3) growing well in secondary normal syngeneic hosts and carrying tumor-specific transplantation antigen (TSTA); and (4) becoming nonimmunogenic and metastatic as a result of repeated immunoselection during their development. The lack of understanding of the precise mechanisms in the development of tumors in thymectomized and/or splenectomized hosts notwithstanding, judging from the results of this experiment alone we may conclude that a sustained repression of the immunological system during carcinogenesis is likely to enhance tumor incidence, and that immunostimulation during tumorigenesis may cause the emergence of nonimmunogenic tumor cell clones. Hence, the development of spontaneously metastasizing tumors is an undesirable consequence of the host immune surveillance mechanism.

2.1.2. Viral Mammary Tumorigenesis

Squartini and associates[19,20] seem to have developed the first spontaneously metastasizing mouse mammary tumors induced by mammary tumor viruses (MuMTV). They reported a difference in "bioactivity" between the C3H and RIII strains of MuMTV in their relative capacity to develop mammary tumors and lung metastases in female BALB/cf mice during 20 months of observation. The C3H virus caused mammary tumors in 47.5% and the RIII strain in 14.6% of the infected mice, despite the fact that the latter yielded far greater quantities of viruses in the milk. The frequency of lung metastases in the tumor-bearing mice was 63.1% for the former and 16.6% for the latter, seemingly occurring via the hematogenous route exclusively, as is the case with most metastasizing murine tumors. The mechanisms of such metastasis are yet to be investigated. The authors postulated that the causative MuMTV might be directly involved in the complex processes leading to the development of secondary tumors in the lung, in addition to the usual mode of tumor cell dissemination from the primary site. Perhaps another critical factor in the development of lung metastasis in these mice is the rather long latency period of these tumors (average of 496 and 517 days, respectively), time enough to undergo various selective processes.

Human herpes simplex virus type 2, which was originally implicated in human cervical cancer, also seems capable of inducing spontaneously metastasizing fibrosarcomas in weanling Syrian hamsters.[21] Fifty-seven percent of these animals developed lung metastases after being injected subcutaneously with virus-transformed hamster embryo fibroblasts that had been passed through newborn hamsters. These metastases also seem to have been the result of direct hematogenous tumor cell dissemination.

2.1.3. Hormonal Mammary Tumorigenesis

Cutts and Noble[22,23] reported that some of the mammary tumors induced in male rats by chronic administration of estrogen were stimulated by androgen and metastasized spontaneously. Further studies are needed to learn the pathogenesis of such tumors, but it is possible that the thymolytic effect of estrogen may have contributed to the development of metastasizing tumor cell clones.

2.1.4. Radiation Mammary Tumorigenesis

Whole-body ionizing radiation is also a potent mammary oncogen.[24] A single dose of 400 roentgens produces mammary adenocarcinomas in more than 30% of young-adult female rats within three months, and this tumor incidence can be increased to 100% by stimulating their mammary glands with either prolactin or estrogen.[25] However, these radiation-induced mammary tumors tend to be hormonally autonomous.[26] We have not found any spontaneously metastasizing, radiation-induced mammary tumors in rodents as yet.

2.1.5. Miscellaneous Metastasizing Tumors

There are several spontaneously metastasizing carcinomas and sarcomas in laboratory animals, including the Walker carcinosarcoma 256 being used by various investigators. However, because the tumors were discovered by chance, the pathogenesis of most of them cannot be traced.

2.2. Characteristics of Spontaneously Metastasizing Rat Mammary Carcinomas

2.2.1. Biological Properties

Upon implantation of viable tumor cells into the right inguinal mammary fat pad of normal syngeneic, young-adult rats, the metastasizing mammary adenocarcinomas spread by either the lymphatic or hematogenous route, or by both, to distant sites. Most of them metastasize via the lymphatic route, beginning with the regional lymph node and eventually involving most lymph nodes, liver, lung, bone marrow, and other parenchymatous organs (Fig. 1). A few disseminate exclusively via the hematogenous route to the lung. Nine of these tumors, representative of different metastasizing characteristics, were selected and are being maintained in our laboratory. Their degree of metastasizing capacity is graded arbitrarily according to the latency and extent of metastasis (Table I). The most virulent strain metastasizes to the axillary lymph node before the transplanted tumor becomes palpable (Fig. 2), whereas the least virulent one produces only microscopic metastasis in the lung after the primary has become very large (more than 30 mm in average diameter). Some of the tumors that metastasize via the lymphatics have a predictable dissemination pattern which follows a precise sequence of involvement, e.g., begins with the regional lymph node, continues to the lymph node chain on the same side, then onto the opposite side, and eventually spreads to the lung, liver, and bone marrow.

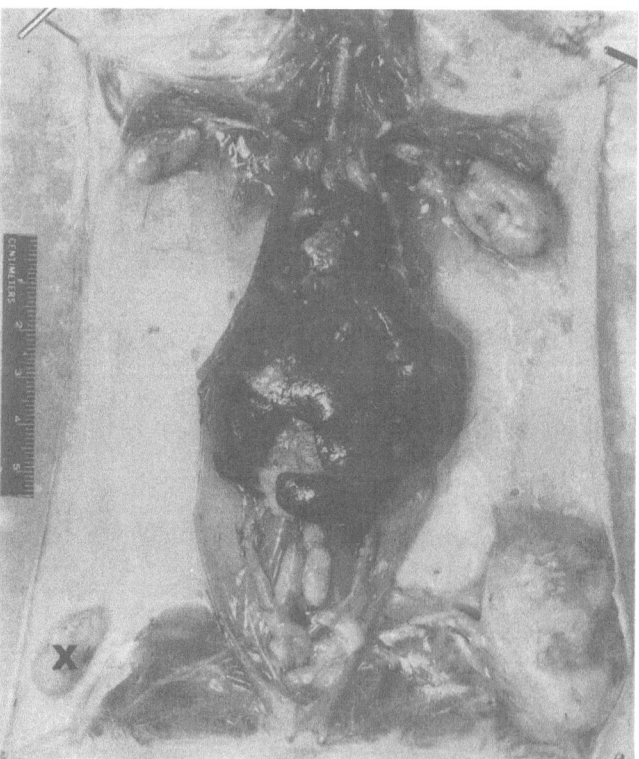

Fig. 1. W/Fu female rat bearing a metastasizing mammary carcinoma (×). Note the widespread metastasis to all lymph nodes and liver. The lung and bones are also involved.

Table I
Characteristics of Established Spontaneously Metastasizing Mammary Carcinomas in W/Fu Rats

Tumor strain	Metastasizing capacity[a]	Metastasizing routes and sites
TMT-50	0–+	Hematogenous; lung only
STMT-058	+–++	Hematogenous and lymphatic; lymph node and lung
MT-449	++	Hematogenous and lymphatic; lymph node and lung
SMT-077	++–+++	Lymphatic; lymph node
DMBA-4	++–+++	Lymphatic and hematogenous; lymph node and lung
DMBA-4R (regressing)	++–+++	Lymphatic and hematogenous; lymph node and lung
SMT-2A	++++	Lymphatic; lymph node, lung, and bone
SMT-2B	++++	Lymphatic; lymph node, lung, liver, bone, and spleen
TMT-081 (solid and ascites)	++++	Hematogenous and lymphatic; lymph node, lung, liver, and spleen

[a] + = slight; ++ = moderate; +++ = marked; ++++ = extensive. Four nonmetastasizing tumors were used as controls.

a. Histology. Under microscopic examination, all metastasizing tumors show an invasive growth pattern, as evidenced by individual or groups of cells infiltrating the soft tissue around the tumor mass (Fig. 3), while the nonmetastasizing tumors grow only expansively, with their border sharply outlined by a thin capsule or compressed fibrofatty tissue (Fig. 4).

b. Estrogen Receptor Protein (ERP). ERP levels were analyzed in four strains of nonmetastasizing rat mammary carcinomas at varying stages of hormone responsiveness. They were found to decrease with the loss of hormone dependency,[27,28] whereas no measurable levels were detected in the metastasizing mammary tumors (Bronn, Kim, and Minton, unpublished data).

c. Tissue Culture. Metastasizing tumor cells seem to have less bonding power or stickiness when cultured with latex particles in suspension, growing singly or in small clusters, than do nonmetastasizing ones which usually adhere to the latex beads, forming cohesive tissue masses.

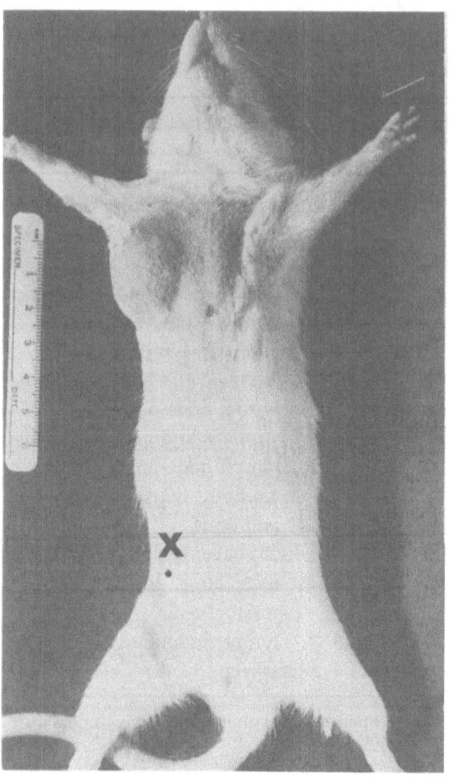

Fig. 2. W/Fu female rate implanted with a highly malignant, metastasizing mammary carcinoma in the right inguinal mammary fat pad (×). The metastatic tumor mass in the right axillary lymph node is already large, while the primary is not yet detectable.

2.2.2. Biochemical Properties

Analysis of plasma membrane marker enzymes of these tumors, e.g., 5'-nucleotidase, alkaline phosphatase, phosphodiesterase I, nucleotide pyrophosphatase, and alkaline RNAase, indicated that their levels are inversely related to the metastasizing capacity and antigen-shedding properties, but directly correlated with the immunogenicity and resistance to metastasis.[5,29,30] In contrast, the level of endogenous glycosyltransferase activity in the tumor cells, e.g., sialyltransferase, galactosyltransferase, and fucosyltransferase,[31–33] is directly correlated with the metastasizing capacity. In other words, the level of plasma membrane marker enzymes represents the amount of antigens remaining on the tumor cell surface, while that of glycosyltransferase represents the rate of antigen synthesis and turnover by the tumor cells. Along with the elevated glycosyltransferase activity in the metastasizing tumor cells, the enzyme levels in the sera of the hosts rise with the growth and dissemination of the tumor.[31,34] In spite of the low levels of 5'-nucleotidase, the metastasizing tumor cells contain two to three times more endogenous cyclic AMP (cAMP) than the nonmetastasizing ones, but the cAMP phosphodiesterase (PDE) levels reflect those of the membrane marker enzymes.[35] The antigen-shedding tumor cells also have an increased lysosomal activity in proportion to the metastasizing capacity.[36]

2.2.3. Characteristics of Tumor Cell-Surface Antigens

All spontaneously metastasizing tumors studied thus far are either weakly immunogenic or nonimmunogenic, particularly those which

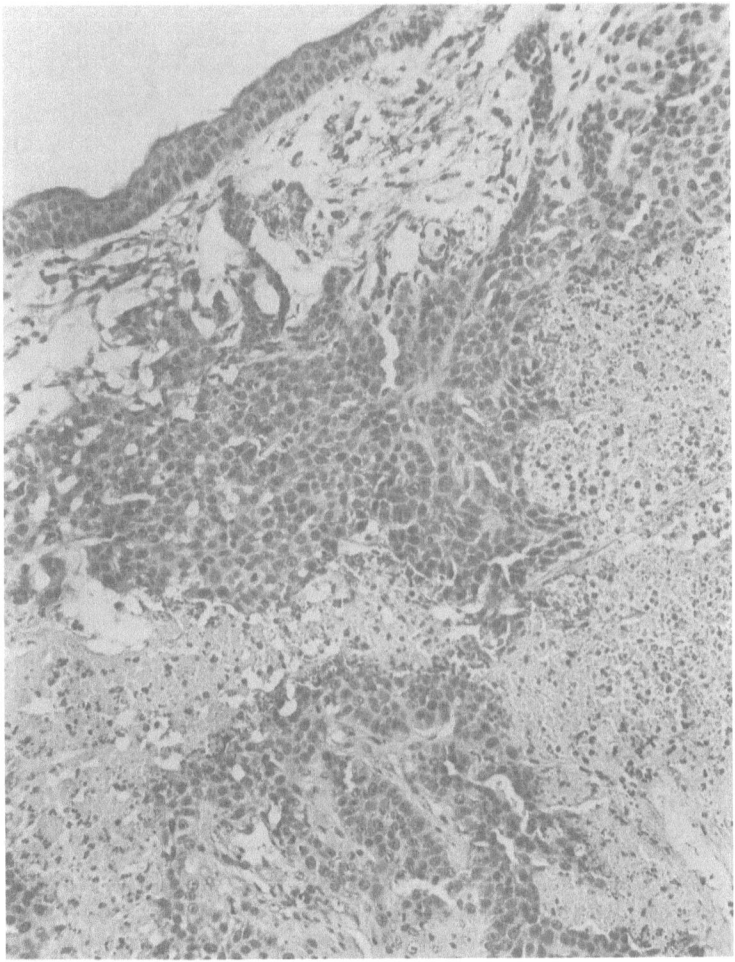

Fig. 3. Photomicrograph of rat skin over a metastasizing, invasive mammary carcinoma. The dermis is infiltrated by irregular nests of tumor cells. Hematoxylin and eosin, ×160.

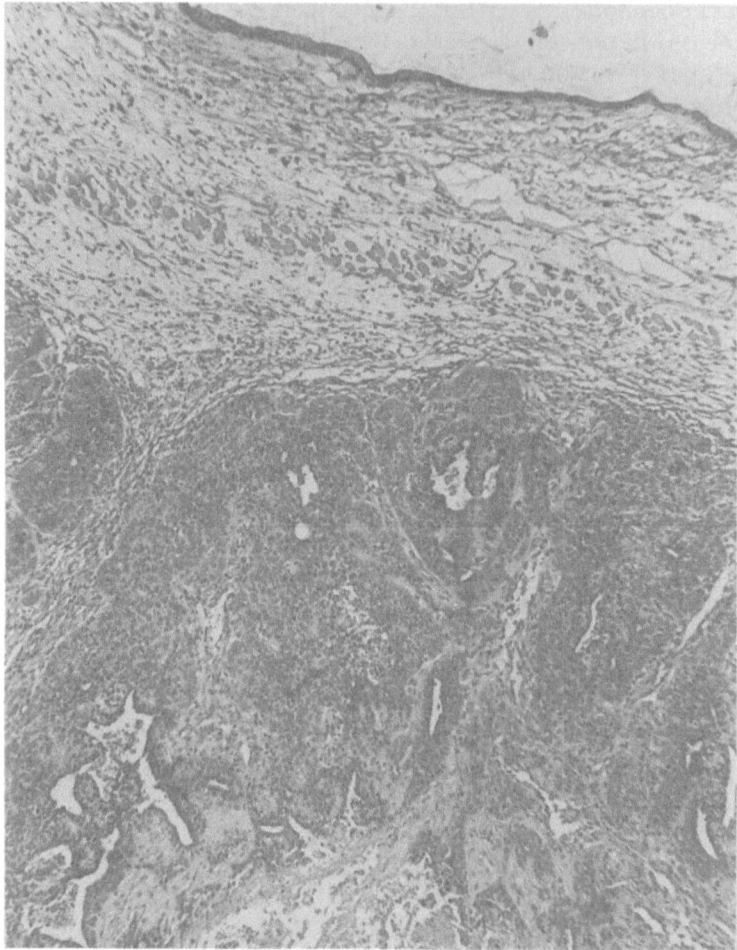

Fig. 4. Photomicrograph of rat skin over a nonmetastasizing mammary carcinoma. The tumor border is sharply delineated and surrounded by some inflammatory cells. Hematoxylin and eosin, ×80.

metastasize via the lymphatic route, whereas, with a few exceptions, most of the nonmetastasizing ones are highly immunogenic. Prior immunization with killed tumor cells protects the host from a corresponding challenge of viable, nonmetastasizing tumor cells, but the same procedure fails to prevent the growth of metastasizing cells. The latter readily shed soluble glycoconjugates (or glycoprotein antigens) from their surface into the systemic circulation of the host, resulting in the loss of their antigen markers and creating an excess of free antigen and antigen–antibody complexes.[29,37,38] The shed antigen can be found in the host sera as early as one week after the tumor implantation, considerably before such tumor is palpable. In contrast, the nonmetastasizing tumor cells seem to retain most of their surface antigens or release small amounts at a much slower rate. These antigens are probably locked in an immune-complex form and are not detected in the host sera at all, or sometimes at very low levels after the tumor becomes extremely large. The soluble glycoprotein antigen from metastasizing tumors, with a molecular weight of 28,000 daltons, cross-reacts with or has the same immunochemical identity as the antigen from normal, hyperplastic rat mammary gland, suggesting that it is an organ-specific antigen.[37,38] This may account for the lack of immunogenicity of these cells. In addition to the low levels of this antigen, the nonmetastasizing tumor cells seem to carry TSTA.[29]

2.2.4. Host Immune Responses

a. T Lymphocyte. The *in vitro* blastogenic response of lymphocytes, isolated by the Ficoll–Hypeque technique from spleen and peripheral blood of metastasizing and nonmetastasizing tumor-bearing rats, to PHA, con A, and bacterial lipopolysaccharide (LPS), showed differential stimulatory patterns as measured by [³H]thymidine incorporation (Kim and Han, unpublished data). The incorporation rate of the spleen cells from nonmetastasizing tumor hosts was much higher than that from the metastasizing ones, but lower than that from normal rats. Somewhat similar results were obtained with the peripheral-blood lymphocytes. These observations seem to indicate that these lymphocytes are functionally different and have an almost opposite reactivity, due perhaps to differential binding of the lymphocyte surface with free antigens or antibodies, or with immune complexes, reflecting different levels of suppressor T-cell activity. The rapid passage of shed antigens from the metastasizing tumors into the systemic circulation via the regional lymph node, before the tumors acquire blood vessels, may saturate and paralyze the lymph node, rendering it immunologically inert.[39]

b. B Lymphocyte. Precipitating antibodies are present, as demonstrated by the standard Ouchterlony radial immunodiffusion technique, in the tenfold concentrated sera from rats that had had a large nonmetastasizing tumor surgically excised two to three weeks before. In some hosts, the tumor need not be excised to induce elevated antibody levels in their sera. In contrast, elevated antibody levels are not detectable in the sera from metastasizing tumor hosts.

c. Macrophage. Macrophages isolated from both groups of tumor-bearing rats also manifested differential functional reactivity *in vitro*. In general, these rats yielded more peritoneal macrophages than normal control rats after an intraperitoneal injection of thioglycolate, with the metastasizing tumor hosts producing the cells more readily than the nonmetastasizing ones. In the standard capillary migration inhibition test for macrophages (MIF test), the peritoneal as well as the large peripheral mononuclear cells from nonmetastasizing tumor hosts, isolated by the Ficoll–Hypeque gradient, migrated as well as did normal control cells or were often slightly stimulated in blank culture media containing no tumor-associated antigens; the macrophages from metastasizing tumor hosts were markedly inhibited in the blank media, indicating that the surface property of these cells had already been altered *in vivo*. On the other hand, when the macrophages were incubated with their respective tumor-associated antigens, the migration of cells from nonmetastasizing tumor hosts was markedly inhibited, while that of cells from the metastasizing hosts was not only restored to the level of normal macrophages, but often stimulated, which may be analogous to "unblocking."[40]

d. *Growth Characteristics in Athymic Nude Mice.* In recent years, various allogeneic and xenogeneic tumors, including highly malignant human cancers, have been successfully transplanted into athymic nude mice. However, it was found that none of these malignant tumors develops metastases.[41] In order to test the relative growth and metastasizing pattern of the rat mammary tumors described here, and to further characterize the soluble, organ-specific antigen of metastasizing tumors as well as that of the plasma membrane-bound, nonmetastasizing rat mammary tumors, two sets of these tumors were implanted subcutaneously into the right mammary fat pad of athymic nude mice of BALB/c background.[42] Surprisingly, the graft of metastasizing rat tumors was either rejected outright or accepted only temporarily for a short period, without developing metastases. The nonmetastasizing rat tumors, on the other hand, were readily accepted by these mice and grew rapidly, producing large tumors and widespread hematogenous metastasis to the lung. These observations suggest that the "T-cell-deficient state" of the nude mouse is effective not only in preventing metastasis, but also in destroying the metastasizing tumor mass itself, while promoting the growth and hematogenous dissemination of the highly immunogenic, nonmetastasizing tumors. It was concluded, therefore, that (1) the soluble surface antigens of metastasizing tumors, which are tolerogenic in the normal syngeneic host, may be "thymus independent," becoming immunogenic in a T-cell-deficient host and evoking a cytotoxic environment against the tumor cells, and (2) the plasma membrane-bound antigens of nonmetastasizing tumors, which are immunogenic in syngeneic hosts, may be "thymus dependent," hence the uninhibited growth and widespread metastasis of these tumors in the T-cell-deficient milieu of nude mice. The creation of an appropriate immunological milieu to meet the specific quality of tumor-associated antigens would seem one of the more promising approaches to the control of human cancer.

3. Natural History of Breast Cancer

3.1. Evolution of Neoplastic State: Selection of Nonimmunogenic Tumor Cells

The neoplastic state evolves from "bad to worse," progressing from structurally well differentiated to poorly differentiated, from functional to nonfunctional, and from hormone dependence to autonomy, accompanied by a steady acceleration of growth rate. This evolutionary pattern is applicable to all cancers, except perhaps to the germ-cell tumors of testis and neuroblastoma. The best example of such a pattern is seen in the chemically induced, nonmetastasizing rat mammary adenocarcinomas[43] and the RIII-MuMTV-induced, pregnancy-dependent mouse mammary tumors.[44]. Primary mammary cancers may carry certain hormonal characteristics and their clinical appearance may sometimes seem abrupt or discontinuous, but this merely represents a phase in the evolutionary sequence arrived at through a gradual but continuous subclinical progression at cellular levels. Furthermore, some tumors may not necessarily go through the entire sequence of evolution within the lifetime of the host, the initial character of the cells having been determined by the balance of forces between carcinogens and physiological control mechanisms at the time of oncogenic exposure and during tumor development. The biological stability of a tumor seems to be dependent on the plurality of stem cells, which is in turn determined by factors such as the type and potency of carcinogens, duration and intensity of exposure, and the hormonal and immunological state of the host. However, acquisition of a degree of autonomy, together with accelerated growth rate and loss of glandular differentiation by tumors, does not lead to the development of metastasizing capacity. None of the rapidly growing, nonmetastasizing rat mammary tumors maintained in our laboratory by successive transplantations[43] has ever become metastatic. As already mentioned, tumor cells must be subjected to repeated immunological pressures during their development in order to select progressively less immunogenic tumor cell clones with the capacity to invade and metastasize. Thus, the progression from immunogenicity to nonimmunogenicity is analogous to that of hormone dependence to autonomy. However, these two processes evolve independently, often causing seemingly discordant biological patterns at random. For exam-

ple, (1) not all nonimmunogenic tumors metastasize[45]; (2) rapidly growing tumors may metastasize faster, but not necessarily wider; (3) metastasizing tumors in animals are usually hormone independent, with rare
exceptions,[46] whereas in man they may be hormone dependent[47–49];
and (4) poorly differentiated tumors always grow faster, but their
growth rate and degree of glandular differentiation are not related to
their metastasizing capacity. When such characteristics are seen in a
random combination, the natural history of human breast cancer becomes complex and often contradictory. More systematic analyses and
rational interpretation of clinical observations on the biological behavior
of human breast cancer are needed.

3.2. Predisposing Conditions for Metastasis

In order to better understand the pattern of metastasis and recurrence of human breast cancer, some of the outstanding, commonly accepted, or suspected conditions inherent in tumors and their microenvi-
ronment, which may be conducive to dissemination, are discussed.

3.2.1. Clinical Conditions

Unlike rodent mammary tumors, the metastasizing properties of
human breast cancer seem to be a built-in characteristic. Therefore, the
conditions leading to metastasis may overlap with the risk factors for
cancer development in women.

a. Age and Menopausal Status. Breast cancer in women 35 years of
age or younger is said to often have histologically poorly differentiated,
more pleomorphic patterns and higher frequency of axillary lymph node
metastases,[50,51] and consequently poorer prognosis,[52–54] than that in
older women. This view, however, is disputed by others.[55–57] In laboratory animals, it is evident that younger ones are more sensitive to various mammary carcinogens (cf. reference 26): only newborn mice are
susceptible to MuMTV, and female rats older than 100 days of age are
resistant to mammary tumorigenesis by either potent chemicals or ionizing radiation. A similar situation may exist in humans, but it would be
difficult to prove.

b. Genetic Factors. The incidence of breast cancer in American
women is not only higher but the tumors are said to be more aggressive
and lethal than those in Japanese women.[58] This could be attributed
more to the difference in dietary habits than to genetic factors. It is well
established that dietary fat increases mammary tumor incidence and
stimulates its growth both in women and laboratory animals.[59,60] The
failure of treatment after potentially curative mastectomy in patients
with negative axillary disease, as well as their lower survival rate,

is also attributed to obesity, perhaps due to an increased estrogen metabolism.[61] Thus, the differences in incidence and malignancy of breast cancer between the two nationalities may not lie in any fundamental dissimilarity in their tumor cells, but rather in the difference of their hormonal microenvironments influenced by dietary habits.

c. *Estrogen Receptor Protein.* ERP assays are used almost routinely with considerable success to discriminate hormone-dependent from hormone-independent breast cancer.[47] However, the ERP content of tumor cells seems to have no bearing on their metastasizing potential. Kiang and Kennedy[48] found positive values in 29% of the primary tumors and 40% of the metastases in breast cancer among premenopausal women, 11 and 14% in paramenopausal, and 61 and 60% in postmenopausal patients, respectively. After a study of ERP levels in multiple tumor specimens from different types of breast cancer, Rosen *et al.*[49] concluded that there is no apparent consistent relationship between the receptor level variations and age, site of the tumor (primary or metastasis), interval between specimens, or the histological features of the tumor tissue. Although none of the metastasizing rat mammary tumors had measurable amounts of ERP, the evidence is insufficient to make any definite conclusions at this time.

3.2.2. Anatomical Conditions

Recently, Fisher *et al.*[62] and McDivitt[63] reviewed the various anatomical considerations for the prognosis of human breast cancer. Some of their criteria have been adopted for the evaluation of established histopathological features that may be associated with the development of metastasis.

a. *Location of Primary Tumors.* When tumors are located in the medial quadrant or central portion of the breast, the frequency of metastases to the internal mammary lymph node increases significantly, which in turn influences the involvement of axillary lymph nodes as well as the tumor recurrence and overall survival rate of the patient.[1] Metastasis to the internal mammary node is even interpreted as a sign of generalized tumor spread.[64] This is probably due to the more strategic location of the internal mammary lymphatic chain in the systemic distribution of tumor cells, rather than to any specific qualities of such cells.

b. *Tumor Size and Growth Rate.* The relationship of primary tumor size to axillary lymph node status was evaluated by Fisher *et al.*[65] and Valagussa *et al.*[1] in five- and ten-year follow-up studies of operable breast cancer treated by radical mastectomy. They found that, in general, the smaller the primary, the less chance of developing node metastasis, with its size directly correlated with the rate of recurrence and patient survival only when the nodes were positive. There was no difference in survival rate between women with the largest and those with the smallest tumors when the nodes were negative. On the other hand, the recurrence rate increased and the survival decreased markedly even in patients with small primary tumors when the nodes were positive.

The tumor growth rate is commonly expressed in terms of the time required for a tumor to double in volume. The tumor "doubling time" may be useful in assessing relative biological behavior or radiosensitivity,[66] for some tumors grow with explosive speed while others are indolent. However, attempts to relate it in terms of metastatic development or recurrence have not been successful.[67] Tubiana et al.[68] calculated the doubling time of many breast cancers and found that more than half of them had metastasized at least two years before the primary became clinically detectable. Citrin et al.[69] further noted positive bone scans in some patients with operable breast cancer, indicating the possibility of early hematogenous spread. Such occult primary tumors are not uncommon.[70–72]

These findings are similar to those in certain strains of metastasizing rat tumors in which extensive regional lymph node metastases develop before the primaries become palpable (Fig. 2). Therefore, it must be concluded that neither the tumor size nor its growth rate exerts any significant influence on the probability of metastatic dissemination.

c. *Histological Type.* In a 30-year follow-up study by Adair et al.[73] of 1458 breast cancer patients who were treated by radical mastectomy, the histological type of the tumors was correlated with long-term survival rates. The longest rates (10 and 30 years) were for patients with comedocarcinoma (77 and 74%), followed in order by those with papillary carcinoma (65 and 65%), medullary (68 and 58%), colloid (72 and 55%), infiltrating lobular (57 and 34%), and, least, poorly differentiated, infiltrating ductal carcinoma (39 and 29%). The favorable survival rates in medullary carcinoma are attributed to the heavy lymphoplasmacytic infiltration around tumor cell nests, suggesting the possible immunogenicity of these tumor cells. When plasma cell reaction was present around the tumor, the survival of patients with even the worst histological type improved significantly. The relatively better prognosis of comedo and colloid carcinomas may be due to their retention of secretory function, though aberrant, for, as a biological rule, cell division ceases when function begins. Because these authors analyzed the histological type of breast cancer based only on the long-term patient survival, it cannot be directly correlated with the metastasizing potential.

d. *Nuclear Grading.* As a means of estimating the degree of malignancy of human breast cancer, Bloom[74] proposed a histological grading system according to the degree of gland formation, nuclear pleomorphism, degree of hyperchromatism, and mitotic rate. Black et al.[75] modified this system into five numerical grades, correlating them with immunological reactions around the tumor and in the regional lymph node, and assessed their effect on survival. They suggested that tumor cells with higher nuclear grade (well differentiated) tend to produce lymphocytic reaction around the primary tumor and cause sinus hystiocytosis in regional lymph nodes, associated with longer survival. These grading systems have not gained many followers due to their reliance on the subjective bias of the analyzers and the quality of tissue sections.

3.3. Patterns of Metastasis

As in most other human carcinomas, the lymphatics are the main route of metastasis in human breast cancer. Hematogenous metastasis, without lymph node involvement, is extremely rare[62] and little is known about its pathogenesis. Nevertheless, some mammary tumors may prefer the latter over the former route, as may be seen in animal models (Table I). In an advanced state, at any rate, the tumor seems to scatter through both routes. In a compilation of the literature on the metastasis of human breast cancer to four key organs,[54,76-79] Gilbert and Kagan[80] found that, according to the autopsy data, such metastasis was most frequent in the bone (50-85%), followed in order by the lung (60%), liver (45-60%), and brain (15-25%). At the time of initial diagnosis and the discovery of axillary disease, the metastatic incidence showed a similar trend, i.e., bone (6%), lung (4%), liver (1%), and brain (less than 1%), suggesting that in the majority of the cases distant metastases follow axillary disease. On the other hand, Fisher et al.,[81] who analyzed 1665 patients with operable breast cancer for the National Surgical Adjuvant Breast Project, reported that there was no significant difference in the failure of treatment or survival rate between women with negative or positive axillary nodes who had undergone radical mastectomy, and those with or without subsequent axillary node dissection following mastectomy, concluding that the axillary lymph node involvement is not the predecessor of distant metastases, but a manifestation of disseminated (but dormant) disease. If such a view is confirmed or accepted, identification of the factors responsible for stimulating the growth of such dormant cells would perhaps open new avenues for the control of metastasis.

4. Ritual of Metastasis

The preliminary steps for all solid tumors to establish secondary colonies in other sites are cellular dispersion, invasion, transportation, and settlement or entrapment.

4.1. Dispersion of Tumor Cells

Unlike leukemias, breast cancer cells must first break down into viable units, small enough to pass through the lymphatics and blood vessels around the tumor, in order to disseminate.

4.1.1. Reduced Cohesiveness and Adhesiveness

In his pioneering work, Coman[82] found that cells from squamous carcinomas of the skin are more readily separated from each other than are normal epidermal cells, and suggested that there is a bonding defect in cancer cells which facilitates their dissemination. This discovery was subsequently confirmed and extended by many investigators, utilizing various physical and chemical means. (cf. references 83–87). However, the reduced adhesiveness may be a property associated with cell-surface changes common to all tumors, including the nonmetastasizing, experimental ones.[88] Generally, as cancer cells evolve toward increasing autonomy and dedifferentiated state, they tend to lose the capacity to form cohesive structures by the absence of tight junctions and microvilli[87,89]; e.g., adenocarcinoma cells, which fail to construct glands, produce only loose aggregates or nests of pleomorphic cells. Since most of these studies were done utilizing nonmetastasizing rodent tumors and corresponding normal tissue, with only a few exceptions,[90] their significance with respect to metastasis is inconclusive. Despite the loss of cohesive force, most undifferentiated tumors in laboratory animals do not metastasize spontaneously. Needless to say, however, the loss of physicochemical bonding is probably the first step required for local tumor cell dispersion.

In association with the reduced adhesiveness, elevated levels of degradative lysosomal enzymes,[36,91–93] which are known to regulate secretion and turnover of nonlysosomal proteins,[94–96] plasma membrane permeability,[83,97] and cell-surface glycoprotein shedding,[29] have been found in and around tumor cells. The increased plasma membrane permeability and related surface changes, characterized as "sublethal autolysis,"[98] are believed to promote the release of various tumor cell products, including tumor-associated antigens, glycosyltransferases, prostaglandins, osteoclast-stimulating factors, immunosuppressive peptides, and tumor angiogenesis factor, in addition to proteases, as will be discussed later.

Among many proteolytic enzymes elaborated by tumor cells, a group of neutral proteases, such as plasminogen activator and collagenase, have drawn a great deal of attention in recent years. *Plasminogen activator*, a constituent of some normal tissues, catalyzes the activation of serum plasminogen to plasmin, which in turn digests fibrinogen, causing fibrinolysis. High levels of this enzyme have been found in experimental tumors of diverse origins[98,99] and in some human cancers,[100] and it is assumed to promote migration and eventual cell metastasis by lysing the fibrin network around them. However, most animal tumors in which this enzyme was found are nonmetastasizing. A preliminary study indicated that there is no significant difference in the plasminogen activator content between the metastasizing and nonmetastasizing rat mammary tumors (Markus and Kim, unpublished data). Thus, it seems as though this enzyme may play a role in the reduction of adhesiveness, but not in the dissemination of tumor cells. *Collagenase*, which is considered more critical in the development of metastasis, has been found in many human cancers.[101–105] Blocking of its activity with a neutral protease inhibitor, i.e., cysteine or aprotinin, has prevented metastasis in experimental animals.[104,105]

4.1.2. Tumor Cell Locomotion

Ameboid movement of tumor cells has long been observed in fresh as well as fixed tumor preparations.[106] Wood[107] recorded cinematographically such movement of the metastasizing rabbit V2 carcinoma cells in and out of blood vessels in the rabbit ear chamber. Recently, Sträuli and Weiss[108] reviewed the literature on the active locomotory movement of cancer cells in relation to the contractile protein system of nonmuscular cells. They thoughtfully concluded that although a great deal of information on the nature of the contractile proteins in a wide variety of cells is available, their relationship to cell movement and tumor cell infiltration is unknown. Active locomotion or invasiveness alone does not necessarily lead to tumor metastasis, for highly invasive basal-cell carcinomas of skin, thymomas, and astrocytomas of the brain seldom metastasize.[109] Therefore, the locomotion of cells cannot be predicted solely from the examination of contractile elements; the matrix in which they migrate, as well as internal and external controlling mechanisms, must also be taken into account. A proteolytic enzyme, such as collagenase, or other degradative enzymes would certainly help to remove natural obstacles in the path of self-propelling tumor cells.[110]

4.2. Invasion

Under the microscope, the tumor growth pattern can be clearly distinguished as *infiltrative* and *expansive*, as exemplified by our rat tumor system (Figs. 3 and 4). The ameboid movement associated with invasiveness can also be characterized as deformability or malleability, for it is an essential property of tumor cells to pass the capillary bed through the narrow endothelial junction by "reverse diapedesis."[111,112]

4.2.1. Lymphatic Invasion

Carr and McGinty[112] described the actual process of invasion of lymphatics by individual tumor cells in the region of tumor implantation. They observed under the electron microscope that tumor cells extend as fingerlike cytoplasmic processes into the open gaps between endothelial cells, and once within the lymphatic vessels they revert to a spherical shape. They further noted that sometimes the endothelial junctions are wide open and several cells can be seen migrating through. However, judging from the localization of radiolabeled bacterial antigen in the lymphoid follicles of popliteal nodes shortly after its injection into the foot pad of rats,[113] not only self-propelling tumor cells, but also any macromolecules spilled into tissue space are likely to find their way to the regional lymph node via the lymphatics. It is possible that soluble or insoluble antigens shed from tumor cells evoke immune responses in the regional lymph node prior to the arrival of viable tumor cells. Since most human breast cancers metastasize mainly by the lymphatic route, the finding of tumor cells within the lymphatic vessels would not be unusual, but Nime et al.[114] give special significance to such occurrence. They reported that about half of the patients with invasive carcinoma who had no axillary node involvement but had microscopic tumor emboli in the intramammary lymphatics eventually developed distant metastases, while those with positive axillary nodes and the emboli subsequently had local recurrence, proposing that the tumor emboli in the intramammary lymphatics, without axillary disease, should be recognized as the sign of potential distant metastases. This would be comparable to tumor cells bypassing anergic regional lymph nodes.

4.2.2. Blood Vessel Invasion

For a long time pathologists have considered blood vessel invasion by the primary tumor as an unfavorable prognostic sign, without concrete supporting evidence, either clinical or pathological. Some have stated that it is prognostically significant only in the presence of concomitant lymph node metastases,[115] while others claim that it is relevant only in the absence of nodal involvement.[116] Fisher et al.[62] reported that only 4.7% of the breast cancer cases reviewed had vascular invasion, with no direct relationship to bad prognosis or short-term treatment failure. Thus, the data linking vascular invasion to prognosis are conflicting, In laboratory animal tumors, exclusive blood vessel invasiveness seems to be more common, for most of the spontaneously metastasizing tumors reported in the literature develop only hematogenous lung metastases.

4.2.3. Tumor Angiogenesis Factor

Vascularization of stroma is essential to support the growth of any cell mass. Certain solid tumors interact with their host tissue to provoke an angiogenic response[117]; and it occurs even when the tumor is separated from the surrounding host stroma by Millipore filters, suggesting that this factor is a diffusible substance. Folkman *et al.*[118] finally isolated from tumor tissues a high-molecular-weight glycoprotein with specific angiogenic activity which stimulates endothelial proliferation, designating it as "tumor angiogenesis factor" (TAF), and they further postulated that it may play an important role in the dissemination of tumor cells.[119] However, most conventional nonmetastasizing rodent tumors seem to produce this substance in varying amounts. Thus, TAF may be essential for maintaining the growth of solid tumors, but not for promoting metastasis. Its effects on the lymphatics are unknown.

4.3. Metastasis

As discussed previously, breast cancer metastasizes almost exclusively via the lymphatics, but the mechanism of such predilection is not clearly understood as yet. A critical analysis of the anatomical and physiological environment of tumor cells, as well as their biological, immunological, and biochemical properties, would contribute toward a more rational interpretation of such phenomena.

4.3.1. Lymph Node Metastasis

Prior to the actual seeding of invasive tumor cells into the subcapsular sinuses of regional lymph nodes, soluble or insoluble tumor-associated antigens shed from the primary tumor may evoke immunological reactions in the node. Initially there may be sinus histiocytosis, mobilization of lymphcoytes into vascular spaces of cortex and medullary sinuses, emergence of immunoblasts in the T-cell zone in conjunction with follicular hyperplasia with reactive center, and appearance of plasma cells in medullary cords.[120,121] The intensity of these reactions may depend on the quality and quantity of the antigen—the greater the immunogenicity, the stronger the reaction—in which case the settlement of tumor cells is prevented. Carr and McGinty[112] have demonstrated that nonspecific immune stimulation of regional lymph nodes with BCG prevents the subcapsular seeding of syngeneic, metastasizing tumor cells in rats. Tsakraklides *et al.*[122] reported that lymphocytic hyperplasia in the regional lymph node is commonly seen among long-term survivors, while lymphocytic depletion is associated with short-term survival in patients with operable breast cancer. Even if some tumor cells are deposited in the node, they may remain dormant for a long time, as observed by Pickren[123] who reported that breast cancer patients with occult metastases in the axillary lymph node have the same favorable prognosis as those with completely negative axillary disease. As the tumor deposit is steadily replenished by increasing numbers of tumor cells released from the primary, it represses the immune reaction of the node.[112,120,121] The tumor cells progressively spread along the lymphatic chains until they converge in the thoracic duct and subclavian vein, or they may directly penetrate venules within the node and enter the venous return. Eventually, they probably join the lesser circulation and develop embolic deposits in the liver and lung, or may traverse the pulmonary vasculature into the greater circulation and gain entry to various organs (Fig. 5). On the other hand, tumor-associated antigens can be found in the blood of metastasizing tumor-bearing rats[37,38] before regional node metastasis is detected, indicating that organ-specific antigen released from the tumor may pass through the node without provoking immune responses, or that large amounts saturate and immunologically paralyze the node,[39] allowing the passage of tumor cells through the node and into the efferent lymphatics unchecked. The effectiveness of lymph nodes as barriers against tumor cell dissemination, therefore, seems to depend entirely on the quality and quantity of tumor-associated antigens draining into them.

4.3.2. Hematogenous Metastasis

The bloodstream is composed of two closed-circuit networks of arteries, capillaries, venules, and veins connected by the heart (Fig. 5). Under normal physiological conditions, only cells with active locomotive power, such as leukocytes, traverse the vascular wall. Viable tumor cells must penetrate the endothelial wall in order to gain entry into the bloodstream. For unknown reasons, the most commonly used metastasizing animal tumors (e.g., Lewis lung carcinoma, rabbit V2 carcinoma, B16 melanoma, and MC3 fibrosarcoma) seem to have this capacity. Malignant tumors in man that arise in close association with the capillary network, such as sarcomas and carcinomas of kidney, liver, endocrine glands, and prostate, can achieve this by means of their own invasive power,[87,109] by being passively pushed into the circulation by the intrinsic pressure of expansive tumor growth, or by inadvertently

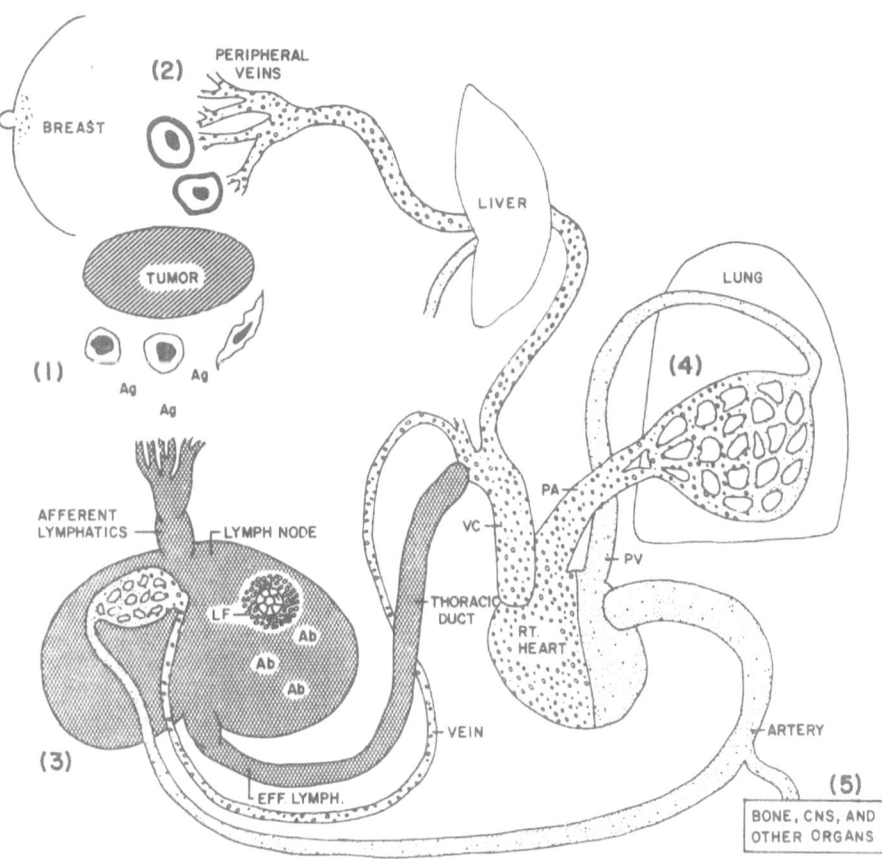

Fig. 5. Metastatic routes and sequence of breast cancer. Antigen-shedding, invasive tumor cells with or without thick glycocalyx (1) may enter into the peripheral vein either actively or passively (2). The shed antigens may stimulate the lymph node to produce antibodies and immune lymphocytes prior to the arrival of viable tumor cells, or they may paralyze it, preparing an immune milieu for their rejection or acceptance. If accepted, the tumor cells may grow and disseminate further through the efferent lymphatics or the postcapillary venules within the node. They may converge in the caval vein and/or the thoracic duct and flow into the right heart (3). In the case of a prolonged right heart failure, some tumor cells in the vena cava may be pushed into the liver. Large tumor cells or cell aggregates may be trapped and establish lung metastases (4), while others may traverse the pulmonary vein into the left heart and embolize other organs by the arterial route (5). Ag: antigens; LF: lymphoid follicles; Ab: antibodies; eff. lymph.: efferent lymphatics; VC: vena cava; PA: pulmonary arteries; PV: pulmonary veins; CNS: central nervous system.

being introduced through trauma. This process may be further facilitated by the abnormal blood vessels or endothelial cells with defective tight junctions found in tumors.[77,124] However, mere entrance of viable tumor cells into the systemic circulation does not assure the establishment of secondary tumor colonies. Single or small groups of tumor cells may flow repeatedly past the lung capillaries, through the left ventricle, and into the greater circulation without being trapped.[125,126] Indeed, viable tumor cells are readily harvested from the venous and arterial blood of cancer patients[127–130] and nonmetastasizing tumor-bearing animals,[126,131] with no apparent manifestation of metastatic disease. The circulating tumor cells must be large enough or form clusters in order to be trapped by the capillaries, or they must have the capacity to adhere to the intima of blood vessels.[132–135] The factors promoting cell-to-cell adhesion or aggregation, therefore, appear to be the critical components for the embolization or development of hematogenous metastases.

5. Mechanisms of Metastasis

Regardless of the metastasizing route, successful establishment of colonies in secondary sites is the culmination of complex interactions between tumor cells and the host. Analysis of these two factors may provide a better understanding of the mechanisms of metastasis.

5.1. Factors Associated with Tumor Cells

So far we have evaluated some of the more pertinent cell-surface changes associated with metastasis, such as cell-to-cell adhesiveness, permeability, and cellular locomotion, as well as altered enzyme activities reflecting those functional changes. In this section, the general dynamics of altered cell-surface components associated with metastasizing capacity are discussed.

5.1.1. Marker Enzymes

a. Plasma-Membrane-Associated Enzymes. As described earlier, when the activity of five commonly used marker enzymes was determined in "purified" plasma membrane preparations, their levels were significantly lower in the metastasizing tumors, decreasing in direct proportion to the metastasizing capacity. In the nonmetastasizing tumors the levels were higher, with the activity seemingly increasing with the immunogenicity of the cells.[29,30] Among the five enzymes, 5′-nucleotidase was the best representative of this phenomenon. Raz et al.[136] reported similar results with six different cell types of normal and transformed fibroblasts grown in vitro and four types of normal and leukemic lymphocytes in vivo. They found a marked decrease of 5'-nucleotidase activity in the malignant cells, as compared to their normal parental cells. This was proportionately correlated with the decrease of cell-surface microviscosity[137] and fluidity of membrane lipids.[138] Since the specific activity of this enzyme is basically determined by the amount of inorganic phosphorus released from the substrate adenosine 5'-monophosphoric acid in cells, its decrease may represent fewer active enzyme units, hence the loss of cell-surface constituents. In women with metastatic breast and other cancers, the serum levels of this enzyme were dramatically elevated,[139,140] but the results of tissue assays have been inconclusive, due probably to the large amounts of stromal components found in most solid tumors (Kim, Chatterjee, and Rossner, unpublished data). Thus, the determination of plasma membrane marker enzymes, particularly 5'-nucleotidase, may be useful to estimate the immunogenicity of tumor cells or the amount of antigens remaining on their surface, provided the tumors are cellular or the stromal contamination is minimized.

b. *Cyclic Nucleotide Phosphodiesterases.* Although the importance of cyclic nucleotides in the growth and differentiation of normal and neoplastic cells is well recognized, analyses of intracellular cAMP levels in various tumor tissues have yielded conflicting results. The cAMP is decreased in established cultured tumor cells[141,142] and its addition to culture media inhibits cell division and partially restores normal characteristics to the tumor cells.[143-145] On the other hand, its levels remain the same or are even elevated in certain human and experimental tumors.[35,146-149] The results of assays of several tumors for the cAMP-degrading enzyme cAMP PDE are also contradictory. Singer et al.[150] studied its activity in human breast carcinomas, benign adenomas, and normal breast tissue and reported that the malignant cells had higher levels of low-K_m enzyme, whereas Cohen et al.[151] found the activity decreased in chemically induced rat mammary tumor cells. We have observed similar patterns in our rat mammary tumor system[35] and postulated that these discrepancies may be due to the fundamental biological differences between metastasizing and nonmetastasizing tumors.

Since adenyl cyclase is a membrane-bound enzyme, metastasizing tumors with diminished surface markers are expected to have low levels of cAMP and cAMP PDE activity, but in actual analyses we found the former relatively high and the latter extremely low.[35] It is generally believed that cyclic nucleotides regulate their own degradation by directly controlling the rate of synthesis of corresponding cyclic nucleotide phosphodiesterases, possibly by way of protein kinases.[152,153] The cAMP metabolism may not proceed in an orderly manner in highly malignant, metastasizing tumor cells, with the impaired cyclic nucleotide generation system causing inappropriate production of PDE which results in accumulation of cAMP, or it is possible that this enzyme plays a more dominant role in the regulation of cAMP. Further analyses of the entire adenyl cyclase system in biologically well-defined experimental tumors are needed to clarify these questions. In addition, studies on the role of cyclic nucleotides in the modulation of lysosomal enzyme release, as seen in the "reverse endocytosis" of leukocytes,[154] are extremely important to establish the interrelationship between cAMP metabolism and the antigen-shedding property of metastasizing tumor cells.

c. Glycosyltransferases. Building carbohydrate moieties into glycoproteins and glycolipids of the plasma membranes is accomplished by the stepwise addition of monosaccharides into their respective nucleotides, with the help of specific glycosyltransferases. Thus, the changes in the metastasizing tumor cell membranes are likely to be reflected in these enzymes. Bosmann and Hall[155] first reported high levels of sialyltransferase activity in invasive human breast and colon cancers, and suggested that such elevations might be responsible for increased synthesis of certain tumor-associated sialoproteins or glycolipids. They further attributed the invasiveness of cancer to the concomitant rise of glycosidases and proteases. In addition to sialyltransferase, high levels of galactosyltransferase and fucosyltransferase were also noted in the serum of breast and other cancer patients by several investigators.[139,156–159] Henderson and Kessel[159] and Kessel et al.[160] also observed that changes in plasma sialyltransferase levels can be directly correlated with the tumor load or the course of the disease. Weiser et al.[161] detected an isoenzyme of galactosyltransferase in the sera of cancer patients, especially those with widespread metastases. We have confirmed and extended these findings by comparing the activity of these three enzymes in the metastasizing rat mammary tumors and their host sera,[31–34] and postulated that these enzymes hyperglycosylate free glycoprotein antigens in the systemic circulation and prolong their half life,[162] compounding antigen excess in the host. Those with high glycosyltransferase activity also had high levels of sialic acid and fucose in their blood.[31,34,163–166] The serum glycoprotein-bound fucose level has been used for some time to assess the prognosis of cancer patients.[163]

Together with our knowledge of the cell-surface glycoproteins, a great deal of information on the altered glycolipid biosynthesis in transformed cells is available.[167] Yogeeswaran et al.[168] reported that a B16 mouse melanoma with high lung-implantation capacity had an increase of cell-surface-exposed gangliosides, along with sialoglycoproteins, as compared to a low-metastasizing variant, although the total lipid- and protein-bound sialic acid was significantly decreased. In addition, Skipski et al.[169] found that the ganglioside patterns in the serum from rats bearing a Morris hepatoma and in the tumor itself were similar, suggesting that the glycolipid components of tumor cell membranes are also released into the bloodstream. These changes in the two major plasma membrane components seem to occur concurrently.

5.1.2. Tumor-Associated Antigens

As we have observed in the experimental rat mammary tumor system, cancer is composed of a mixture of different cell clones,[43] and such heterogeneity often expresses itself biologically by producing a variety of immunologically cross-reacting, tumor-associated antigens in individual tumors.

a. Oncofetal Antigens. The reexpression of embryonal characteristics on the surface of cells that have undergone malignant transformation has been demonstrated in a variety of human and animal tumors. In human breast cancer, the most widely investigated oncofetal antigens are carcinoembryonic antigen (CEA) of gastrointestinal carcinomas,[170] α-fetoproteins (α-FP) of hepatomas and testicular tumors,[171] human chorionic gonadotropin (HCG), α_1-acid glycoprotein (AGP),[172] and pregnancy-associated α-macroglobulin (PAM),[173] although the last three may be better characterized as "organ-specific" antigens. Most of the oncofetal antigens seem to cross-react among human cancers and they are being used almost routinely to detect and follow the progression of breast cancer, with considerable success.[174-178] These antigens are generally nonimmunogenic in the autochthonous host and their identification depends entirely on the use of antisera raised in xenogeneic hosts. Experimental animal tumors, on the other hand, are often found to carry tumor-specific antigen immunogenic to autochthonous or syngeneic hosts[179] and, in addition, the metastasizing rat mammary tumors produce large amounts of organ-specific, nonimmunogenic, soluble antigen[29,37,28] resembling that of human cancers.

b. Blood Group Substances. The search for breast-cancer-specific antigens in humans has not been successful. Recently, however, Springer et al.[180] discovered an N-like human blood group substance in the serum and ascitic fluid of mice bearing the Haushka subline of TA3 mammary adenocarcinoma which inhibited hemagglutination by *Vicia graminea* lectin. They later isolated the MN blood group substance precursors in both malignant and benign tumor tissues in women,[181] and subsequently found that all malignant tumors, but none of the benign ones, contained an additional Thomsen–Friedenreich (T)-like glycoprotein antigen which reacted to *Arachis hypogaea* lectin.[182,183] They also noted that the anti-T antibody, which is present in all normal human sera, was severely depressed in breast cancer patients. In the screening of a large group of women, those with low anti-T titer were later found to have breast cancer, and after mastectomy the titer rose. Such blood group substances were also recovered in large amounts from the tissue culture fluid of the established human breast cancer cell line BOT-2.[184] Thus, it seems as though a human breast-cancer-specific antigen complex, and naturally occurring antibody, may at last be available.

c. Miscellaneous Tumor Cell Products. In addition to the enzymes and antigens derived from mammary cancers, there are several other tumor-associated substances that are used for assessing prognosis of human breast cancer. These include ferritin, α-casein, C-reactive proteins, and calcitonin,[177,178] as well as urinary hydroxyproline, polyamines, and nucleosides.[177,185] However, most of them are often elevated in nonneoplastic diseases as well and, therefore, have a limited value as biological markers for cancer.

5.1.3. Prostaglandins

Prostaglandins (PGs) are ubiquitous biological mediators which modulate many important cellular functions through cAMP. There is ample evidence indicating that they are produced by certain human and animal tumors and cause various cancer-related phenomena such as cell detachment, vasodilatation and increased blood flow, hypercalcemia, immune depression, platelet aggregation, and metastasis.[154,186–191]

a. Cell Detachment. Weissman *et al.*[154] have shown that PGs, cyclic nucleotides, and colchicine influence the release of lysosomal hydrolases in the "reverse endocytosis" model system. It is postulated that a similar mechanism may be involved in the extrusion from tumor cells of the hydrolytic enzymes associated with reduced adhesiveness, active locomotory movement, or invasiveness.

b. Vasodilatation and Blood Flow. Inflammatory reaction is generally characterized as hyperemia, exudation of plasma into tissue space, and swelling. It is also believed to be mediated by PGs, particularly prostaglandin E_1 (PGE_1). Williams and Peck[192] reexamined the mode of PG action in inflammation by measuring separately the increased blood flow and plasma exudation in rabbit skin, and concluded that PG mediates increase of plasma exudation by vasodilatation, which provides greater blood-exchange area in the vessel wall, rather than by promoting vascular permeability. By whatever mechanism, tumor-cell-generated PGs are likely to influence extravasation of circulating tumor cells, as well as vascular invasion. Indeed, blood vessel invasion by tumor cells is more frequently seen in inflamed tissue.[62]

c. *Hypercalcemia.* Next to the lymph node, bone is the site most commonly affected by metastatic human breast cancer[80] Hypercalcemia is also more frequently associated with breast cancer than with any other malignancy, including multiple myeloma.[193] Tumor deposits in bone are always hematogenous in origin, and as they settle in the marrow, a diffusable substance is released to mobilize osteoclasts for bone resorption.[77,194] Osteolytic sterol was isolated from a lipid fraction of both malignant and benign human breast tissue,[195,196] indicating that it is not specific. However, the osteoclast-activating factor or osteolytic principle was recognized as PG by bioassay and chromatographic analysis.[197] The critical role of PG in osteolysis was further substantiated by the inhibition or retardation of bone resorption with anti-PG compounds, such as aspirin and indomethacin.[198] The finding of a high concentration of PG-like material in "hypercalcemia-prone" human breast cancer by Bennett *et al.*[199] may not be coincidental. There are discrepant observations on this matter and readers are referred to an excellent synopsis on osteolytic metastases which appeared as an editorial in *Lancet.*[200] Kibbey *et al.*,[201] who analyzed prostaglandin E_2 (PGE_2) levels and the activity of microsomal PGE_2 synthetase in some of the metastasizing and nonmetastasizing rat mammary tumors listed in Table I, found the levels much lower in the former, contradicting the conclusions of Bennett and associates. The osteolysis by tumor-derived PG is perhaps augmented locally by inflammatory cells which are also known to produce osteolytic factors. The earlier expectations of controlling osseous metastatic breast cancer in women with aspirin and indomethacin have yet to be realized.

d. *Immune Depression.* Plescia *et al.*[189] suggested that production of PG by certain animal tumors may be a mechanism whereby host immune responses are somehow subverted, for PGE_2 from tumors increases cAMP in T lymphocytes, abrogating their cytotoxic function against the tumor and resulting in the enhancement of its growth.[202-204] Harvey *et al.*[205] failed to correlate circulating PG levels with delayed hypersensitivity skin reaction against various recall antigens or dinitrochlorobenzene (DNCB) sensitization. This does not exclude the possibility of PGs acting "locally," for peripheral PGs are known to be rapidly inactivated with one circulatory pass through the lung. Such an assumption, however, has also been ruled out by Mortel *et al.*,[206] who reported low levels of PG in the tumor bed of women with gynecological malignancy, and by Demers *et al.*,[207] who found elevated circulating PG levels in groups of cancer and non-cancer patients with positive delayed hypersensitivity skin reaction and hypercalcemia. They concluded that PGs do not correlate with the nonspecific depression of cell-mediated immunity, nor do they modify host–tumor interaction in man.

    e. Platelet Aggregation. It has been reported that PGE_1 inhibits platelet aggregation, while PGE_2 stimulates it. There also seems to be a considerable species variation in the effect of PGE series on platelet functions.[190] Therefore, the interrelationship between various PGs elaborated by neoplastic cells, and their direct role in platelet aggregation in the development of metastases, cannot be generalized. Nevertheless, the role of platelet aggregation in the development of lung metastasis seems to be widely accepted.

5.1.4. Immunosuppressive and Cytotoxic Peptides

    Two tumor-associated substances, which may influence metastasis, were recently isolated from malignant effusions and plasma of cancer patients.

    a. Immunosuppressive Peptides. Nonspecific suppression of delayed hypersensitivity reaction is known to occur in patients with advanced cancer. The mechanism responsible for this phenomenon is not fully understood, but it has been suggested that it may be the direct result of the presence of immunosuppressive factors in the serum.[208-210] Occhino et al.[211] isolated a peptide fraction from the serum α-globulin of cancer patients, which has immunosuppressive activity, and it appears in higher concentrations in cancer serum than in normal serum.[210] Badger et al.[212] also found a similar immunosuppressive activity in malignant effusions from advanced cancer patients with pleural or peritoneal involvement. Although the origin of this factor has not been determined, it is postulated that an active substance may be produced, or induced, by tumor cells and excreted into the body fluid, facilitating dissemination of cancer. This substance is probably biologically similar to the serum "blocking factor"[40] which has been identified as tumor-associated antigens and antigen–antibody complexes.[29]

    b. Galactosyltransferase Glycopeptide Acceptor. Podolsky and Weiser[213] reported the isolation of a low-molecular-weight acceptor for galactosyltransferase activity from the sera and malignant effusions of advanced cancer patients during the development of metastasis. The purified acceptor acted as substrate for normal and cancer-associated galactosyltransferase isoenzymes, but had a higher affinity for the latter. This substance inhibited the growth of BHKpy tumors in hamsters and in tumor cell cultures, apparently through its function as a substrate for galactosyltransferase. Thus, Podolsky et al. related its tumor-inhibitory capacity with the suppression of enzyme shedding by tumor cells.[214]

Confirmation of these findings would provide new perspectives on the control mechanism of cell-surface-antigen shedding.

5.2. Host Factors in Metastasis

5.2.1. Platelets and Coagulation

Since O'Meara[215] recognized the coagulative property of cancer cells by the presence of fibrin network at the tumor periphery, numerous investigators reported that the platelet-aggregating activity of tumor cells causes their vascular lodgment and survival during the process of metastasis.[216] This notion was strengthened by observations of thrombocytopenic agents causing reduction of lung metastases by blood-borne tumor cells.[217-219] Most of the work was based on the artificial induction of pulmonary embolization by the intravenous injection of tumor cells, often in allogeneic hosts, but the general theorem can still be supported by a less artificial experimental system, e.g., surgical amputation of a tumor-bearing rodent's limb, which also causes the development of hematogenous lung metastases.[220,221] Increased release of platelets into the bloodstream, brought about by surgical trauma and elevated antibody levels through the removal of a primary tumor that had been serving as an "antibody sink," has been said to cause cross-linking of tumor cells in the circulation and their eventual entrapment in the pulmonary arteries.[134,222] The attachment of serum growth-factor-containing platelet aggregates to such cells may further promote their proliferation.[223,224] Gasic et al.[225] reported that the aggregating principle resides in the plasma membrane vesicles shed by cultured tumor cells. The quality of coagulation disorders induced by a large number of tumor cells injected intravenously may be quite different from that caused by the slow release of cells into the bloodstream by metastasizing tumors.[226] The thrombogenic properties of tumor cells may also be different in the venous and arterial compartments, for most of the experimental metastases associated with platelet aggregation seem to occur in the lesser circulation. In the rat mammary tumors that metastasize via the lymphatics, a large number of tumor cells can be harvested from the abdominal aorta of the host,[126] indicating that they traverse the pulmonary vasculature freely into the arterial circulation without being trapped. It is possible that these cells have a reduced platelet-aggregating capacity. In human mammary carcinoma, plasminogen activator seems to be relatively more critical than platelets in the development of metastases, as suggested by the association of the high in vitro fibrinolytic activity of these tumors with their greater invasiveness and lymph node involvement.[227] The platelet-aggregating property, necessary for the passive vascular entrapment of cells, is perhaps more pronounced in the ordinary, nonmetastasizing animal tumors. Thus, the thrombogenic response by the host seems to depend on the surface quality of tumor cells.

5.2.2. Cell-Mediated Immunity

Depressed cell-mediated immunity in breast cancer patients, as demonstrated by various *in vivo* and *in vitro* tests, is generally recognized as an advanced state of the disease. Such tests are used in conjunction with routine diagnostic procedures to estimate the immunological potential of the patient or to assess the extent of malignancy.[228-231] Apart from the gross immune depression due to replacement of hematolymphopoietic organs by metastatic tumors, the subclinical immune suppression is believed to begin with the interaction between tumor-associated antigens and T lymphocytes, with the number of cells decreasing prior to any detectable signs of metastasis.[232,233]

a. *Blocking Factors.* Serum factors are among the most widely accepted mechanisms through which tumor cells escape immunological destruction by the cytotoxic lymphocytes of the host. They are capable of blocking the cytotoxic effect of sensitized lymphocytes against tumor cells *in vitro*, as demonstrated first by the Hellströms[234] with the serum from mice bearing a progressively growing Moloney sarcoma (progressor). They further confirmed this finding with many human and animal tumors and their host sera, and designated the factors as "blocking antibodies." Later, however, this identity of the blocking factors came under dispute: Halliday and Miller[235] suggested that they were "enhancing antibodies," based on their leukocyte adherence inhibition test; Bonsal and Sjögren[236] proposed them as soluble tumor antigens; and, finally, Sjögren and Hellström, along with their colleagues,[237,238] concluded that they were antigen–antibody complexes. The reason behind such an inconsistency may be in the qualitative variations of tumor cell-surface antigens in man and animals: Highly immunogenic, stable surface antigens are likely to produce antibody excess in the host, as seen in most conventional tumor-bearing animals; less stable antigens are shed, together with antibodies, as immune complexes; and the soluble antigens of metastasizing tumor cells create the state of antigen excess in the circulation. The apparent inconsistency notwithstanding, the activity of the blocking factors can be directly correlated with tumor burden, extent of metastatic spread, and clinical stage in breast cancer patients.[231,239] In the sera from highly metastasizing mammary–tumor-bearing rats and a mouse with squamous-cell carcinoma,[240] only soluble tumor-associated antigens were found, with no detectable antibodies, while those from the nonmetastasizing tumor-bearing rats had high levels of tumor-specific antibodies. The subversion of T-lymphocyte function in malignant tumor hosts may be accomplished by soluble, T-independent antigens, masking the surface of the T lymphocytes and rendering them immunologically unresponsive or tolerant. It is well established that purified human IgG can be made highly tolerogenic to mice by deaggregating or solubilizing it.[241,241] Zighelboim et al.[243] reported that soluble alloantigen extract prepared from EL-4 tumors neither generated cell-mediated cytotoxic lymphocytes against ^{51}Cr-labeled EL-4 target cells in the spleen of BALB/c mice nor produced complement-dependent cytotoxic antibodies in their sera. Thus, this immune escape mechanism, as manifested by cancer cells releasing soluble antigens to block cell-mediated immune response, resembles the manner by which protozoic parasites evade host immune destruction.[244,245]

b. T-Lymphocyte-Deficient State. Immunosuppressive treatments, such as whole-body or local irradiation, antilymphocytic serum, and potent antitumor drugs, will lead to the development of metastases, wider dissemination of localized secondary tumors, and shorter survival of cancer patients and tumor-bearing animals.[246-249] More specifically, however, a sustained removal of T lymphocytes would cause blood-borne tumor cells, which had been prevented from establishing secondary lesions by cell-mediated immunity, to embolize in the lung. This was demonstrated by Eccles and Alexander,[249] who reported that the drainage of thoracic duct lymph from rats, either bearing or after excision of an immunogenic sarcoma, caused increased lung metastases, and that similar results could be achieved even when removing only the thoracic duct fluid and returning the cells to the host. Further, Rose[250] reported that the continuous drainage of thoracic duct fluid, with intravenous return of the cells, from rats preimmunized with various antigens caused marked generalized lymphadenopathy and as much as a 100-fold increase of specific antibody levels in their sera. The enhancement of passive lung metastases in *athymic nude mice* by the nonmetastasizing, highly immunogenic rat mammary tumors,[42] therefore, may be caused not only by the deprivation of T lymphocytes, but also by the increased tumor-specific antibody levels which may help the circulating antigen-bearing tumor cells to aggregate.

5.2.3. Humoral Immunity

Antitumor antibodies against human breast cancer have been demonstrated on the tumor cell surface by various techniques.[251-256] However, attempts to correlate the serum immunoglobulin levels with the clinical course of breast cancer patients have not been successful.[257,258] Such inconclusive observations are understandable, for the level of anti- body response is determined by the degree of immunogenicity of tumor cells, amount of soluble antigen shed by them into the circulation, and immunocompetence of the host. The progressive elevation of serum IgG in breast cancer patients with metastases, as observed by Dostálová et al.,[259,260] may be a situation similar to that of a hamster lymphoma in which abrogation of "concomitant immunity" caused the development of metastases in the host by enhancing antibodies,[261] or to the promo- tion of lung metastases in immunocompetent mice by Lewis tumors.[262] On the other hand, it has been noted that antitumor antibodies are often detected in the sera of patients with or shortly after the surgical removal of a small localized tumor, and that there is an inverse relationship between the level of cytotoxic antibodies and tumor load.[263] It has also been suggested that the presence of circulating antitumor antibodies is responsible for the prevention of metastasis.[264] Whether antitumor an- tibodies are stimulatory or inhibitory in the development of metastases seems to depend entirely on the quality of tumor cell-surface antigens, be they T dependent or independent.

5.2.4. Macrophages

The macrophage has reemerged as one of the most critical compo- nents in tumor immunology with respect to its role in the prevention of metastasis. The number of macrophages found in tumor tissues is said to be inversely correlated with the metastasizing capacity of tumor cells,[265,266] and infusion of specifically activated macrophages can either prevent or reduce artificial lung metastases in mice caused by an in- travenous injection of viable tumor cells.[267] Even in metastasizing fib- rosarcoma of rats, an intralesional injection of BCG causes heavy infiltra- tion of macrophages around the tumor cells, resulting in the prevention of lung metastasis.[268] Macrophages are also known to kill tumor cells either specifically or nonspecifically.[269,270] In our metastasizing rat mammary tumors, the impaired in vitro migratory capacity of peritoneal macrophages[40] seems to indicate that their soluble tumor antigens are also capable of disarming the killer macrophage.

6. Summary and Conclusions

Recognition of the fundamental differences between human and animal cancers is the most important prerequisite to interpretation and analysis of laboratory data derived from experimental tumor models.

This is particularly true in the study of metastasis, which is almost the rule in human cancers, whereas in animals it is the exception. The reason behind such difference, as we perceive it, is that human cancer is usually a late event in life, likely to have come through repeated host selective pressures, while most experimental tumors in laboratory animals are the product of human expediency to fulfill our scientific anxiety in the shortest possible time. Would, then, subjecting animal cells to simulated recurrent immunoselective pressures, during a prolonged carcinogenic process, produce tumors that behave like human cancer? Such laboratory contrivance has been successful in the development of spontaneously metastasizing rat mammary adenocarcinomas with many of the qualities of human breast cancer. Thus, it seems as though malignant tumors in man are the undesirable by-product of the host immune surveillance mechanism, and, in this sense, this mechanism becomes a double-edged sword, cutting down transformed cells it recognizes as foreign, but leaving intact the ones it does not; or perhaps it even encourages them to injure the host itself.

Such a tumor model has given us the opportunity to study the mechanism of metastasis by comparing these tumors to the nonmetastasizing, but otherwise identical, conventional rat mammary tumors and, hopefully, to learn their biochemical, immunological, and biological peculiarities. This may help us to understand the factors influencing metastasis of human breast cancer. The most outstanding characteristic of the metastasizing rat tumor cells is that they seem to have extremely unstable plasma membrane structures, which causes them to constantly shed incompletely assembled membrane constituents, with concomitant renewal of the loss. Such membrane instability may permit the leakage of various degradative lysosomal enzymes ordinarily meant for the physiological cell renewal or homeostatic control mechanism. These enzymes may then help not only in weakening and breaking down cell-to-cell bonds in the tumor mass, but also in clearing the path for dispersion of freed cells. The locomotive property of these cells is probably a manifestation of the plasma membrane's instability. With the loss and rearrangement of membrane constituents, the transformed cells lose their identity and evade the cell-mediated immune surveillance system. The dissociated plasma membrane constituents include glycoprotein and glycolipid antigens, surface marker enzymes, glycosyltransferases, glycoses, and some degradative enzymes. Some of these substances play havoc with the host defense system, resulting in the dissemination and establishment of secondary tumor cell colonies. Fundamentally, therefore, the quality of the tumor cell-surface antigens and their degree of solubility or nonimmunogenicity are likely to determine to what extent they subvert the host immune machinery. On the other hand, modification of the host immune system itself may allow nonmetastasizing tumor cells to embolize. It is hoped that these theoretical considerations, formulated mostly from our experimental tumor model, will facilitate the interpretation and analysis of clinical and laboratory findings related to the metastases of human breast cancer and their eventual control.

I have attempted to bring together as much relevant information as possible in developing a cohesive central theme on the mechanism of metastases in breast cancer. Consequently, some important work by other investigators dealing with the fundamental aspects of metastases, but not related to breast cancer, may have been omitted, or, in some cases, misquoted. I kindly beg their indulgence.

ACKNOWLEDGMENTS: The author's work reported here was supported in part by American Cancer Society Grant PDT-28 and U.S. Public Health Service, National Cancer Institute Grant R01CA-24215.

7. References

1. P. Valagussa, G. Bonadonna, and U. Veronesi, Pattern of relapse and survival following radical mastectomy. Analysis of 716 consecutive patients, *Cancer* **41**, 1170–1178 (1978).
2. B. Fisher, N. Slack, D. Katrich, and N. Wolmark, Ten year follow-up results of patients with carcinoma of the breast in a co-operative clinical trial evaluating surgical adjuvant chemotherapy, *Surg. Gynecol. Obstet.* **140**, 525–534 (1975).
3. E. Silverberg, Cancer statistics 1977, *A Cancer Journal for Clinicians* **27**, 26–41 (1977).
4. R. T. Prehn, The relationship of tumor immunogenicity to the concentration of the inducing oncogen, *J. Natl. Cancer Inst.* **55**, 189–190 (1975).
5. U. Kim, Metastasizing mammary carcinomas in rats: Induction and study of their immunogenicity, *Science* **67**, 72–74 (1970).
6. U. Kim, Pathogenesis of spontaneously metastasizing mammary carcinomas in rats, *Gann Monogr.* **20**, 73–81 (1977).
7. G. Haughton and A. C. Whitmore, Genetics, the immune response and oncogenesis, *Transplant. Rev.* **28**, 75–97 (1976).
8. J. F. A. P. Miller, G. A. Grant, and F. J. C. Roe, Effect of thymectomy on the induction of skin tumours by 3,4-benzopyrene, *Nature* **199**, 920–922 (1963).
9. Y. Nishizuka, K. Nakakuki, and M. Usui, Enhancing effect of thymectomy on hepatotumorigenesis in Swiss mice following neonatal injection of 20-methylcholanthrene, *Nature* **205**, 1236–1238 (1965).
10. H. Balner and H. Dersjant, Neonatal thymectomy and tumor induction with methylcholanthrene in mice, *J. Natl. Cancer Inst.* **36**, 513–521 (1966).
11. G. Grant, F. J. C. Roe, and M. C. Pike, Effect of neonatal thymectomy on incidence of papillomata and carcinomata by 3,4-benzopyrene in mice, *Nature* **210**, 603–604 (1966).
12. K. Nomoto and K. Takeya, Immunologic properties of methylcholanthrene-induced sarcomas of neonatally thymectomized mice, *J. Natl. Cancer Inst.* **42**, 445–453 (1969).

13. P. K. Kalpaktsoglou, E. J. Yunis, and R. A. Good, Early splenectomy and survival of inbred mice, *Nature* **215**, 633–634 (1967).

14. L. Kubai and R. Auerbach, Neonatal splenectomy: Absence of runting in mice, *Nature* **217**, 460 (1968).

15. J. K. Moody and N. D. Reed, Neonatal splenectomy and survival of mice, *Nature* **218**, 1056–1057 (1968).

16. D. M. Jacobs and W. Byrd, Adult thymectomy results in loss of T-dependent mitogen response in mouse spleen cells, *Nature* **255**, 153–155 (1975).

17. F. Squartini, Mouse mammary tumorigenesis by mammary tumor virus in the absence of thymus, spleen or both, in: *Immunological Parameters of Host–Tumor Relationship* (D. W. Weiss, ed.), pp. 26–35, Academic Press, New York (1971).

18. E. Bonmassar, E. Menconi, A. Goldin, and G. Cudkowicz, Escape of small number of allogenic lymphoma cells from immune surveillance, *J. Natl. Cancer Inst.* **53**, 475–479 (1974).

19. F. Squartini and M. Bistocchi, Bioactivity of C3H and RIII mammary tumor viruses in virgin female BALB/c mice: Brief communication, *J. Natl. Cancer Inst.* **58**, 1845–1847 (1977).

20. M. Bistocchi, M. Nuti, and F. Squartini, Quantitative comparison on milk-released C3H and RIII mammary tumor viruses in infected BALB/c hosts, *Tumori* **63**, 535–542 (1977).

21. R. Duff, E. Doller, and F. Rapp, Immunologic manipulation of metastases due to Herpesvirus transformed cells, *Science* **180**, 79–81 (1973).

22. J. H. Cutts and R. L. Noble, Estrogen-induced mammary tumors in the rat. I. Induction and behavior of tumors, *Cancer Res.* **24**, 1116–1123 (1964).

23. J. H. Cutts, Unusual response to androgen of estrogen dependent mammary tumors, *J. Natl. Cancer Inst.* **42**, 485–488 (1969).

24. C. J. Shellaberger, V. P. Bond, and E. P. Cronkite, Studies on radiation-induced mammary gland neoplasia in the rat. IV. The response of females to a single dose of sublethal total-body gamma radiation as studied until first appearance of breast neoplasia or death of the animals, *Radiat. Res.* **13**, 242–249 (1960).

25. K. Yokoro, J. Furth, and N. Haran-Ghera, Induction of mammotropic pituitary tumors by X-rays in rats and mice. The role of mammotropes in development of mammary tumors, *Cancer Res.* **21**, 178–186 (1961).

26. U. Kim and J. Furth, The role of prolactin in carcinogenesis, *Vitam. Horm. (N. Y.)* **34**, 107–136 (1976).

27. R. Bronn, U. Kim, L. Divecchia, W. E. Kibbey, and J. P. Minton, Estrogen receptor in hormonally progressive mammary tumors, *J. Surg. Oncol.* **9**, 595–601 (1977).

28. M. Ip, R. Molholland, F. Rosen, and U. Kim, Mammary cancer: Selective action of the estrogen receptor complex, *Science* **203**, 361–363 (1979).

29. U. Kim, A. Baumler, C. Carruthers, and K. Bielat, Immunological escape mechanism in spontaneously metastasizing mammary tumors, *Proc. Natl. Acad. Sci. U. S. A.* **72**, 1012–1016 (1975).

30. S. K. Chatterjee, U. Kim, and K. Bielat, Plasma membrane associated enzymes of mammary tumours as the biochemical indicators of metastasizing capacity. Analyses of enriched membrane fractions, *Br. J. Cancer* **33**, 15–26 (1976).

31. R. Bernacki and U. Kim, Concomitant elevation in sialyltransferase activity and sialic acid content in rats with metastasizing mammary tumors, *Science* **195**, 577–580 (1977).

32. S. K. Chatterjee and U. Kim, Galactosyltransferase activity in metastasizing and nonmetastasizing rat mammary carcinomas and its possible relationship with tumor cell surface antigen shedding, *J. Natl. Cancer Inst.* **58**, 273–280 (1977).

33. S. K. Chatterjee and U. Kim, Fucosyltransferase activity in metastasizing and nonmetastasizing rat mammary carcinomas, *J. Natl. Cancer Inst.* **61**, 151–162 (1978).

34. U. Kim and S. K. Chatterjee, Possible role of glycosyltransferase in the surface antigen shedding mechanisms in spontaneously metastasizing rat mammary carcinomas, *Proc. Am. Assoc. Cancer Res.* **17**, 179 (1976).

35. S. K. Chatterjee and U. Kim, Adenosine-3',5'-cyclic monophosphate levels and adenosine-3',5'-cyclic monophosphate phosphodiesterase activity in metastasizing and nonmetastasizing rat mammary carcinomas, *J. Natl. Cancer Inst.* **54**, 181–186 (1975).

36. M. Tunis, U. Kim, and C. Carruthers, Correlation of an enzyme profile with the metastasizing capacity of rat mammary carcinomas, *Proc. Am. Assoc. Cancer Res.* **14**, 80 (1973).

37. S. K. Ghosh, A. L. Grossberg, U. Kim, and D. Pressman, Identification and purification of an organ specific, tumor membrane-associated antigen from a spontaneously metastasizing rat mammary carcinoma, *Immunochemistry* **15**, 345–352 (1978).

38. S. K. Ghosh, A. L. Grossberg, U. Kim, and D. Pressman, A tumor associated, organ specific antigen in rat mammary carcinomas, present at high levels in metastatic and at low levels in non-metastatic tumors, *J. Natl. Cancer Inst.* **62**, May (1979).

39. U. Kim, Pathogenesis of lung metastasis, in: *Symposium on Lung Metastasis* (L. Weiss and H. A. Gilbert, eds.), pp. 76–90 G. K. Hall & Co., Boston (1978).

40. U. Kim and G. Montessori, Patterns of spleen cell migration *in vitro* in spontaneously metastasizing and nonmetastasizing mammary tumor hosts: Possible immune escape mechanism, *Proc. Am. Assoc. Cancer Res.* **16**, 155 (1975).

41. J. Rygaard, *Thymus & Self, Immunobiology of the Mouse Mutant Nude*, John Wiley & Sons, New York (1973).

42. U. Kim, V. H. Freedman, and S.-I. Shin, Selective inhibition and stimulation of xenogeneic tumor growth and metastasis in athymic nude mice, *Proc. Am. Assoc. Cancer Res.* **19**, 155 (1978).

43. U. Kim and M. J. Depowski, Progression from hormone dependence to autonomy in mammary tumors as an *in vivo* manifestation of sequential clonal selection, *Cancer Res.* **35**, 2068–2077 (1975).

44. L. Foulds, Mammary tumours in hybrid mice: Growth and progression of spontaneous tumours, *Br. J. Cancer* **3**, 345–375 (1949).

45. R. W. Baldwin, Immunological aspects of chemical carcinogenesis, *Adv. Cancer Res.* **18**, 1–75 (1973).

46. Y. Harada, Induction of metastasizing carcinoma in rats and their biological characteristics, *Acta Pathol. Jpn.* **25**, 451–461 (1975).

47. W. L. McGuire, P. P. Carbone, M. E. Sears, and G. C. Escher, Estrogen receptors in human breast cancer: An overview, in: *Estrogen Receptors in Human Breast Cancer* (W. L. McGuire, P. P. Carbone, and E. P. Vollmer, eds.), pp. 1–7, Raven Press, New York (1975).

48. D. Kiang and B. J. Kennedy, Factors affecting estrogen receptors in breast cancer, *Cancer* **40**, 1571–1576 (1977).

49. P. P. Rosen, C. J. Menendez-Botet, J. A. Urban, A. Fracchia, and M. K. Schwartz, Estrogen receptor protein (ERP) in multiple tumor specimens from individual patients with breast cancer, *Cancer* **39**, 2194–2200 (1977).

50. J. Rouessé, G. Contesso, J. Génin, D. Sarazin, J. Weiler, and F. May-Levin, Les adénocarcinomes du sein chez les femmes de moins de trente ans, *Bull. Cancer (Paris)* **59**, 41–60 (1972).

51. A. Wallgren, C. Silfverswärd, and A. Hultborn, Carcinoma of the breast in women under 30 years of age, *Cancer* **40**, 916–923 (1977).

52. H. J. Morris and H. B. Taylor, Carcinoma of the breast in women less than thirty years old, *Cancer* **26**, 953–959 (1970).

53. T. G. J. Brightmore, W. P. Greening, and I. Hamlin, An analysis of clinical and histopathological features in 101 cases of carcinoma of breast in women under 35 years of age, *Br. J. Cancer* **24**, 644–669 (1970).

54. C. D. Haagensen, *Diseases of the Breast,* 2nd Edition, W. B. Saunders, Philadelphia (1971).

55. N. Treves and A. I. Holleb, A report of 549 cases of breast cancer in women 35 years of age or younger, *Surg. Gynecol. Obstet.* **107**, 271–283 (1958).

56. D. M. Birks, G. M. Crawford, I. G. Ellison, and F. R. C. Johnstone, Carcinoma of the breast in women 30 years of age or less, *Surg. Gynecol. Obstet.* **137**, 21–25 (1973).

57. J. Gogas and G. Skalkeas, Prognosis of mammary carcinoma in young women, *Surgery* **78**, 339–342 (1975).

58. E. L. Wynder, T. Kajitani, J. Kuno, J. C. Lucas, A. De Palo, and J. Farrow, A comparison of survival rates between American and Japanese patients with breast cancer, *Surg. Gynecol. Obstet.* **117**, 196–200 (1963).

59. F. deWaard, Breast cancer incidence and nutritional status with particular reference to body weight and height, *Cancer Res.* **35**, 3351–3356 (1975).

60. K. K. Carrol, Experimental evidence of dietary factors and hormone-dependent cancers, *Cancer Res.* **35**, 3374–3383 (1975).

61. W. L. Donegan, A. J. Hartz, and A. A. Rimm, The association of body weight with recurrent cancer of the breast, *Cancer* **41**, 1590–1594 (1978).

62. E. Fisher, R. Gregorio, and B. Fisher, The pathology of invasive breast cancer, *Cancer* **36**, 1–85 (1975).

63. R. W. McDivitt, Breast carcinoma, *Hum. Pathol.* **9**, 3–21 (1978).

64. W. L. Donegan, The influence of untreated internal mammary metastases upon the course of mammary cancer, *Cancer* **39**, 533–538 (1977).

65. B. Fisher, N. H. Slack, and I. D. Bross, Cancer of the breast: Size of neoplasm and prognosis, *Cancer* **24**, 1071–1080 (1969).

66. K. Breur, Growth rate and radiosensitivity of human tumours. II. Radiosensitivity of human tumours, *Eur. J. Cancer* **2**, 173–188 (1966).

67. A. W. Pearlman, Breast cancer—Influence of growth rate on prognosis and treatment evaluation. A study based on mastectomy scar recurrences, *Cancer* **38**, 1826–1833 (1976).

68. M. Tubiana, P. Chauvel, A. Renaud, and E. P. Malaise, Growth rate and natural history of human breast cancers, *Bull. Cancer* **62**, 341–358 (1975).

69. D. L. Citrin, R. G. Bessent, W. R. Greig, N. J. McKellar, C. Furnival, and L. H. Blumgart, Application of 99$_{TC}$M phosphate bone scan to the study of breast cancer, *Br. J. Surg.* **62**, 201–204 (1975).

70. E. H. Pierce, H. K. Gray, and M. B. Dockerty, Surgical significance of isolated axillary adenopathy, *Ann. Surg.* **145**, 104–107 (1957).

71. L. Feuerman, J. N. Attie, and B. Rosenberg, Carcinoma in axillary lymph nodes as an indicator of breast cancer, *Surg. Gynecol. Obstet.* **114**, 5–8 (1962).

72. R. Ashikari, P. P. Rosen, J. A. Urban, and T. Senoo, Breast cancer presenting as an axillary mass, *Ann. Surg.* **183**, 415–417 (1976).

73. F. Adair, J. Berg, L. Joubert, and G. F. Robbin, Long-term follow-up of breast cancer patients: The 30-year report, *Cancer* **33**, 1145–1150 (1974).

74. H. T. G. Bloom, Prognosis in carcinoma of the breast, *Br. J. Cancer* **4**, 259–289 (1950).

75. M. M. Black, S. R. Opler, and F. D. Speer, Survival in breast cancer cases in relation to structure of primary tumor and regional lymph nodes, *Surg. Gynecol. Obstet.* **100**, 543–551 (1955).

76. R. A. Willis, *The Spread of Tumours in the Human Body,* 3rd Edition, Butterworths, London (1973).

77. W. L. Harnett, A statistical report on 2529 cases of cancer of the breast, *Br. J. Cancer* **2**, 212–239 (1948).

78. J. W. Turner and H. L. Jaffer, Metastatic neoplasms, *Am. J. Roentgenol.* **43**, 479–492 (1973).

79. E. Viadana, I. D. Bross, and J. W. Pickren, An autopsy study of some routes of dissemination of cancer of the breast, *Br. J. Cancer* **27**, 336–340 (1973).

80. H. A. Gilbert and A. R. Kagan, Metastases: Incidence, detection, and evaluation without histologic confirmation, in: *Fundamental Aspects of Metastasis* (L. Weiss, ed.), pp. 385–405, North-Holland Publishing Co., Amsterdam (1976).

81. B. Fisher, E. Montague, C. Redmond, B. Barton, D. Borland, E. R. Fisher. and other NSABP investigators, Comparison of radical mastectomy with alternative treatments for primary breast cancer: A first report of results from a prospective randomized clinical trial, *Cancer* **39**, 2827–2839 (1977).

82. D. R. Coman, Decreased mutual adhesiveness, a property of cells from squamous cell carcinomas, *Cancer Res.* **4**, 625–629 (1944).

83. B. Sylvén, Biochemical and enzymatic factors involved in cellular detachment, in: *Chemotherapy of Cancer Dissemination and Metastasis* (S. Garattini and G. Franchi, eds.), pp. 129–136, Raven Press, New York (1973).

84. L. Weiss, Biophysical aspects of the metastatic cascada, in: *Fundamental Aspects of Metastasis* (L. Weiss, ed.), pp. 51–70, North-Holland Publishing Co.; Amsterdam (1976).

85. P. Sträuli, The spread of cancer in the organism, facts and problems, *Naturwissenschaften* **64**, 403–409 (1977).

86. E. J. Ambrose, The surface properties of tumor cells, in: *Biology of Cancer* (E. J. Ambrose and F. J. C. Roe, eds.), pp. 27–57, Halsted Press, John Wiley & Sons, New York (1975).

87. G. C. Easty, Invasion by cancer cells, in: *Biology of Cancer* (E. J. Ambrose and F. J. C. Roe, eds.), pp. 58–73, Halsted Press, John Wiley & Sons, New York (1975).

88. R. Roblin, I. N. Chou, and P. H. Black, Proteolytic enzymes, cell surface changes and viral transformation, *Adv. Cancer Res.* **22**, 203–259 (1975).

89. U. Kim and K. Bielat, Structural changes in microvilli of mammary adenocarcinoma cells associated with progression from hormone dependence to autonomy, *Fed. Proc. Fed. Am. Soc. Exp. Biol.* **30**, 397 (1971).

90. N. S. McNutt, R. A. Herschberg, and R. S. Weinstein, Further observations on the occurrence of nexuses in benign and malignant human cervical epithelium, *J. Cell Biol.* **51**, 805–825 (1971).

91. A. R. Poole, Tumor lysosomal enzymes and invasive growth, in: *Lysosomes in Biology and Pathology* (J. T. Dingle, ed.), Vol. 3, pp. 303–337, North-Holland Publishing Co., Amsterdam (1973).

92. H. B. Bosmann, G. F. Bieber, A. E. Brown, K. R. Case, D. M. Gersten, T. W. Kimmerer, and A. Lione, Biochemical parameters correlated with tumor cell implantation, *Nature* **246**, 487–489 (1973).

93. Z. Werb, Lysosomes as modulators of cellular functions. Influence on the synthesis and secretion of non-lysosomal materials, *Front. Biol.* **45**, 127–156 (1976).

94. A. L. Goldberg, J. D. Kowit, and J. D. Etlinger, Studies of the selectivity and mechanisms of intracellular protein degradation, in: *Proteolysis and Physiological Regulation* (D. W. Ribbons and K. Brew, eds.), pp. 313–333, Academic Press, New York (1976).

95. H. L. Segal, Mechanism and regulation of protein turnover in animal cells, *Curr. Top. Cell. Regul.* **11**, 183–201 (1976).

96. R. Goldman, Ion distribution and membrane permeability in lysosomal suspension, *Front. Biol.* **45**, 309–336 (1976).

97. A. C. Spataro, H. R. Morgan, and H. B. Bosmann, Neutral protease activity of Rous sarcoma (RSV) transformed chick embryo fibroblast, *J. Cell Sci.* **21**, 407–413 (1976).

98. D. B. Rifkin and R. Pollack, Protease produced by normal and malignant cells in culture, in: *Proteolysis and Physiological Regulation* (D. W. Ribbons and K. Brew, eds.), pp. 263–285, Academic Press, New York (1976).

99. D. B. Rifkin, J. N. Loeb, G. Moore, and E. Reich, Properties of plasminogen activators formed by neoplastic human cell cultures, *J. Exp. Med.* **139**, 1317–1328 (1974).

100. D. B. Rifkin and R. Pollack, Production of plasminogen activators by established cell lines of mouse origin, *J. Cell Biol.* **73**, 47–55 (1977).

101. M. H. Dresden, S. A. Heilman, and J. D. Schmidt, Collagenolytic enzymes in human neoplasms, *Cancer Res.* **32**, 993–996 (1972).

102. Y. Yamanishi, E. Maeyens, M. K. Dabbous, H. Ohyama, and K. Hashimoto, Collagenolytic activity in malignant melanoma: Physico-chemical studies, *Cancer Res.* **33**, 2507–2512 (1973).

103. K. Hashimoto, Y. Yamanishi, E. Maeyens, M. K. Dabbous, and T. Kanazaki, Collagenolytic activities of squamous cell carcinoma of the skin, *Cancer Res.* **33**, 2790–2801 (1973).

104. N. R. Campbell, P. C. Reade, and B. G. Radden, Effect of cysteine on the survival of mice with transplanted malignant thymoma, *Nature* **251**, 158–159 (1974).

105. T. Giraldi, C. Nisi, and G. Sava, Lysosomal enzyme inhibitors and antimetastatic activity in the mouse, *Eur. J. Cancer* **13**, 1321–1323 (1977).

106. H. T. Enterline and D. R. Coman, The ameboid motility of human and animal neoplastic cells, *Cancer* **3**, 1033–1038 (1950).

107. S. Wood, Jr., Pathogenesis of metastasis formation observed *in vivo* in the rabbit ear chamber, *Arch. Path.* **66**, 550–568 (1958).

108. P. Sträuli and L. Weiss, Cell locomotion and tumor penetration. Report on a workshop of the EORTC cell surface project group, *Eur. J. Cancer* **13**, 1–12 (1977).

109. R. L. Carter, Metastasis, in: *Biology of Cancer* (E. J. Ambrose and F. J. C. Roe, eds.), pp. 74–95, Halsted Press, John Wiley & Sons, New York (1975).

110. L. Strauch, The role of collagenases in tumor invasion, in: *Tissue Interactions in Carcinogenesis* (D. Tarin, ed.), pp. 399–433, Academic Press, New York (1973).

111. I. Zeidman, The fate of circulating tumor cells. I. Passage of cells through capillaries, *Cancer Res.* **21**, 38–39 (1961).

112. I. Carr and F. McGinty, Neoplastic invasion and metastasis within the lymphoreticular system, in: *The Reticuloendothelial System in Health and Disease* (S. Reichard, M. Escobar, and H. Friedman, eds.), pp. 319–329, Plenum Press, New York (1976).

113. R. S. Weiser, Q. N. Myrvik, and N. N. Pearsall, *Fundamentals of Immunology*, Lea & Febiger, Philadelphia (1970).

114. F. A. Nime, P. P. Rosen, H. T. Thaler, R. Ashikari, and J. A. Urban, Prognostic significance of tumor emboli in intramammary lymphatics in patients with mammary carcinoma, *Am. J. Surg. Pathol.* **1**, 25–30 (1977).

115. J. R. Bell, G. H. Friedell, and I. S. Goldenberg, Prognostic significance of pathologic findings in human breast carcinoma, *Surg. Gynecol. Obstet.* **129**, 258–262 (1969).

116. S. J. Kister, S. C. Sommers, C. D. Haagensen, and E. Cooley, Re-evaluation of blood vessel invasion as a prognostic factor in carcinoma of the breast, *Cancer* **19**, 1213–1216 (1966).

117. B. A. Warren and P. Shubik, The growth of the blood supply to melanoma transplants in the hamster cheek pouch, *Lab. Invest.* **15**, 464–478 (1966).

118. J. Folkman, E. Merler, C. Abernathy, and G. Williams, Isolation of a tumor factor responsible for angiogenesis, *J. Exp. Med.* **133**, 275–288 (1971).

119. J. Folkman, Tumor angiogenesis, in: *Cancer, A Comprehensive Treatise* (F. F. Becker, ed.), Vol. 3, pp. 355–388, Plenum Press, New York (1975).

120. P. G. Herman, C.-S. Kim, M. A. B. de Sousa, and H. Z. Mellins, Microcirculation of the lymph node with metastases, *Am. J. Pathol.* **85,** 333–348 (1976).

121. C. Van de Velde and I. Carr, Lymphatic invasion and metastasis, *Experientia* **33,** 837–843 (1977).

122. V. Tsakraklides, P. Olson, J. H. Kersey, and R. A. Good, Prognostic significance of the regional lymph node histology in cancer of the breast, *Cancer* **34,** 1259–1267 (1974).

123. J. W. Pickren, Significance of occult metastases—Breast cancer, *Cancer* **14,** 1266–1271 (1961).

124. A. G. Ide, R. A. Harvey, and S. L. Warren, Role played by trauma in the dissemination of tumor fragments by the circulation, *Arch. Pathol.* **28,** 851–860 (1939).

125. I. Zeidman and J. M. Buss, Transpulmonary passage of tumor cell emboli, *Cancer Res.* **12,** 731–733 (1952).

126. U. Kim, Factors controlling metastasis of experimental breast cancer, *Cancer Res.* **26,** 461–464 (1966).

127. G. E. Moore, A. Sandberg, and J. R. Shubarg, Clinical and experimental observations on the occurrence and fate of tumor cells in the blood stream, *Ann. Surg.* **148,** 580–587 (1957).

128. J. D. Griffiths and A. J. Salsbury, *Circulating Cancer Cells,* C. C. Thomas, Springfield, Illinois (1965).

129. R. A. Malmgren, Studies of circulating tumor cells in cancer patients, in: *Mechanisms of Invasion of Cancer* (P. Derick, ed.), pp. 108–117, Springer-Verlag, New York (1967).

130. A. L. Salsbury, The significance of the circulating cancer cell, *Cancer Treatment Rev.* **2,** 55–72 (1975).

131. T. P. Butler and P. M. Gullino, Quantitation of cell shedding into efferent blood of mammary carcinoma, *Cancer Res.* **35,** 512–516 (1975).

132. W. H. Knisely and M. S. Mahaley, Relationship between size and distribution of "spontaneous" metastases and three sizes of intravenously injected VX2 carcinoma, *Cancer Res.* **18,** 900–905 (1958).

133. L. A. Liotta, J. Kleinerman, and G. M. Saidel, The significance of hematogenous tumor cell clumps in the metastatic process, *Cancer Res.* **36,** 889–894 (1976).

134. I. Glaser, Cell–cell recognition, *Trends Biochem. Sci.* **1,** 84–86 (1976).

135. P. A. W. Edwards, Differential cell adhesion may result from nonspecific interactions between cell surface glycoproteins, *Nature* **271,** 248–249 (1978).

136. A. Raz, J. C. Collard, and M. Inbar, Decrease in 5′-nucleotidase activity in malignant transformed and normal stimulated cells, *Cancer Res.* **38,** 1258–1262 (1978).

137. M. Inbar and M. Shinitzky, Decrease in microviscosity of lymphocyte surface membranes associated with stimulation induced by concanavalin A, *Eur. J. Immunol.* **5,** 166–170 (1975).

138. M. Inbar, I. Yuli, and A. Raz, Contact-mediated changes in the fluidity of membrane lipids in normal and malignant transformed mammalian fibroblasts, *Exp. Cell Res.* **105,** 325–335 (1977).

139. C. Ip and T. Dao, Alteration in serum glycosyltransferases and 5′-nucleotidase in breast cancer patients, *Cancer Res.* **38,** 723–728 (1978).

140. N. K. Kim, W. G. Yasmineh, E. F. Freier, A. I. Goldman, and A. Theologides, Value of alkaline phosphatase, 5′-nucleotidase, γ-glutamyltransferase, glutamate dehydrogenase activity in serum in diagnosis of metastasis to the liver, *Clin. Chem.* **23,** 2034–2038 (1977).

141. J. R. Sheppard, Difference in the cyclic adenosine 3′,5′-monophosphate levels in normal and transformed cells, *Nature (London) New Biol.* **236,** 14–16 (1972).

142. I. Pastan and G. S. Johnson, Cyclic AMP and the transformation of fibroblasts, *Adv. Cancer Res.* **19**, 303–326 (1974).

143. M. L. Heidrick and W. L. Ryan, Cyclic nucleotides on cell growth *in vitro*, *Cancer Res.* **30**, 376–378 (1970).

144. L. A. Smets, Contact inhibition of transformed cells incompletely restored by dibutyryl cyclic AMP, *Nature (London) New Biol.* **239**, 123 (1972).

145. R. Van Wijk, W. D. Wicks, and K. Clay, Effects of derivatives of cyclic 3′,5′-adenosine monophosphate on the growth, morphology and gene expression of hepatoma cells in culture, *Cancer Res.* **32**, 905–911 (1972).

146. F. R. Butcher, D. F. Scott, V. R. Potter, and H. P. Morris, Endocrine control of cyclic adenosine 3′,5′-monophosphate levels in several Morris hepatomas, *Cancer Res.* **32**, 2135–2140 (1972).

147. R. Chayoth, S. M. Epstein, and J. B. Field, Glucagon and prostaglandin E_1 stimulation of cyclic adenosine 3′,5′-monophosphate levels and adenylate cyclase activity in benign hyperplastic nodules and malignant hepatomas of ethionine-treated rats, *Cancer Res.* **33**, 1970–1974 (1973).

148. E. W. Thomas, F. Murad, W. B. Looney, and H. P. Morris, Adenosine 3′,5′-monophosphate and guanosine 3′,5′-monophosphate: Concentration in Morris hepatomas of different growth rates, *Biochim. Biophys. Acta* **297**, 564–567 (1973).

149. J. P. Minton, T. Wisenbaugh, and R. H. Matthews, Elevated cyclic AMP levels in human breast cancer tissue, *J. Natl. Cancer Inst.* **53**, 283–284 (1974).

150. A. L. Singer, R. P. Sherwin, A. S. Dunn, and M. M. Appleman, Cyclic nucleotide phosphodiesterases in neoplastic and nonneoplastic human mammary tissues, *Cancer Res.* **36**, 60–68 (1976).

151. L. A. Cohen, D. Straka, and P.-C. Chan, Cyclic nucleotide phosphodiesterase activity in normal and neoplastic rat mammary cells grown in monolayer culture, *Cancer Res.* **36**, 2007–2012 (1976).

152. H. R. Bourne, G. M. Tomkins, and S. Dion, Regulation of phosphodiesterase synthesis. Requirement for cyclic adenosine monophosphate-dependent protein kinase, *Science* **181**, 952–954 (1973).

153. M. M. Appleman, W. J. Thompson, and T. R. Russell, Cyclic nucleotide phosphodiesterases, *Adv. Cyclic Nucleotide Res.* **3**, 65–98 (1973).

154. G. Weissman, I. Goldstein, and S. Hoffstein, Prostaglandins and the modulation of cyclic nucleotides by lysosomal enzyme release, *Adv. Prostaglandin Thromboxane Res.* **2**, 803–814 (1976).

155. H. B. Bosmann and T. C. Hall, Enzyme activity in invasive tumors of human breast and colon, *Proc. Natl. Acad. Sci. U.S.A.* **71**, 1833–1837 (1974).

156. D. Kessel and J. Allen, Elevated plasma sialyltransferase in the cancer patient, *Cancer Res.* **35**, 670–672 (1975).

157. M. Bhattacharya, S. K. Chatterjee, and J. J. Barlow, Uridine 5′-diphosphate-galactose glycoprotein galactosyltransferase activity in the ovarian cancer patients, *Cancer Res.* **36**, 2096–2101 (1976).

158. D. Kessel, T. H. Chou, and M. Henderson, Determinants of fucosyltransferase levels in plasma of the cancer patients, *Proc. Am. Assoc. Cancer Res.* **17**, 16 (1976).

159. M. Henderson and D. Kessel, Alterations in plasma sialyltransferase levels in patients with neoplastic disease, *Cancer* **39**, 1129–1134 (1977).

160. D. Kessel, M. K. Samson, P. Shah, J. Allen, and L. H. Baker, Alterations in plasma sialyltransferase associated with successful chemotherapy of a disseminated tumor, *Cancer* **38**, 2132–2134 (1976).

161. M. M. Weiser, D. K. Podolsky, and K. Isselbacker, Cancer-associated isoenzyme of serum galactosyltransferase, *Proc. Natl. Acad. Sci. U.S.A.* **73**, 1319–1322 (1976).

162. J. Lunney and G. Ashwell, A hepatic receptor of avian origin capable of binding specifically modified glycoproteins, *Proc. Natl. Acad. Sci. U.S.A.* **73**, 341–343 (1976).

163. M. K. Wallack, A. S. Brown, E. F. Rosato, S. Rubin, J. L. Johnson, and F. E. Rosato, Serum fucose as a monitor for recurrent malignancy, *J. Surg. Oncol.* **10**, 39–44 (1978).

164. J. J. Barlow and P. H. Dillard, Serum protein-bound fucose in patients with gynecologic cancers, *Obstet. Gynecol.* **39**, 727–734 (1972).

165. A. Hadjivassiliou, A. Castanaki, G. Hristou, and B. Lissaios, The diagnostic value of protein bound serum fucose in cancer of the breast, *Surg. Gynecol. Obstet.* **140**, 239–240 (1975).

166. T. Tatsumura, H. Sato, A. Mori, Y. Komori, K. Yamamoto, G. Fukatani, and S. Kuno, Clinical significance of fucose level in glycoprotein fractions of serum in patients with malignant tumors, *Cancer Res.* **37**, 4101–4103 (1977).

167. P. H. Fishman and R. O. Brady, Biosynthesis and function of gangliosides, *Science* **194**, 906–915 (1976).

168. G. Yogeeswaran, B. S. Stein, and H. Sebastian, Altered cell surface organization of gangliosides and sialyl glycoproteins of mouse metastatic melanoma variant lines selected *in vivo* for enhanced lung implantation, *Cancer Res.* **38**, 1336–1344 (1978).

169. V. P. Skipski, N. Katopodis, J. S. Prendergast, and C. C. Stock, Gangliosides in blood serum of normal rats and Morris hepatoma 5123tc-bearing rats, *Biochem. Byophys. Res. Commun.* **67**, 1122–1127 (1975).

170. P. Gold and S. O. Freedman, Demonstration of tumor-specific antigens in human colonic carcinomata by immunological tolerance and absorption techniques, *J. Exp. Med.* **121**, 439–462 (1965).

171. G. I. Abeler, Production of embryonal serum α-globulin by hepatomas: Review of experimental and clinical data, *Cancer Res.* **28**, 1344–1350 (1968).

172. J. G. Roberts, J. W. Keyser, and M. Baum, Serum α_1-acid glycoprotein as an index of dissemination in breast cancer, *Br. J. Surg.* **62**, 816–819 (1975).

173. W. H. Stimson, Variations in the level of a pregnancy associated α-macroglobulin in patients with cancer, *J. Clin. Pathol.* **28**, 868–871 (1975).

174. D. C. Tormey, T. P. Waalkes, D. Ahmann, C. W. Gehrke, R. W. Zumwatt, J. Snyder, and H. Hansen, Biochemical markers in cancer of the breast. I. Incidence of abnormalities of CEA, hCG, three polyamines and three minor nucleosides, *Cancer* **35**, 1095–1100 (1975).

175. D. C. Tormey, T. P. Waalkes, and R. M. Simon, Biological markers in breast carcinoma. II. Clinical correlations with human chorionic gonadotrophin, *Cancer* **39**, 2391–2396 (1977).

176. D. C. Tormey, T. P. Waalkes, J. J. Snyder, and R. M. Simon, Biological markers in breast carcinoma. III. Clinical correlations with carcinoembryonic antigen, *Cancer* **39**, 2397–2404 (1977).

177. P. Franchimont, P. F. Zangerle, J. C. Hendrick, A. Reuter, and C. Colin, Simultaneous assays of cancer associated antigens in benign and malignant breast diseases, *Cancer* **39**, 2806–2812 (1977).

178. R. C. Coombes, T. J. Powles, J. C. Gazet, H. T. Ford, A. G. Nash, J. P. Sloan, C. J. Hillyard, P. Thomas, J. W. Keyser, D. Marcus, N. Zinberg, W. H. Stimson, and A. M. Neville, A biochemical approach to the staging of human breast cancer, *Cancer* **40**, 937–944 (1977).

179. L. J. Old and E. A. Boyse, Immunology of experimental tumors, *Annu. Rev. Med.* **15**, 167–186 (1964).

180. G. F. Springer, J. F. Codington, and R. W. Jeanloz, Surface glycoprotein from a mouse tumor cell as specific inhibitor of anti-human blood-group N agglutinin, *J. Natl. Cancer Inst.* **49**, 1469–1470 (1972).

181. G. F. Springer, P. R. Desai, and I. Banatwala, Blood group MN antigens and precursors in normal and malignant human breast glandular tissue, *J. Natl. Cancer Inst.* **54**, 335–339 (1975).

182. G. F. Springer, P. R. Desai, and E. F. Scanlon, Blood group MN precursors as human breast-carcinoma-associated antigens and "naturally" occurring human cytotoxins against them, *Cancer* **37**, 169–176 (1976).

183. V. Friedenreich, *The Thomsen Hemagglutination Phenomenon*, Levin & Munksgaard, Copenhagen (1930).

184. J. H. Anglin, Jr., M. P. Lerner, and R. E. Nordquist, Blood group-like activity released by human mammary carcinoma cells in culture, *Nature* **269**, 254–255 (1977).

185. K. B. Woo, T. P. Waalkes, D. L. Ahmann, D. C. Tormey, C. W. Gehrke, and V. T. Olivero, A quantitative approach to determining disease response during therapy using multiple biologic markers. *Cancer* **41**, 1685–1703 (1978).

186. T. J. Williams and M. J. Peck, Simultaneous measurement of local plasma exudation and blood flow changes induced by intradermal injection of vasoactive substances, using [^{131}I]albumen and ^{133}Xe, *J. Physiol. (London)* **254**, 48–58 (1976).

187. A. H. Tashjian, Jr., E. F. Veolkel, P. Goldhaber, and L. Levine, Prostaglandins, calcium metabolism and cancer, *Fed. Proc. Fed. Am. Soc. Exp. Biol.* **33**, 81–86 (1974).

188. H. Seyberth, G. V. Segre, J. L. Morgan, G. J. Sweetman, J. T. Potts, and J. A. Oates, Prostaglandins as mediators of hypercalcemia associated with certain types of cancer, *New Engl. J. Med.* **293**, 1278–1283 (1975).

189. O. J. Plescia, A. H. Smith, and K. Grinwich, Subversion of immune system by tumor cells and role of prostaglandins, *Proc. Natl. Acad. Sci. U.S.A.* **72**, 1848–1851 (1975).

190. M. Johnson and P. W. Ramwell, Implication of prostaglandins in hematology, in: *Prostaglandins and Cyclic AMP* (R. H. Kahn and W. E. M. Lands, eds.), pp. 275–304, Academic Press, New York (1973).

191. R. H. Kahn and W. E. M. Lands (eds.), *Prostaglandins and Cyclic AMP*, Academic Press, New York (1973).

192. T. J. Williams and M. J. Peck, Role of prostaglandin-mediated vasodilatation in inflammation, *Nature* **270**, 530–532 (1977).

193. O. H. Warwick, E. R. Yendt, and J. S. Olin, The clinical features of hypercalcemia associated with malignant disease, *Can. Med. Assoc. J.* **85**, 719–723 (1961).

194. C. S. B. Galasko, Mechanisms of bone destruction in development of skeletal metastases, *Nature* **263**, 507–508 (1976).

195. G. S. Gordan, T. J. Cantino, and L. Erhardt, Osteolytic sterol in human breast cancer, *Science* **151**, 1226–1228 (1966).

196. M. J. Mellies, T. T. Ishikawa, C. J. Glueck, and J. D. Crissman, Phytosterols and cholesterol in malignant and benign breast tumors, *Cancer Res.* **37**, 3034–3036 (1977).

197. C. S. B. Galasko and A. Bennett, Relationship of bone destruction in skeletal metastases to osteoclast activation and prostaglandins, *Nature* **263**, 508–510 (1976).

198. T. J. Powles, S. A. Clark, D. M. Easty, G. C. Easty, and A. M. Neville, The inhibition by aspirin and indomethacin of osteolytic tumour deposits and hypercalcemia in rats with Walker tumour, and its possible application to human breast cancer, *Br. J. Cancer* **28**, 316–321 (1973).

199. A. Bennett, E. M. Charlier, A. M. McDonald, J. S. Simpson, I. F. Stamford, and T. Zebro, Prostaglandins and breast cancer, *Lancet* **2**, 624–626 (1977).

200. Editorial, Osteolytic metastases, *Lancet* **2**, 1063–1064 (1976).

201. W. F. Kibbey, D. G. Bronn, and J. P. Minton, Prostaglandins and metastasis, *Lancet* **1**, 101 (1978).

202. C. S. Henney and L. M. Lichtenstein, The role of cyclic AMP in the cytolytic activity of lymphocytes, *J. Immunol.* **107**, 610–615 (1971).

203. T. B. Strom, C. B. Carpenter, M. R. Garovoy, K. F. Austen, J. P. Merrill, and M. Kaliner, The modulating influence of cyclic nucleotides upon lymphocyte-mediated cytotoxicity, *J. Exp. Med.* **138**, 381–393 (1973).

204. J. Watson, R. Epstein, and M. Cohn, Cyclic nucleotides as intracellular mediators of the expression of antigen-sensitive cells, *Nature* **246**, 405–409 (1973).

205. H. A. Harvey, J. C. Allegra, L. M. Demers, J. R. Luderer, D. E. Brenner, J. J. Trautlein, D. S. White, M. A. Gillin, and A. Lipton, Immunosuppression and human cancer: Role of prostaglandins, *Cancer* **39**, 2362–2364 (1977).

206. R. Mortel, J. C. Allegra, L. M. Demers, H. A. Harvey, J. Trautlein, W. Nahas, D. White, M. A. Gillin, and A. Lipton, Plasma prostaglandins across the tumor bed of patients with gynecologic malignancy, *Cancer* **39**, 2201–2203 (1977).

207. L. M. Demers, J. C. Allegra, H. A. Harvey, A. Lipton, J. R. Luderer, R. Mortel, and D. E. Brenner, Plasma prostaglandins in hypercalcemia patients with neoplastic disease, *Cancer* **39**, 1559–1562 (1977).

208. W. F. Sample, H. R. Gertner, and P. B. Chretien, Inhibition of phytohemagglutinin-induced lymphocyte transformation by serum from patients with carcinoma, *J. Natl. Cancer Inst.* **46**, 1291–1297 (1971).

209. E. J. Field and E. A. Caspary, Lymphocyte sensitisation in advanced malignant disease: A study of serum lymphocyte depressive factor, *Br. J. Cancer* **26**, 164–173 (1972).

210. A. H. Glasgow, R. B. Nimberg, J. O. Menzoian, I. Saporoschetz, S. R. Cooperband, K. Schmid, and J. A. Mannick, Association of anergy with an immunosuppressive peptide fraction in the serum of patients with cancer, *New Engl. J.Med.* **291**, 1263–1267 (1974).

211. J. C. Occhino, A. H. Glasgow, S. R. Cooperband, J. A. Mannick, and K. Schmid, Isolation of an immunosuppressive peptide fraction from human plasma, *J. Immunol.* **110**, 685–694 (1973).

212. A. M. Badger, S. R. Cooperband, V. J. Merluzzi, and A. H. Glasgow, Immunosuppression activity of ascitic fluid from patients with cancer metastatic to the peritoneum, *Cancer Res.* **37**, 1220–1228 (1977).

213. D. K. Podolsky and M. M. Weiser, Detection, purification, and characterization of a human cancer-associated galactosyltransferase acceptor, *Biochem. J.* (in press).

214. D. K. Podolsky, M. M. Weiser, and K. J. Isselbacher, Inhibition of the growth of transformed cells and tumors by an endogenous acceptor of galactosyltransferase, *Proc. Natl. Acad. Sci. U.S.A.* **75**, 4426–4430 (1978).

215. R. A. Q. O'Meara, Coagulative properties of cancer, *Irish J. Med. Sci.* **394**, 474–479 (1958).

216. Y. N. Lee, Experimental studies of metastases. A review, *Mo. Med.* **65**, 36–39; 123–128; 205–210 (1968).

217. G. J. Gasic, T. B. Gasic, and C. C. Stewart, Antimetastatic effects associated with platelet reduction, *Proc. Natl. Acad. Sci. U.S.A.* **61**, 46–52 (1968).

218. B. Hagmar, Experimental tumor metastases and blood coagulability, *Acta Path. Microbiol. Scand. Suppl.* 211 (1970).

219. H. Gastpar, Inhibition of cancer cell stickiness by anticoagulants, fibrinolytic drugs, and pyrimido-pyrimidine derivatives, *Hematol. Rev.* **3**, 1–51 (1972).

220. A. S. Ketcham, H. Wexler, and N. Mantel, The effect of removal of a "primary" tumor on development of spontaneous metastases. I. Development of standardized experimental technic, *Cancer Res.* **19**, 940–944 (1959).

221. L. Ivarsson, Pulmonary metastasis formation after trauma, *Acta Chir. Scand.* **463**, 1–46 (1976).

222. E. E. Clifton and D. Agostino, Factors affecting the development of metastatic cancer. Effects of alteration in clotting mechanism, *Cancer* **15**, 276–283 (1962).

223. N. Kohler and A. Lipton, Platelets as a source of fibroblast growth-promoting activity, *Exp. Cell Res.* **87**, 297–301 (1974).
224. R. Ross, J. Glomset, B. Kariya, and L. Harker, A platelet-dependent serum factor that stimulates the proliferation of arterial smooth muscle cells *in vitro*, *Proc. Natl. Acad. Sci. U.S.A.* **71**, 1207–1210 (1974).
225. G. J. Gasic, D. Boettiger, J. L. Catalfamo, T. B. Gasic, and G. J. Stewart, Aggregation of platelets and cell membrane vesiculation by rat cells transformed in vitro by Rous sarcoma virus, *Cancer Res.* **38**, 2950–2955 (1978).
226. A. Poggi, N. Polentarutti, M. B. Donati, G. de Gaetano, and S. Garattini, Blood coagulation changes in mice bearing Lewis lung carcinoma, a metastasizing tumor, *Cancer Res.* **37**, 272–277 (1977).
227. H. I. Peterson, I. Kjartansson, K. Korsan-Bengtsen, C. M. Rudenstam, and L. Zettergren, Fibrinolysis in human malignant tumor, *Acta Chir. Scand.* **139**, 219–223 (1973).
228. T. Nemoto, T. Han, J. Minowada, V. Angkur, A. Chamberlain, and T. L. Dao, Cell-mediated immune status of breast cancer patients: Evaluation by skin tests, lymphocyte stimulation, and counts of rosette-forming cells, *J. Natl. Cancer Inst.* **53**, 641–645 (1974).
229. M. Flores, J. H. Marti, N. Grosser, J. K. MacFarlane, and D. M. P. Thomson, An overview: Antitumor immunity in breast cancer assayed by tube leukocyte adherence inhibition, *Cancer* **39**, 494–505 (1977).
230. A. E. Papatestas, G. J. Lesnick, G. Genkins, and A. H. Aufses, Jr., The prognostic significance of peripheral lymphocyte counts in patients with breast carcinoma, *Cancer* **37**, 164–168 (1976).
231. A. E. Bray and P. G. Holt, Serum blocking factor as an index of metastatic spread following primary tumor excision, *Eur. J. Cancer* **11**, 855–860 (1975).
232. R. B. Herberman, Immunologic approaches to the diagnosis of cancer, *Cancer* **37**, 549–562 (1976).
233. A. S. Levin, V. S. Byers, H. H. Fudenberg, J. Wybran, A. J. Hackett, J. O. Johnston, and L. E. Spitler, Osteogenic sarcoma—Immunologic parameters before and during immunotherapy with tumor-specific transfer factors, *J. Clin. Invest.* **55**, 487–499 (1975).
234. K. E. Hellström and I. Hellström, Lymphocyte-mediated cytotoxicity and blocking serum activity to tumor antigens, *Adv. Immunol.* **18**, 209–277 (1974).
235. W. J. Halliday and S. Miller, Leukocyte adherence inhibition. A simple test for cell-mediated tumor immunity and serum blocking factors, *Int. J. Cancer* **9**, 477–483 (1972).
236. S. Bonsal and H. O. Sjögren, Correlation between changes in antitumor immune parameters and tumor growth in rats, *Fed. Proc. Fed. Am. Soc. Exp. Biol.* **32**, 165–172 (1973).
237. H. O. Sjögren, I. Hellström, S. C. Bonsal, and K. E. Hellström, Suggestive evidence that the "blocking antibodies" of tumor bearing individuals may be antigen–antibody complexes, *Proc. Natl. Acad. Sci. U.S.A.* **68**, 1372–1375 (1971).
238. J. Tamerius, J. Nepom, I. Hellström, and K. E. Hellström, Tumor associated blocking factors: Isolation from sera of tumor bearing mice, *J. Immunol.* **116**, 724–730 (1976).
239. R. H. Yonemoto, T. Fujisawa, and S. R. Waldman, Effect of serum blocking factors on leukocyte adherence inhibition in breast cancer patients: Specificity and correlation with tumor burden, *Cancer* **41**, 1289–1297 (1978).
240. R. J. Jamasbi, P. Nettesheim, and S. J.Kennel, Detection of circulating tumor antigens in mice carrying a highly metastatic pulmonary squamous cell carcinoma, *Int. J. Cancer* **21**, 387–394 (1978).

241. D. W. Dresser and N. A. Mitchison, The mechanism of immunological paralysis, *Adv. Immunol.* **8**, 129–181 (1968).

242. W. O. Weigle, D. G. Sieckmann, M. V. Doyle, and J. M. Chiller, Possible role of suppressor cells in immunological tolerance, *Transplant. Rev.* **26**, 186–205 (1975).

243. J. Zighelboim, B. Bonavida, V. S. Rao, and J. L. Fahey, Blocking activity induced by soluble alloantigens, *J. Immunol.* **112**, 433–435 (1974).

244. R. J. M. Wilson, Soluble antigens as blocking antigens, in: *Ciba Foundation Symposium on Parasites in the Immunized Host: Mechanisms of Survival*, pp. 185–203, Associated Scientific Publishers, New York (1974).

245. B. M. Ogilvie and R. J. M. Wilson, Evasion of the immune response by parasites, *Br. Med. Bull.* **32**, 177–181 (1976).

246. H. B. Hewitt and E. R. Blake, Facilitation of nodal metastasis from a non-immunogenic murine carcinoma by previous whole-body irradiation of tumour recipients, *Br. J. Cancer* **36**, 23–34 (1977).

247. E. J. Stanbridge, L. R. Boulger, C. R. Franks, J. A. Garrett, D. E. Reeson, D. Bishop, and F. T. Perkins, Optimal conditions for the growth of malignant human and animal cell populations in immunosuppressed mice, *Cancer Res.* **35**, 2203–2212 (1975).

248. J. Stjernswärd, Decreased survival related to irradiation postoperatively in the early operable breast cancer, *Lancet* **2**, 1285–1286 (1974).

249. S. Eccles and P. Alexander, Immunologically mediated restraint of latent tumour metastases, *Nature* **257**, 52–53 (1975).

250. S. Rose, Augmentation of immune activity by elimination of antibody and its implication in cancer, *J. Surg. Oncol.* **5**, 137–166 (1973).

251. E. S. Priori, G. Seman, L. Dmochowski, H. S. Gallagher, and D. E. Anderson, Immunofluorescent studies on sera of patients with breast carcinoma, *Cancer* **28**, 1462–1471 (1971).

252. E. M. Edynak, Y. Hirshaut, M. Bernhard, and G. Trempe, Fluorescent antibody studies of human breast cancer, *J. Natl. Cancer Inst.* **48**, 1137–1143 (1972).

253. J. G. Sinkovics, W. J. Reeves, and J. R. Cabiness, Cell- and antibody-mediated immune reactions of patients to culture cells of breast carcinoma, *J. Natl. Cancer Inst.* **48**, 1145–1149 (1972).

254. C. R. Boehm, B. J. Boehm, and L. J. Humphrey, The natural history of the antibody response to breast cancer antigens, *Clin. Exp. Immunol.* **16**, 31–40 (1974).

255. M. J. K. Hudson, L. J. Humphrey, F. A. Mantz, and P. A. Morse, Jr., Correlation of circulating serum antibody to the histological findings in breast cancer, *Am. J. Surg.* **128**, 756–763 (1974).

256. R. E. Nordquist, F. B. Schafer, N. E. Manning, D. R. Ishmael, and A. F. Hoge, Antitumor antibodies in human breast cancer sera as detected by fixed cell immunofluorescence and living cell membrane immunofluorescence assays, *J. Lab. Clin. Med.* **89**, 257–261 (1977).

257. M. M. Roberts, E. M. Bathgate, and A. Stevenson, Serum immunoglobulin levels in patients with breast cancer, *Cancer* **36**, 221–224 (1975).

258. D. Y. Wang, P. R. Goodwin, R. D. Bulbrook, and J. L. Hayward, Plasma immunoglobulin levels in patients with breast cancer. *Cancer* **39**, 2190–2193 (1977).

259. O. Dostálová, E. Schön, M. Wagnarová, J. Jelinek, and V. Wagner, Serum immunoglobulin levels in cancer patients. II. Serum immunoglobulins and stage of tumor progression. *Neoplasma* **23**, 95–102 (1977).

260. O. Dostálová, V. Wagnarová, E. Schön, V. Wagner, and J. Jelinek, Serum immunoglobulin levels in cancer patients. III. Immunoglobulin levels and metastases of malignant tumors. *Neoplasma* **24**, 177–191 (1977).

261. R. K. Gershon, R. L. Carter, and K. Kondo, Immunologic defenses against metas-

tases: Impairment by excision of an allotransplanted lymphoma, *Science* **159**, 646–648 (1968).

262. C. Carnaud, B. Hoch, and N. Trainin, Influence of immunologic competence of the host on metastases induced by the 3LL Lewis tumor in mice, *J. Natl. Cancer Inst.* **52**, 395–399 (1974).

263. F. Avis, I. Avis, J. P. Hindsley, Jr., and G. Haughton, Interactions of cancer cells with antibodies and other humoral factors, in: *Fundamental Aspects of Metastasis* (L. Weiss, ed.), pp. 191–204, North-Holland Publishing Co., Amsterdam (1976).

264. M. G. Lewis, The role of circulating antibody in the control of metastases, *J. Clin. Pathol.* **27**, Suppl. 7, 83–93 (1974).

265. S. A. Eccles and P. Alexander, Macrophage content of tumours in relation to metastatic spread and host immune reaction, *Nature* **250**, 667–669 (1974).

266. G. W. Wood and G. Y. Gillespie, Studies on the role of macrophages in regulation of growth and metastasis of murine chemically induced fibrosarcomas, *Int. J. Cancer* **16**, 1022–1029 (1975).

267. I. J. Fidler, Macrophage deficiency in tumor bearing animals: Control of experimental metastasis with macrophages activated *in vitro*, in: *The Macrophage in Neoplasia* (M. A. Fink, ed.), pp. 245–257, Academic Press, New York (1976).

268. L. A. Liotta, J. Kleinerman, and G. M. Saidel, Mechanism of Bacillus Calmette-Guérin-induced suppression of metastases in a poorly immunogenic fibrosarcoma, *Cancer Res.* **36**, 3255–3259 (1976).

269. R. Evans and P. Alexander, Mechanisms of extracellular killing of nucleated mammalian cells by macrophages, in: *Immunobiology of the Macrophage* (D. S. Nelson, ed.), pp. 535–576, Academic Press, New York (1976).

270. J. B. Hibbs, Jr., R. R. Taintor, H. A. Chapman, and J. B. Weinberg, Macrophage tumor killing: Influence of the local environment, *Science* **197**, 279–282 (1977).

Mechanism of Regression in Hormone-Dependent Mammary Carcinomas

PIETRO M. GULLINO

1. Introduction

Ovariectomy, hypophysectomy, and adrenalectomy, either singly or in combination, can appreciably alter the growth rate of human mammary carcinomas in 30 to 40% of patients. The modification may range from growth arrest for a variable period of time to shrinkage or total disappearance of the tumor. Spontaneous or induced mammary carcinomas of experimental animals behave as the human counterpart. The objective of this chapter is to analyze the events that occur within mammary carcinomas regressing after the hormonal status of the host has been altered. An understanding of these events may offer some clues for the therapeutic induction of tumor regression.

Abbreviations Used in This Chapter: cAMP—cyclic adenosine 3′,5′-monophosphate; dibutyryl cAMP—$N^6,O^{2'}$-dibutyryl cyclic adenosine 3′,5′-monophosphate; DMBA—primary, hormone-dependent, dimethylbenz(α)anthracene-induced mammary carcinoma in Sprague–Dawley female rats; MTW9—transplantable, mammotropin-dependent mammary carcinoma in Wistar/Furth female rats; W256—transplantable, hormone-independent Walker 256 mammary carcinoma.

PIETRO M. GULLINO • Laboratory of Pathophysiology, National Cancer Institute, National Institutes of Health, Bethesda, Maryland 20014.

2. Pathophysiology of the Regressing Tumor

2.1. Morphology

The regression process of hormone-dependent mammary carcinomas conforms to a sequence of events common to several tissues
undergoing controlled cell death. None of the structural changes recognizable in the regressing tumor can be considered as a specific consequence of hormonal deprivation. However, tissue destruction during
hormone-dependent regression follows some of the general patterns
that are more characteristic of shrinkage necrosis or apoptosis[1-3] than of
ischemic coagulative necrosis.[4-7]

The term "coagulative necrosis" describes the histologic aspect of
the parenchyma. It is most frequently related to the vagaries of tumor
blood supply and involves an entire sector of tissue, mainly the center;
it can be found in almost every tumor, mammary carcinomas included,
regardless of their hormone dependency. As shown by Tannock[8] in a
mouse mammary tumor, massive cell death will occur at a predictable
distance from functioning blood vessels. Cells close to the vessel proliferate and dislodge surrounding cells. The distance between the vessel
and the region where cell necrosis is morphologically evident is almost
100 μm, which Thomlinson and Gray[9] observed to coincide roughly with
the limit of oxygen diffusion. Whether the cause of cell death is due only
to a lack of oxygen remains to be ascertained; however, it seems reasonable to assume that coagulative necrosis is not a hormone-related event
but rather is dependent on the general inability of the vascular system to
maintain an environment compatible with cell survival in the face of
continuous cell proliferation.

Apoptosis consists of tissue alterations where cell-limited processes
of digestion prevail, and regression appears to evolve as a programmed
phenomenon. Most of the structural changes characteristic of apoptosis
are found in regressing hormone-dependent mammary tumors. Cytoplasm "loosening" is one of the earliest morphologic events described as
an indication of impending cell death. The cell appears to "condense"
and its association with neighboring cells is altered, probably by a process of dehydration.[1] Thereafter, the following events occur in a variable sequence: disappearance of ribosomes with disruption of the endoplasmic reticulum, mitochondrial damage represented most often by
swelling and disappearance of the membranous structure, extensive in-
dentations of the plasma membrane resulting in fragmentation of the
cytoplasm, and clumping of nuclear chromatin with an increase in electron opacity of both the nucleus and cytoplasm. MTW9, a transplantable

mammary carcinoma of the rat that regresses promptly after elimination of mammotropins,[10-14] closely repeats these events.

Atrophy and hydropic degeneration are two other structural features that are more commonly seen in 7,12-dimethylbenz(α)anthracene (DMBA)-induced mammary carcinomas regressing after ovariectomy. Atrophy is more visible in tumors with adenomatous and papillary structures. The epithelial cells are stretched over the stroma, often endothelial-like in appearance, with flattened nuclei and only one-half the cytoplasm present in growing tumors. It might be noted that in cells of the adrenal cortex, atrophy produced by hypophysectomy involves loss of template activity secondary to DNA damage.[15] No similar observation has been made for the mammary epithelium. Hydropic changes are usually confined to the cytoplasm and localized in single cells that appear like inflated balloons among normal-appearing cells. Cysts may be present and are most often found in DMBA-induced tumors.

Lymphocytic infiltrates of the type seen in transplant rejection or in the regression of hormone-unrelated tumors, such as sarcomas produced by Moloney virus,[16-18] are not seen during regression of hormone-dependent mammary carcinomas. When diffuse atrophy of the epithelial component occurs, the number of mononuclear cells of the stroma may appear to be increased on standard histologic sections but it is impossible to establish whether this is the actual case or just an effect of shrinkage.

When apoptosis is the predominant event in regression, a large number of cells become fragmented. Peculiar characteristics of these fragments are the preservation of the plasma membrane and the rapid phagocytosis by the surrounding neoplastic cells.[3] The cellular fragmentation observed in histologic sections may be the consequence of intensive blebbing as observed in cultured cells before death approaches (zeiosis).[19] The zeiotic bleb apparently begins as a change in the morphology of the plasma membrane followed by extrusion of the cytoplasm. Retraction of the bleb begins with alterations of the endoplasmic reticulum which later disappears, having an aggregation of what appears to be polysomes in a pool of electron-transparent matrix enclosed by the cell membrane.[20,21]

The morphologic picture of regressing tumors with prevalent apoptosis is characterized by the presence of phagosomes in many neoplastic cells. Differentiation between auto- and heterophagosomes becomes difficult in these cases. The phagocytic capacity of neoplastic cells must be kept in mind when the morphology of regressing tumors is studied and the role of macrophages is evaluated.

In growing tumors one can find all the same morphologic events as described in regressing tumors, the difference being mostly in their frequency. It is deceiving, however, to believe that the number of regressing cells visible on a histologic section can reflect the extent of cell destruction and turnover occurring in the tumor. The turnover time of a cell population depends on cell death and on removal of cellular debris. This last event is usually rapid but has little morphologic evidence. Lastly, in describing pathologic changes in cell populations that undergo an apparent programmed death, one has the impulse to draw up a timetable in which the structural changes are placed in order of appearance, with the implication that earlier events are causally related to later events. While such a "timetable" may be a useful guide, one must be aware that it may also be misleading until the mechanism of regression is better understood.

2.2. Cell Loss

Tumor growth results from a prevalence of cell accumulation over destruction. At least three factors are involved in this process: cell cycle time, cell growth fraction, and rate of cell loss. The labeled-mitosis technique[22–27] permits estimation of both the time interval during which a group of cells completes one full mitotic cycle and the fraction of cells within a population that are considered to be proliferating because they incorporate a DNA precursor. The rate of cell loss is an indirect value, measured by the discrepancy between the expected growth rate (calculated from the cell cycle and growth fraction) and the observed growth rate *in vivo*. This last factor changes with time and a retardation of growth is usually observed as the tumor mass increases. Cell loss is best expressed as the ratio between the rate constant of cell loss and cell production. Steel[28,29] calls this value the loss factor; it has the advantage of being independent of population size, which usually varies during the period of study.

For most human tumors, the cell loss has been estimated to be between 54% and 99% of cell production.[28,30,31] For rat mammary tumors induced by DMBA, Steel calculated[32] from the data of Simpson-Herren and Lloyd[33] a cell loss factor of 86%. In spontaneous C3H mammary tumors, cell loss factors of 69% and 79% were calculated and the rate of cell loss per hour was estimated to be 0.75% and 1.27%, respectively, of the total cell population.[29] In Ehrlich ascites tumors, the cell loss factor increased with time and was estimated to be 18% at day 1 but 70% at day 7 after implant. The rate of cell loss per hour, however, did not change appreciably: 1.39% at day 1 and 1.27% at day 7 after transplant.[34] This finding cannot be generalized. For a transplanted fibrosarcoma studied by Frindel et al.,[35] Steel calculated that the fraction of tumor cells lost per hour increased from about 0 at day 3 after transplant to 55% of the rate of cell production at day 20.[36]

The relative impact of cycle time, growth fraction, and cell loss on deceleration of growth rate as tumor size increased was studied by Lala[37] in Ehrlich ascites tumors. He concluded that a gradual prolongation of each stage of the mitotic cycle and a progressive transition of cells into a resting state were the two events with major impact on growth deceleration. An analysis of published data convinced Lala[38] that for a variety of ascites tumors the progressive increase in the duration of the cell cycle was the major factor contributing to growth deceleration as tumor volume increased, while the decline in the growth fraction contributed in some but not in other tumors, and the increase in the rate of cell loss seemed to play a minor role.

The model of ascites tumor growth does not appear to be applicable to solid tumors. Studies on cell population kinetics of tumors grown in both solid and ascites forms[35,39-42] indicated that a decrease in the growth fraction was the prevalent event in determining growth deceleration of solid tumors, while changes in the cell cycle were less prominent than in the ascites model and cell loss played a role mostly when tumors were rather large. The only direct determination of cell loss via blood that I know of was obtained in our laboratory for MTW9. With an immunologic approach to estimate the number of neoplastic cells in the efferent tumor blood, the cell loss was evaluated at $3-4 \times 10^6$/g per 24 hr and did not increase during hormone-induced regression of the tumor. [43]

Tumor shrinkage, as the end result of cell loss, is magnified by the rapid decline of the cell growth fraction as soon as hormones are removed. Upon continuous infusion of labeled precursors, incorporation into DNA of MTW9 mammary carcinomas was about one-third that of the control at the end of 24 hr from hormone removal, one-fifth at the end of 48 hr, and practically nil at the end of the third day.[44] The thymidine labeling index of DMBA-induced mammary carcinomas rapidly declined after ovariectomy and both the S phase and the intermitotic time of the few dividing cells were prolonged.[45]

If one compares the growth of a tumor to the increment in volume of a fluid in a container provided with an inlet pouring at a rate slightly superior to the drainage, hormone removal acts both on the input (cell reproduction) and the output (cell loss). The role of hormones in maintaining high levels of cell reproduction is beyond the scope of this discussion. The influence of hormones on determining cell loss appears to be related mainly to lysis by digestion. Cell loss by migration out of the tumor, via efferent blood, has been shown in at least one experimental system to be negligible.[43] One of the first questions to answer is whether cell loss after hormone withdrawal results from metabolic derangement of the tissue.

2.3. Metabolism

The metabolic requirement of mammary tumors regressing after hormonal deprivation of the host has been studied mainly to ascertain whether reduction of the cell growth fraction and cell death could be related to metabolic deficiencies. The role of blood supply was evaluated *in vivo* using a tumor preparation that permitted direct measurement for several hours of the total volume of blood passing through the tumor.[46] On the average, regressing tumors had as good a blood supply as growing ones. For instance, blood flow of growing MTW9 mammary carcinomas was 6.5 ± 1.2 ml/hr per gram and 6.7 ± 0.4 in the regressing counterpart. The range of variability in blood flow among tumors of a similar size was also about the same whether measured during growth or regression.[47]

The consumption of oxygen and glucose *in vivo* was taken as an index of the overall tumor metabolic activity and it was found that during regression MTW9 rat mammary carcinomas had the same consumption as the growing counterpart on a weight basis. This implied that regression required as much energy as growth and that during tumor shrinkage the pericellular structures retained the ability to perform their basal physiological functions. This last possibility was tested experimentally by two approaches. The sizes of the vascular, interstitial, and cellular compartments were measured in primary DMBA-induced tumors and in transplantable MTW9. The vascular space measured with high-molecular-weight dextran was found to be about 5% of tumor size in MTW9 and 10% in DMBA carcinomas; the interstitial space measured with ^{24}Na was about 43% and 59%, respectively; and the cellular space was calculated from the difference to be in the order of 50% and 31%, respectively. When the same measurements were repeated in tumors regressed to one-half the original size, the relative proportion of the compartment sizes was not significantly changed.[47] Tumor shrinkage therefore occurred as a coordinated event with preservation of the basic physiologic compartments. The efficiency of the physiologic structures was tested by comparing the oxygen-utilizing capacity of growing and regressing MTW9 carcinomas *in vivo*.[47-50] Tumors that had regressed to about one-half the original size removed about 50% of the oxygen brought by the afferent blood. When this blood supply was reduced to one-half or one-third, the oxygen-removal capacity of the tumor increased to 80–85% of the oxygen received; but when the physiologic level of the blood supply was doubled, the oxygen-removal ratio decreased to about 25% of the input.[44,47] Thus, a decreased supply was compensated for by an increased removal, and vice versa, but utilization was kept at physiologic levels. This behavior of regressing MTW9 carcinomas was the same as that of the growing counterpart. Therefore, the efficiency in regulating a basic physiologic function such as oxygen removal from blood was preserved during regression. Whether the results obtained with these models can be generalized to all hormone-dependent mammary carcinomas remains an open question. It seems reasonable to conclude, however, that gross metabolic deficiencies are undetectable in tumors at the onset or during hormone-induced regression and, therefore, their role is not likely to be a determinant one in tissue destruction.

3. Tissue Destruction during Regression

3.1. Phagocytosis

Cells with cytoplasmic phagosomes are present in both growing and regressing mammary carcinomas but a systematic comparison of their relative number as regression progresses has not been made. Morphologic examination of randomly selected areas suggests, however, that regressing tumors have a higher content of phagocytosing cells. MTW9 carcinoma is a particularly representative model in this respect since during growth phagocytes are relatively rare but at the end of the first week of regression almost all cells contain phagosomes in their cytoplasms.[47]

The role of macrophages in hormone-dependent tumor regression has not been properly explored. The acquisition of a phagocytic capacity by neoplastic cells, however, has been well recognized.[3] Consequently, it is difficult to distinguish morphologically a phagocyte that has migrated into the tumor from a neoplastic cell with phagocytic activity.

In the last few years the cytotoxicity of activated macrophages against neoplastic cells has been studied extensively.[51,52] One of the primary objectives was to define the conditions necessary for "activating" the macrophage to kill the neoplastic cell. Impetus for this work was provided by the observation that macrophages could be cytotoxic against neoplastic BALB/3T12 fibroblasts but not against normal BALB/3T3 fibroblasts. [53-55] In most of this work, a macrophage was defined as a cell present in the peritoneal exudate and obtained by a variety of treatments, e.g., thioglycollate, peptone, *Toxoplasma* infection, etc. Tumor-localized macrophages have been characterized[56-59] as cells (1) able to adhere to glass after tissue dispersion with hydrolytic enzymes, (2) resistant to detachment by trypsinization, (3) lysed by antimacrophage serum and complement, (4) having Fc receptors, and (5) able to phagocytize opsonized sheep erythrocytes. Following these criteria, the content of macrophages found in human mammary carcinomas varied from 0 to 30%[60] and in experimental tumors such as rat sarcomas from 3% to 55%.[58,61] No correlation with tumor type or growth rate was apparent. However, the metastasizing capacity of transplantable rat sarcomas was found to be low when a large number of macrophages were found in the tumors.[61-64] Human mammary carcinomas known to have metastasized contained less than 10% of macrophages whereas carcinomas without evidence of metastasis at surgery had a widely varying number of macrophages.[60] The opinion that an elevated concentration of macrophages reduces the chances of metastasis has some supporting evidence. However, the diagnostic application of this concept specifically to the evaluation of sinus histiocytosis in axillary lymph nodes of mammary carcinomas has been less fruitful than expected.[65-67]

The containment of metastases should be related to the cytotoxic capacity of macrophages. In fact, macrophages specifically activated *in vitro* against B16 melanoma were able to reduce the number of pulmonary metastases when injected intravenously into mice that had received a melanoma transplant 48 hr earlier.[68,69] Peritoneal macrophages are not cytotoxic to neoplastic cells under physiologic conditions. Tumoricidal potential, however, can be induced in macrophages with a variety of treatments and can be evaluated by the interaction between phagocytes and neoplastic cells *in vitro*.[55] In fact, the tumoricidal capacity is defined not by the induction procedure but by the specificity of the effect. As an example, mice injected with BCG or *Toxoplasma* produced peritoneal macrophages that in culture were strongly cytotoxic to neoplastic fibroblasts when tested within 24 hr of initial culture. After 72 hr, however, the tumoricidal capacity was lost. Addition of peritoneal lymphocytes plus tuberculin restored the cytopathic action but addition of lymphocytes or tuberculin alone failed to restore cytotoxicity.[70] This example brings to light two major components of the tumoricidal activity of macrophages, one specifically linked to antigenic determinants and involving lymphocytes, and the second nonspecific.[55,70-77] Studies on the interactions among inducing antigens, sensitized lymphocytes, activated macrophages, and effects of various environmental conditions on macrophage cytotoxicity[78,79] provided results that were most often applicable only to the experimental system used and offered little assurance of their validity *in vivo*. Unfortunately, hormone-dependent mammary carcinomas have not been utilized in this work. To my knowledge a comparison of macrophage behavior during growth and regression has only been made in sarcomas produced by Moloney virus.[16-18] In this system, however, regression is characterized by a massive cellular infiltration of an inflammatory type that is totally different both in morphology and pathologic behavior from that found in hormone-induced regression where an inflammatory type of cellular infiltrate is absent.

The mechanism of cell killing by macrophages has been studied extensively by Keller.[76] He distinguished between a cytostatic and a cytocidal effect[80] and estimated the cytostatic effect by the depression in growth rates of a variety of cell populations in culture, using the incorporation of labeled precursors as a marker. Despite the limitation of the methodology, it appears that macrophages can induce growth depression of rapidly replicating cells. Moreover, evidence that cytostasis is mediated by a soluble factor secreted by macrophages is accumulating [81-86] although a purified product is not yet available and the reproducibility of results using supernatants of macrophage cultures is not satisfactory. A cytolytic or cytocidal effect appears to require a close proximity between macrophage and target cell. [87-89] Zbar et al. [90,91] described two steps in macrophage-induced cytolysis: The first step concerning cell recognition is specific and depends on sensitized lymphocytes; the second step concerning cell destruction is nonspecific. The promotion of cell destruction by close contact implies transfer of macrophage products into the target cell. Indeed, Hibbs[92] and Bucana et al.[93] have presented evidence suggesting that macrophages inject lysosomes into the target cells. Currie and Basham,[54] however, pointed out that cell contact was necessary for a lytic effect only when the culture media had a high serum concentration; in media with low serum content the selective lysis of tumor cells was mediated by a soluble supernatant factor. Melsom et al.[94,95] observed lysis of erythrocytes produced by a factor of small molecular weight, dependent on SH groups for its action and released by macrophages activated simply by cultivation on glass or plastic. In this as in many other circumstances, the environment may have a determinant role in shaping the cell response. The relevance of the in vitro observations to the in vivo situation cannot be evaluated at this time, particularly in reference to hormone-dependent mammary carcinomas.

The phagocytic capacity of the neoplastic cells is so prominent in these tumors that it is difficult to distinguish bona fide macrophages from phagocytosing neoplastic cells. Comprehensive studies of the effect of infiltrating macrophages on the biological properties of hormone-dependent mammary carcinomas are not available. What are the macrophages doing in the tumor? There is evidence to support a restraining effect on tumor growth but the specificity of this action and the conditions that may limit its effectiveness in vivo are still unclear. [96] In particular, the influence of hormones on the properties of macrophages and lymphocytes present in hormone-dependent mammmary carcinomas is unknown. One must also keep in mind an old observation that has been confirmed for a variety of tumors, namely that aortic infusion of inert carbon particles produces very little phagocytosis in the tumor as compared to organs such as liver and spleen. [47] *In vivo*, the capacity of tumor phagocytes to incorporate inert particles is very low; indeed the test suggests that tumor phagocytes are unable to phagocytize. The "paralyzing" effect of neoplastic cells on macrophages is still a puzzling event. [52]

3.2. Lysis of Tissue Components

A comparison between the gross chemical composition of growing and regressing mammary carcinomas was carried on with the main objective of determining whether conspicuous differences of a general nature were evident.[44,47,97] In two experimental systems, primary DMBA-induced and MTW9 transplantable tumors, tissues were analyzed when tumors had regressed to about one-half their original size of 3–4 g. When referred to tissue weight, the content of collagen and DNA was 32–40% larger in regressing than in the growing counterparts, the water content remained unchanged, and all other components were reduced to a varying degree. When referred to DNA content, the concentration of RNA was about 30% lower during regression in both experimental systems but the loss of proteins was more pronounced in MTW9 than in DMBA tumors: 40% of total proteins and 53% of phosphoproteins in the former as compared with 19% and 35%, respectively, in the latter. Loss of phospholipids was about 30% in both tumor types but a sharp difference was observed in the triglyceride content. Regressing MTW9 had about 30% fewer triglycerides than the growing counterpart whereas regressing DMBA accumulated triglycerides to about twice the amount measured in the growing tumors. This was the largest difference observed between the two systems.[47] Ratios of DNA, RNA, and protein content of nuclear and cytoplasmic fractions revealed differences within 20% for MTW9 and 25% for DMBA. Thus the relative proportion of these fractions was not drastically altered by regression.

Since glucose is a metabolite used in large amounts by tumors *in vivo*,[49] continuous intravenous infusion of [U-D^{14}C]glucose for periods varying from 24 to 96 hr was utilized to test the ability of regressing tumors to incorporate a basic substrate in different cell components. In both DMBA and MTW9 carcinomas, label incorporation into DNA fell rapidly and was practically nil at 72 hr in MTW9 and at 96 hr in DMBA. During the same period of time, incorporation into RNA and protein of both nuclear and cytoplasmic fractions was still substantial but quite different in the two tumor types. When expressed as specific activity, regressing MTW9 incorporated from two- to fivefold less label than growing tumors, but regressing DMBA incorporated as much label as the growing counterpart. When ratios of specific activities were compared for various tissue fractions, no difference in label distribution was observed in regressing versus growing DMBA; in MTW9, however, there was a significant difference in RNA and protein contents of both nuclear and cytoplasmic fractions.[44]

The overall impression derived from these measurements as well as from changes in gross chemical composition, blood supply, size of compartments, and utilization of metabolites during regression was that tumor shrinkage after hormone removal involved not only an arrest of cell proliferation but also a complex modification in the turnover of the cell population with prevalence of lysis over reproduction as the end result.

The extent of the lytic process was demonstrated by an increase of 40% to 60% of the free amino acid level in the efferent blood of regressing as compared to growing tumors. When this increment was related to blood flow and degree of shrinkage for each tumor, it became clear that most of the tumor proteins had to be hydrolyzed up to the amino acid level before being eliminated via the efferent blood.[97] This finding is in accord with the observation that macrophages catabolized [^{131}I]albumin to [^{131}I]monoiodotyrosine as the only detectable radioactive fragment[98] and with studies showing that lysosomal membranes were permeable to free amino acids, much less permeable to dipeptides, and almost impermeable to larger peptides.[99]

The involvement of lysosomes in tissue digestion is a well-known event.[100,101] The increment of lysosomal activity during regression has been shown in mammary tumors both after nonspecific tissue damage, i.e., radiations,[102-105] and after hormone removal.[106-108] In this last case, the increment in activity of lysosomal enzymes (acid phosphatase, β-glucuronidase, β-galactosidase, arylsulfatase, cathepsin, and acid ribonuclease) corresponded to an increase in the number of enzyme molecules per gram of tumor.[107,108] To my knowledge, the turnover rate has been measured only for acid ribonuclease in MTW9 and DMBA tumors.[109,110] Within 24 hr after hormone removal, the half life of the enzyme decreased from 7.8 to 2.6 days, enzyme production increased 15-fold, and accumulation in the tissue doubled the enzyme concentration per gram of tumor. The increment in synthesis of these enzymes is in accord with the high energy consumption found during regression.[47]

The work described above was done on whole tumor homogenates and it was obviously important to establish whether the enzymatic activities were localized within or outside the cells. To this end the interstitial fluid of tumors was collected *in vivo* with a microchamber developed in our laboratory.[46] Lysosomal enzyme activity was only found in whole tumor homogenates but never in tumor interstitial fluid. Nor were lysosomal enzymes found to be present either during tumor growth or regression. Lysosomal enzymes were also absent from the normal sub-cutaneous interstitial fluid. However, when supernatants of tumor homogenates were introduced into the subcutaneous space, fluid sampled from the micropore chamber had an elevated activity, indicating that the enzymes could have been measured if present in active forms. Thus, absence of lysosomal enzyme activity in tumor interstitial fluid collected *in vivo* was interpreted to indicate that digestion was an endocellular process and spillage of lysosomal enzymes outside the cells was a negligible event during hormone-dependent tumor regression.[97] Woessner[111] reached similar conclusions in his studies on involution of the lactating gland.

The elevation of lysosomal activity during mammary tumor regression can be interpreted in at least two ways: as an indication that lysosomes have been activated to destroy the neoplastic cells or that lysosomes are simply expanding their physiologic activity because more substrates are made available as a consequence of hormone removal. Aggressive lysis by lysosomes could be induced by breakage or leakage of the limiting membrane and "spilling" of lytic enzymes into the cytoplasm. [102] The possibility of such an event during an induced hormonal imbalance is sustained by several types of observations: Progesterone changes the permeability of rat liver lysosomes[112]; one day after hypophysectomy clear damage of mitochondrial cristae can be seen in the cells of the zona fasciculata of the adrenals[15]; and lysosomes isolated from liver and muscle of adrenalectomized rats are more "fragile" as indicated by increased levels of free catheptic activity.[113] Indeed, the ratio of free to bound lysosomal enzyme activities in regressing mammary carcinomas is higher than in growing tumors.[109] This is usually interpreted to indicate that lysosomal enzymes not encapsulated within a membrane and "activated" are more abundant during regression. Moreover, factors that labilize and stabilize lysosomes have been found in serum.[114,115]

Against the hypothesis that cell lysis results from lysosomal "attack" are the observations of plasma membrane preservation during the digestion of regressing cells or cell fragments,[3] the lack of enzyme "spilling" into the extracellular fluid,[107] and the increment of free-to-bound ratios in lysosomal enzyme activity appearing only 72 hr after hormone removal when tumors like MTW9 already showed measurable shrinkage. [107,109] None of these conditions should be expected to occur if regression was due to an active digestion by lysosomes pouring lytic enzymes into the cell or its environment. Consequently, the hypothesis seems justified that an increment in both the number of lysosomes and the activity of lysosomal enzymes might be the effect, not the cause, of events triggering regression. Alterations produced by hormone removal may result in increased availability of substrates, which require a higher workload for lysosomes. In support of this hypothesis are the observations that steroids can bind to proteins and induce structural changes.[116-118] Consequently, deprivation of steroids, as in ovariectomy, may influence the structure of proteins and change their half lives, since degradative rates are determined by protein conformation.[119] Evidence has been found by two groups[120,121] that more labile proteins are structurally suited to adhering to membranes rich in lipids; thus penetration into lysosomes should be facilitated, since lipoproteins constitute about one-half of the lysosomal proteins.[122] Within the lysosome, proteins that deviate from normal conformation are rapidly hydrolyzed. The work of Capecchi et al.[123] provides a good example. Mouse L-cell variants lacking hypoxanthine–guanine phosphoribosyltransferase were able to produce proteins that could still react against the purified enzyme. In many of these mutants the inactive protein was degraded up to 20 times faster than the wild-type enzyme and the degradative rates were inversely proportional to the levels of cross-reacting material. Since this rapidly degraded protein reacted with the wild-type enzyme, the observation of Capecchi et al.[123] also suggests that the degradative system of L cells may recognize relatively minor variations from the normal conformation. In fact, different subunits within a multimeric protein have shown distinct half lives, as Fritz et al.[124] described for hepatic isozymes of lactate dehydrogenase. Irreversible damage of major consequence to the cell can be obtained through alteration of a few key proteins. For instance, most enzymes of cholesterol biosynthesis have half lives of 8–12 hr but the rate-limiting enzyme, hydroxymethylglutaryl-CoA reductase, has a half life of 3 hr. The 12 liver proteins with the shortest reported half lives catalyze either the first or the rate-limiting step in metabolic pathways; therefore metabolic control can be accurately monitored by the rapid change in the concentration of these short-lived proteins and errors in their synthesis can rapidly impair cell function and survival.[119,125]

　　　In an attempt to evaluate whether this kind of event could occur during hormone-dependent regression, experiments in our laboratory showed that within 24 hr of hormone withdrawal, cytosol proteins of MTW9 became more easily degraded by trypsin, α-chymotrypsin, or subtilisin BPN.[126] Labilization of cytosol proteins occurred much earlier than any change in the level of protein synthesis or in most of the lysosomal enzyme activities. The increased susceptibility to proteolysis could not be explained by the presence of endogenous proteases or by the destruction of the exogenous proteases used in the assay or by the presence of protease inhibitors in the homogenate, nor could it be modified by preincubation with dithiothreitol, prolactin, 17β-estradiol, progesterone, or hydrocortisone. Moreover, the pattern of leucine incorporation into cytosol proteins differed between growing and regressing MTW9 mammary carcinomas and this difference was localized in three bands of the electrophoretic pattern. This change in pattern appeared within 6 hr after hormone removal, or about 4 hr after prolactin levels in the blood were below the concentration needed by MTW9 to grow.[127] To my knowledge, these are the first indications that hormonal deprivation of the host may induce regression of mammary carcinomas via an effect on the catabolic component in the protein turnover of the cell population.

4. cAMP and Hormone-Dependent Tumor Regression

The hypothesis that phagocytosis and morphologic evidence of tissue lysis are relatively late events in the course of tumor regression implies that specific conditions triggering these events should operate at an earlier stage. Our laboratory concentrated on cAMP as a possible participant in these triggering events since Gericke and Chandra[128] first and Keller[129] later reported growth inhibition of a lymphosarcoma and W256 mammary carcinoma, respectively, by cAMP treatment. Growth inhibition, as represented by inability to form solid tumors in the hamster cheek pouch, was also described for human neoplastic cells when 1 mM cAMP was present in the growing medium before transplantation.[130] Cho-Chung et al.[131-133] studied the growth-inhibiting effect of cAMP derivatives on a series of mammary carcinomas and concluded that one subcutaneous injection of 10 mg/day per 200-g rat of dibutyryl cAMP was sufficient to produce growth arrest of the hormone-dependent DMBA and MTW9 mammary carcinomas. The same dibutyryl cAMP treatment was also able to arrest growth in about 30% of W256, a hormone-independent mammary carcinoma. Some W256 carcinomas in particular regressed completely within two weeks from the start of dibutyryl cAMP treatment. By retransplanting one of these tumors in an untreated animal as soon as shrinkage was observed, one could perpetuate a line of W256 carcinomas regressing constantly after dibutyryl cAMP treatment. Thus, models to study the relationship, if any, between hormone- and/or cAMP-induced regression of mammary carcinomas became available.

The first indication that a relationship existed between steroids and cAMP during regression was provided by the observation that both castration and dibutyryl cAMP injections were inducing a sharp increment of acid RNase activity and quantity within a few hours from initiation of treatment.[109,110] The presence of high levels of cAMP in the tumor was not sufficient to explain the induction of regression since W256 carcinomas, both responsive and unresponsive to dibutyryl cAMP treatment, had similar increments in cAMP levels. Published data also do not give any firm indication that cAMP levels and neoplastic conditions can be correlated *in vivo*.[134].

A relatively large amount of work has been dedicated to the enzymes responsible for the cAMP level in tumors, i.e., adenylate cyclase and cAMP phosphodiesterase. Hepatomas were mostly studied and correlations were sought between neoplastic transformation and levels of activity, or specific localization on cell membranes, or responsiveness to activators such as NaF, glucagon, prostaglandin E_1, etc. Differences were found between normal and neoplastic tissues, but no clear picture emerged linking specific alterations of the two enzymes with the neoplastic transformation.[134] Cho-Chung and Newcomer[135] investigated kinetic properties and regulation of basal activities of both adenylate cyclase and cAMP phosphodiesterase in mammary carcinomas. W256, regressing or not under dibutyryl cAMP treatment, had the same basal adenylate cyclase activity. However, response to stimulation by NaF or prostaglandin E_1 was larger and lasted longer in dibutyryl cAMP-responsive versus -unresponsive tumors. The stimulating effect was due to an increase in V_{max} since there was no significant effect on the K_m for substrates. Although differences in the behavior of adenylate cyclase and cAMP phosphodiesterase suggested that these enzymes play an important role in dibutyryl cAMP responsiveness of W256, it was the study of cAMP-binding proteins that yielded data relevant to the understanding of the regression mechanism.[136]

In eukaryotic systems cAMP operates through enzymatic phosphorylation of proteins via cAMP-dependent protein kinase.[137] This enzyme has been purified from various sources and consists of a catalytic and a regulatory subunit. When cAMP binds to the regulatory subunit, the catalytic locus is activated to promote phosphorylation. In mammary carcinomas, the kinase activity has been found to be lower than in normal tissue[138,139] and, in particular, the stimulating effect of cAMP was weaker.[136,140] Daniel *et al.*[141] were the first to observe a correlation between deficiency of cAMP-binding protein and resistance of S49 lymphosarcoma cells to the lethal effects of dibutyryl cAMP. Coffino and associates[142-146] expanded these observations by analyzing mutants of S49 lymphosarcoma cells resistant to dibutyryl cAMP. They found that some mutant populations had no detectable cAMP-binding or protein kinase activity, some had kinase with reduced apparent affinity for cAMP (K_m), and others had wild-type kinase but with reduced function (V_{max}). Purification of dissociated regulatory and catalytic subunits of the protein kinase followed by reconstruction of the holoenzyme indicated that K_m mutants had an alteration of the regulatory subunit, the binding site for cAMP. In W256 mammary carcinomas the interdependence between alteration of cAMP-binding protein and resistance to alkylating agents was reported by Tisdale and Phillips.[147] Cho-Chung et al.[140] expanded this work and showed that two types of cAMP-binding proteins were present in both dibutyryl cAMP-responsive and -unresponsive W256 but binding capacity was highest at pH 6.5 for dibutyryl cAMP-responsive W256 and at pH 4.5 for cAMP-unresponsive W256. Heat denaturation (50°C), after presaturation of binding sites, destroyed binding capacity much more readily in unresponsive than responsive W256 carcinomas. In fact, a striking coincidence was found between heat stability of binding sites and regression induced by dibutyryl cAMP.[148]

When the cAMP-binding capacity and the protein kinase activity were evaluated in the cytosol and nuclei of regressing W256 analyzed at various intervals after dibutyryl cAMP treatment, evidence was found of a transfer of the cAMP + binding-protein complex from the cytoplasm into the nuclei.[149] This transfer, however, occurred only in W256 regressing after dibutyryl cAMP treatment, not in the unresponsive W256 carcinomas. The intracellular redistribution of cAMP-binding proteins and protein kinase activity after cAMP treatment has also been observed in other tissues.[150,151] The point to stress here is the sharp difference between responsive and unresponsive W256 carcinomas in the nuclear transfer of cAMP + receptor complex. This lack of nuclear accumulation appeared to be associated with an alteration of the complex itself.[152] In a cell-free system, when nuclei of responsive or unresponsive W256 carcinomas were incubated with the cAMP + binding-protein complex from the cytosol of dibutyryl cAMP-responsive W256, accumulation within the nuclei was always observed, regardless of their origin. However, when the same nuclei were incubated with the cAMP + binding protein derived from the cytosol of unresponsive W256, accumulation was not observed, regardless of the origin of the nuclei. Thus, lack of nuclear accumulation of the cAMP + binding-protein complex does not depend on the nuclei but on the complex itself.

The transfer of cAMP + binding-protein complex into the nuclei is followed by the appearance of a phosphorylated nonhistone nuclear protein.[153] The following experiment sustains the statement: The nuclear pellet from a hormone-dependent DMBA-induced mammary carcinoma was incubated with [γ^{33}P]-ATP; the protein kinases of these nuclei phosphorylated nuclear proteins that migrated in acrylamide gels as a single, multispiked peak. When the same experiment was repeated using nuclei from DMBA tumors growing in rats treated with dibutyryl cAMP for a few days until regression was measurable, the phosphorylated proteins of the nucleus constituted two distinct peaks. One was located in the same position observed with nuclei from growing tumor, although almost 40% smaller, and the second was a multispiked peak and less mobile. When purified nuclei from a DMBA growing tumor were isolated and then incubated in the presence of cAMP, the second peak of phosphorylated proteins did not appear on the gel, suggesting that the presence of cytoplasm was necessary at the time of cAMP treatment. The cAMP + binding-protein complex had to migrate into the nuclei before phosphorylation of the regression-related proteins could occur.

An important extension of this observation reinforced the probability that a common mechanism of action was involved in mammary tumor regression induced either by dibutyryl cAMP treatment or castration. The nuclear pellet isolated from primary DMBA-induced mammary carcinomas that had regressed after castration to about one-half their original size was able to phosphorylate nuclear proteins moving in two major peaks, as seen in DMBA tumors regressing under dibutyryl cAMP treatment. Moreover, when the regressing tumor was induced to regrow by injections of 17β-estradiol, the slow-moving peak of phosphorylated proteins disappeared just as it did in the tumor when dibutyryl cAMP treatment was interrupted.[153]

The hypothesis of an interdependency of regression induced in W256 by dibutyryl cAMP treatment and regression obtained after castration in primary mammary carcinomas induced by DMBA was further strengthened by comparing cAMP- and estrogen-binding activities.[154,155] During the first 24 hr following castration, total protein content of DMBA tumors did not change appreciably, whereas cAMP content doubled, and cAMP-binding activity doubled in the cytosol and tripled in the nuclei. Six days after ovariectomy the cAMP content of the regressing tumor was fourfold the original level, the binding activity of the nuclei was increased fivefold over the growing counterpart, while the cAMP bound to the cytosol was decreasing because of the transfer into the nuclei. The pattern for estrogen-binding proteins changed in the opposite direction. In sucrose gradients, as expected, the cytosol of growing tumors showed two major fractions sedimenting at 4 S and 8 S whereas the nuclear fraction contained an estrogen-binding component of a 5 S species. As regression progressed after ovariectomy, the estrogen-binding activity decreased in both the nuclei and cytosol by

80% and 50%, respectively, while binding of cAMP increased. Injections of 17β-estradiol induced tumor regrowth and reversed the trend: Estrogen receptor levels increased and cAMP binding decreased. In a few (12%) DMBA tumors that failed to regress after ovariectomy, cAMP- and estrogen-binding activities remained unchanged.[154] It is important to remember that 17β-estradiol promotes growth of regressing DMBA tumors, but dibutyryl cAMP injected with 17β-estradiol blocks growth.[131,133]

The evidence for steroid and cAMP interaction during regression of mammary carcinomas is based on three events that occur in hormone-dependent tumor models after either ovariectomy or dibutyryl cAMP treatment: (1) phosphorylation of nonhistone nuclear proteins, (2) interdependence of the increase or decrease in the concentration of estrogen- or cAMP-binding proteins, and (3) a sharp change in turnover of acid ribonuclease within a few hours after castration or dibutyryl cAMP treatment. These observations also sustain the opinion that tumor regression can be achieved not only by interfering with the cell reproduction but also by appropriate manipulations of the catabolic component of cell turnover.

5. Physiologic Remodeling, Programmed Cell Death, and Tumor Regression

Death of cells is a regular event in morphogenesis and the means whereby embryonal and larval organs are eliminated at the time of metamorphosis. An earlier generation of biologists emphasized a kind of chance causality for many events involving cell death, i.e., death produced by pressure during morphogenetic movements, death resulting from "losing" the competition for energy sources, etc. Morphologic analysis of regressing tissues offered the basis for placing the phagocyte in the assassin's role and present-day immunologic studies have revived this view. Modern fashion emphasizes the occurrence of cellular death during physiologic remodeling of tissues as being not so much the consequence of chance but rather an event in the execution of a program that is initiated by intrinsic or extrinsic factors. The hypothesis of cell death as a programmed event suggests a sequence of steps and invites a comparison of apparently unrelated phenomena, all part of a process ending in cell lysis. As a result of studies on several biologic systems from insects to vertebrates, a set of generalizations gradually emerged, obviously with limitations. The collapse of cell populations in a wide variety of morphogenetic events, from the development of mutants in

Drosophila [156-158] to the cataclysmic events in amphibian metamorphosis [159-161] or the destruction of neurons without synaptic connections in vertebrates, [162,163] occurs in the absence of obviously toxic stimuli. Acutely killed cells undergo a markedly different type of death by coagulative necrosis in contrast to apoptosis, as previously mentioned. A second generalization, applicable in a wide range of conditions where a "physiologic cell death" occurs, is that a sudden removal of vital supplies does not occur. Although beating a retreat, the cell population does it in an organized and physiologic manner. A third generalization is that RNA and protein synthesis very often occur at the beginning of involution. This appears to be a crucial event since antimetabolites that alter RNA and protein synthesis also alter the course of such different processes as the collapse of the tadpole tail [164] and the lysis of thymocytes treated with glucocorticoid. [165] A fourth generalization concerns the role of phagocytosis and lysosomes in tissue involution. In many tissues, from vertebrates to insects, when cell death is a major event, mobilization of phagocytes and lysosomal activity appears more often to be a secondary event following conditions that "invite" lysosomal attack. [166] The idea that lysosomes actually rupture and release enzymes to initiate the lytic process has now fallen out of vogue.

All four generalizations described above can be applied to hormone-dependent mammary tumor regression. Cell destruction occurs in the absence of obviously toxic stimuli, while metabolic supplies are well preserved. Tumor shrinkage occurs as a coordinated event and a high level of RNA and protein synthesis can be observed at the beginning of regression. Lysosomal involvement appears to be more of a "mopping-up" type of operation than the cause of regression. Cyclic AMP plays a role in the triggering of tumor regression as evidenced by: (1) growth arrest and regression following dibutyryl cAMP treatment of the host, (2) antagonistic change in concentrations of estrogen and cAMP receptors during regression, and (3) appearance of phosphorylated proteins in the nuclei following both ovariectomy and dibutyryl cAMP treatment. Whether or not these events are part of a program is unclear. However, the acceleration of cell lysis observed during hormone-dependent regression of mammary carcinomas appears to result from an amplification of the still mysterious signals that control tissue catabolism in general.

ACKNOWLEDGMENT: I wish to thank my collaborators over the years and Ms. U. Walz for her contribution to the preparation of this chapter.

6. References

1. J. F. R. Kerr, Shrinkage necrosis: A distinct mode of cellular death, *J. Pathol.* **105**, 13–20 (1971).
2. J. F. R. Kerr and J. Searle, The digestion of cellular fragments within phagolysosomes in carcinoma cells, *J. Pathol.* **108**, 55–58 (1972).
3. J. F. R. Kerr, A. H. Wyllie, and A. R. Currie, Apoptosis: A basic biological phenomenon with wide-ranging implications in tissue kinetics, *Br. J. Cancer* **26**, 239–257 (1972).
4. G. Majno, M. LaGattuta, and T. E. Thompson, Cellular death and necrosis; chemical, physical and morphologic changes in rat liver, *Virchows Arch. Pathol. Anat.* **333**, 421–465 (1960).
5. J. D. Judah, K. Ahmed, and A. E. M. McLean, Pathogenesis of cell necrosis, *Fed. Proc. Fed. Am. Soc. Exp. Biol.* **24**, 1217–1221 (1965).
6. A. U. Arstila and B. F. Trump, Studies on autophagocytosis. The formation of autophagic vacuoles in the liver after glucagon administration, *Am. J. Pathol.* **53**, 687–733 (1968).
7. B. F. Trump and F. L. Ginn, The pathogenesis of subcellular reaction to lethal injury, in: *Methods and Achievements in Experimental Pathology* (E. Bajusz and G. Jasmin, eds.), Vol. 4, pp. 1–29, S. Karger, New York (1969).
8. I. F. Tannock, The relation between cell proliferation and the vascular system in a transplanted mouse mammary tumour, *Br. J. Cancer* **22**, 258–273 (1968).
9. R. H. Thomlinson and L. H. Gray, The histological structure of some human lung cancers and the possible implications for radiotherapy, *Br. J. Cancer* **9**, 539–549 (1955).
10. U. Kim and J. Furth, Relation of mammotropes to mammary tumors. IV. Development of highly hormone dependent mammary tumors. *Proc. Soc. Exp. Biol. Med.* **105**, 490–492 (1960).
11. R. M. MacLeod, M. S. Allen, and V. P. Hollander, Hormonal requirements for the growth of mammary adenocarcinoma (MTW9) in rats, *Endocrinology* **75**, 249–258 (1964).
12. R. M. MacLeod, M. S. Allen, and V. P. Hollander, Studies on the influence of mammo-somatotropic tumor (MtTW5) on the metabolism of mammary tumor (MTW9) and adipose tissue, *Endocrinology* **75**, 259–265 (1964).
13. E. J. Diamond, M. Giladi, S. Khan, and V. P. Hollander, Estradiol binding in ovariectomy-responsive and -nonresponsive rat mammary carcinoma, *Cancer Res.* **37**, 1852–1856 (1977).
14. B. L. Powell, E. J. Diamond, S. Koprak, and V. P. Hollander, Prolactin binding in ovariectomy-responsive and ovariectomy-nonresponsive rat mammary carcinoma, *Cancer Res.* **37**, 1328–1332 (1977).
15. T. T. Tchen, S. W. Chan, T. H. Kuo, K. M. Mostafapour, and V. H. Drzewiecki, Studies on the adrenal cortex of hypophysectomized rats: A model for abnormal cellular atrophy and death, *Mol. Cell. Biochem.* **15**, 79–87 (1977).
16. S. W. Russell and C. G. Cochrane, The cellular events associated with regression and progression of murine (Moloney) sarcomas, *Int. J. Cancer* **13**, 54–63 (1974).
17. S. W. Russell, W. F. Doe, and C. G. Cochrane, Macrophages in regressing and progressing Moloney sarcomas, in: *The Macrophage in Neoplasia* (M. A. Fink, ed.), pp. 199–204, Academic Press, New York (1976).
18. S. W. Russell, W. F. Doe, and C. G. Cochrane, Number of macrophages and distribution of mitotic activity in regressing and progressing Moloney sarcomas, *J. Immunol.* **116**, 164–166 (1976).
19. I. Costero and C. M. Pomerat, Cultivation of neurons from the adult human cerebral and cerebellar cortex, *Am. J. Anat.* **89**, 405–465 (1951).

20. M. Bessis, Studies on cell agony and death: An attempt at classification, in: *Cellular Injury* (A. V. S. de Reuck and J. Knight, eds.), pp. 287–328, Little, Brown and Co., Boston (1964).

21. Z. H. Price, The micromorphology of zeiotic blebs in cultured human epithelial (HEp) cells, *Exp. Cell Res.* **48**, 82–92 (1967).

22. H. Quastler and F. G. Sherman, Cell population kinetics in the intestinal epithelium of the mouse, *Exp. Cell Res.* **17**, 420–438 (1959).

23. M. L. Mendelsohn, The growth fraction: A new concept applied to tumors, *Science* **132**, 1496 (1960).

24. M. L. Mendelsohn, F. C. Dohan, Jr., and H. A. Moore, Jr., Autoradiographic analysis of cell proliferation in spontaneous breast cancer of C3H mouse. I. Typical cell cycle and timing of DNA synthesis, *J. Natl. Cancer Inst.* **25**, 477–484 (1960).

25. M. L. Mendelsohn, Autoradiographic analysis of cell proliferation in spontaneous breast cancer of C3H mouse. III. The growth fraction, *J. Natl. Cancer Inst.* **28**, 1015–1029 (1962).

26. D. E. Wimber and H. Quastler, A ^{14}C- and ^{3}H-thymidine double labeling technique in the study of cell proliferation in *Tradescantia* root tips, *Exp. Cell Res.* **30**, 8–22 (1963).

27. P. K. Lala, M. A. Maloney, and H. M. Patt, Measurement of DNA-synthesis time in myeloid–erythroid precursors, *Exp. Cell Res.* **38**, 626–634 (1965).

28. G. G. Steel, Cell loss as a factor in the growth rate of human tumours, *Eur. J. Cancer* **3**, 381–387 (1967).

29. G. G. Steel, Cell loss from experimental tumours, *Cell Tissue Kinet.* **1**, 193–207 (1968).

30. O. H. Iverson, Kinetics of cellular proliferation and cell loss in human carcinomas. A discussion of methods available for *in vivo* studies, *Eur. J. Cancer* **3**, 389–394 (1967).

31. S. B. Refsum and P. Berdal, Cell loss in malignant tumours in man, *Eur. J. Cancer* **3**, 35–236 (1967).

32. G. G. Steel, The cell cycle in tumours: An examination of data gained by the technique of labelled mitoses, *Cell Tissue Kinet.* **5**, 87–100 (1972).

33. L. Simpson-Herren and H. H. Lloyd, Kinetic parameters and growth curves for experimental tumor systems, *Cancer Chemother. Rep. Pt. 1* **54**, 143–174 (1970).

34. P. K. Lala and H. M. Patt, Cytokinetic analysis of tumor growth, *Proc. Natl. Acad. Sci. U.S.A.* **56**, 1735–1742 (1966).

35. E. Frindel, A. J. Valleron, F. Vassort, and M. Tubiana, Proliferation kinetics of an experimental ascites tumour of the mouse, *Cell Tissue Kinet.* **2**, 51–65 (1969).

36. G. G. Steel, *Growth Kinetics of Tumours: Cell Population Kinetics in Relation to the Growth and Treatment of Cancer*, Clarendon Press, Oxford (1977).

37. P. K. Lala, Measurement of S period in growing cell populations by a graphic analysis of double labeling with ^{3}H- and ^{14}C-thymidine, *Exp. Cell Res.* **50**, 459–463 (1968).

38. P. K. Lala, Studies on tumor cell population kinetics, in: *Methods in Cancer Research* (H. Busch, ed.), Vol. 6, pp. 3–95, Academic Press, New York (1971).

39. F. D. Bertalanffy, R. Schacter, J. Ali, and J. C. Ingimundson, Mitotic rate and doubling time of intraperitoneal and subcutaneous Ehrlich ascites tumors, *Cancer Res.* **25**, 685–691 (1965).

40. E. Frindel, E. P. Malaise, E. Alpen, and M. Tubiana, Kinetics of cell proliferation of an experimental tumor, *Cancer Res.* **27**, 1122–1131 (1967).

41. I. F. Tannock, A comparison of cell proliferation parameters in solid and ascites Ehrlich tumors, *Cancer Res.* **29**, 1527–1534 (1969).

42. P. K. Lala, Factors controlling growth of Ehrlich ascites tumors in ascites and solid forms, *Proc. Can. Fed. Biol. Soc.* **13**, 6 (1970).

43. T. P. Butler and P. M. Gullino, Quantitation of cell shedding into efferent blood of mammary adenocarcinoma, *Cancer Res.* **35**, 512–516 (1975).

44. P. M. Gullino, F. H. Grantham, I. Losonczy, and B. Berghoffer, Mammary tumor regression. III. Uptake and loss of substrates by regressing tumors, *J. Natl. Cancer Inst.* **49**, 1675–1684 (1972).

45. L. Simpson-Herren and D. P. Griswold, Jr., Studies of the cell population kinetics of induced and transplanted mammary adenocarcinoma in rats, *Cancer Res.* **33**, 2415–2424 (1973).

46. P. M. Gullino, Techniques for the study of tumor physiopathology, in: *Methods in Cancer Research* (H. Busch, ed.), Vol. 5, pp. 45–91, Academic Press, New York (1970).

47. P. M. Gullino, F. H. Grantham, I. Losonczy, and B. Berghoffer, Mammary tumor regression. I. Physiopathologic characteristics of hormone-dependent tissue, *J. Natl. Cancer Inst.* **49**, 1333–1348 (1972).

48. P. M. Gullino, F. H. Grantham, and A. H. Courtney, Utilization of oxygen by transplanted tumors *in vivo*, *Cancer Res.* **27**, 1020–1030 (1967).

49. P. M. Gullino, F. H. Grantham, and A. H. Courtney, Glucose consumption by transplanted tumors *in vivo*, *Cancer Res.* **27**, 1031–1040 (1967).

50. P. M. Gullino, F. H. Grantham, A. Courtney, and I. Losonczy, Relationship between oxygen and glucose consumption by transplanted tumors *in vivo*, *Cancer Res.* **27**, 1041–1052 (1967).

51. G. Currie, Immunological aspects of host resistance to the development and growth of cancer, *Biochim. Biophys. Acta* **458**, 135–165 (1976).

52. P. Alexander, The functions of the macrophage in malignant disease, *Annu. Rev. Med.* **27**, 207–224 (1976).

53. J. B. Hibbs, Jr., Macrophage nonimmunologic recognition: Target cell factors related to contact inhibition, *Science* **180**, 868–870 (1973).

54. G. A. Currie and C. Basham, Activated macrophages release a factor which lyses malignant cells but not normal cells, *J. Exp. Med.* **142**, 1600–1605 (1975).

55. J. B. Hibbs, Jr., The macrophage as a tumoricidal effector cell: A review of *in vivo* and *in vitro* studies on the mechanism of the activated macrophage nonspecific cytotoxic reaction, in: *The Macrophage in Neoplasia* (M. A. Fink, ed.), pp. 83–111, Academic Press, New York (1976).

56. W. Rosenau and H. D. Moon, Cellular reactions to methylcholanthrene-induced sarcomas transplanted to isogenic mice, *Lab. Invest.* **15**, 1212–1224 (1966).

57. D. S. Nelson, *Macrophages and Immunity* Chap. 8, pp. 211–246, North-Holland Publishing Co., Amsterdam (1969).

58. R. Evans, Macrophages in syngeneic animal tumours, *Transplantation* **14**, 468–473 (1972).

59. R. Evans, Preparation of pure cultures of tumor macrophages, *J. Natl. Cancer Inst.* **50**, 271–273 (1973).

60. C. L. Gauci and P. Alexander, The macrophage content of some human tumours, *Cancer Lett.* **1**, 29–32 (1975).

61. S. A. Eccles and P. Alexander, Macrophage content of tumours in relation to metastatic spread and host immune reaction, *Nature* **250**, 667–669 (1974).

62. G. W. Wood and G. Y. Gillespie, Studies on the role of macrophages in regulation of growth and metastasis of murine chemically induced fibrosarcomas, *Int. J. Cancer* **16**, 1022–1029 (1975).

63. C. L. Gauci, The significance of the macrophage content of human tumours, *Recent Results Cancer Res.* **56**, 122–130 (1976).

64. I. Lauder, W. Aherne, J. Stewart, and R. Sainsbury, Macrophage infiltration of breast tumours: A prospective study, *J. Clin. Pathol.* **30**, 563–568 (1977).

65. M. M. Black and F. D. Speer, Sinus histiocytosis of lymph nodes in cancer, *Surg. Gynecol. Obstet.* **106**, 163–175 (1958).

66. G. H. Friedell, E. A. Soto, S. Kumaoka, O. Abe, J. L. Hayward, and R. D. Bulbrook,

Sinus histiocytosis in British and Japanese patients with breast cancer, *Lancet* **2**, 1228–1229 (1974).

67. R. W. McDivitt, Breast carcinoma, *Hum. Pathol.* **9**, 30–21 (1978).
68. I. J. Fidler, Immune stimulation–inhibition of experimental cancer metastasis, *Cancer Res.* **34**, 491–498 (1974).
69. I. J. Fidler, Inhibition of pulmonary metastasis by intravenous injection of specifically activated macrophages, *Cancer Res.* **34**, 1074–1078 (1974).
70. J. B. Hibbs, Jr., Activated macrophages as cytotoxic effector cells. II. Requirement for local persistence of inducing antigen, *Transplantation* **19**, 81–87 (1975).
71. G. A. Granger, Mechanisms of lymphocyte-induced cell and tissue destruction *in vitro, Am. J. Pathol.* **60**, 469–481 (1970).
72. R. Keller and V. E. Jones, Role of activated macrophages and antibody in inhibition and enhancement of tumour growth in rats, *Lancet* **2**, 847–849 (1971).
73. B. W. Papermaster, O. A. Holterman, D. Rosner, E. Klein, and T. Dao, Regressions produced in breast cancer lesions by a lymphokine fraction from a human lymphoid cell line, *Res. Commun. Chem. Pathol. Pharmacol.* **8**, 413–416 (1974).
74. P. B. Blair and M.-A. Lane, Non-T cell killing of mammary tumor cells by spleen cells: Secretion of antibody and recruitment of cells, *J. Immunol.* **115**, 184–189 (1975).
75. J. B. Hibbs, Jr., Role of activated macrophages in nonspecific resistance to neoplasia, *J. Reticuloendothel. Soc.* **20**, 223–231 (1976).
76. R. Keller, Cytostatic and cytocidal effects of activated nonimmune macrophages, in: *The Macrophage in Neoplasia* (M. A. Fink, ed.), pp. 149–164, Academic Press, New York (1976).
77. O. Stutman, Correlation of *in vitro* and *in vivo* studies of antigens relevant to the control of murine breast cancer, *Cancer Res.* **36**, 739–747 (1976).
78. H. A. Chapman, Jr. and J. B. Hibbs, Jr., Modulation of macrophage tumoricidal capability by components of normal serum: A central role for lipid, *Science* **197**, 282–285 (1977).
79. J. B. Hibbs, Jr., R. R. Taintor, H. A. Chapman, Jr., and J. B. Weinberg, Macrophage tumor killing: Influence of the local environment, *Science* **197**, 279–282 (1977).
80. R. Keller, Susceptibility of normal and transformed cell lines to cytostatic and cytocidal effects exerted by macrophages, *J. Natl. Cancer Inst.* **56**, 369–374 (1976).
81. D. S. Nelson, Production by stimulated macrophages of factors depressing lymphocyte transformation, *Nature* **246**, 306–307 (1973).
82. S. R. Waldman and A. A. Gottlieb, Macrophage regulation of DNA synthesis in lymphoid cells: Effects of a soluble factor from macrophages, *Cell. Immunol.* **9**, 142–156 (1973).
83. J. Calderon, R. T. Williams, and E. R. Unanue, An inhibitor of cell proliferation released by cultures of macrophages, *Proc. Natl. Acad. Sci. U.S.A.* **71**, 4273–4277 (1974).
84. J. Calderon and E. R. Unanue, Two biological activities regulating cell proliferation found in cultures of peritoneal exudate cells, *Nature* **253**, 359–361 (1975).
85. J. Calderon, J.-M. Kiely, J. L. Lefko, and E. R. Unanue, The modulation of lymphocyte functions by molecules secreted by macrophages. I. Description and partial biochemical analysis, *J. Exp. Med.* **142**, 151–164 (1975).
86. R. Keller, Major changes in lymphocyte proliferation evoked by activated macrophages, *Cell. Immunol.* **17**, 542–551 (1975).
87. R. Evans and P. Alexander, Cooperation of immune lymphoid cells with macrophages in tumour immunity, *Nature* **228**, 620–622 (1970).
88. R. Evans and P. Alexander, Mechanism of immunologically specific killing of tumour cells by macrophages, *Nature* **236**, 168–170 (1972).
89. J. B. Hibbs, Jr., L. H. Lambert, Jr., and J. S. Remington, Possible role of macrophage

mediated nonspecific cytotoxicity in tumour resistance, *Nature (London) New Biol.* **235**, 48–50 (1972).

90. B. Zbar, H. T. Wepsic, T. Borsos, and H. J. Rapp, Tumor-graft rejection in syngeneic guinea pigs: Evidence for a two-step mechanism, *J. Natl. Cancer Inst.* **44**, 473–481 (1970).

91. B. Zbar, H. T. Wepsic, H. J. Rapp, L. C. Stewart, and T. Borsos, Two-step mechanism of tumor graft rejection in syngeneic guinea pigs. II. Initiation of reaction by a cell fraction containing lymphoctyes and neutrophils, *J. Natl. Cancer Inst.* **44**, 701–717 (1970).

92. J. B. Hibbs, Jr., Heterocytolysis by macrophages activated by bacillus Calmette-Guérin: Lysosome exocytosis into tumor cells, *Science* **184**, 468–471 (1974).

93. C. Bucana, L. C. Hoyer, B. Hobbs, S. Breesman, M. McDaniel, and M. G. Hanna, Jr., Morphological evidence for the translocation of lysosomal organelles from cytotoxic macrophages into the cytoplasm of tumor target cells, *Cancer Res.* **36**, 4444–4458 (1976).

94. H. Melsom, G. Kearney, S. Gruca, and R. Seljelid, Evidence for a cytolytic factor released by macrophages, *J. Exp. Med.* **140**, 1085–1096 (1974).

95. H. Melsom, T. Sanner, and R. Seljelid, Macrophage cytolytic factor. Some observations on its physicochemical properties and site of action, *Exp. Cell Res.* **94**, 221–226 (1975).

96. J. S. Haskill, J. W. Proctor, and Y. Yamamura, Host responses within solid tumors. I. Monocytic effector cells within rat sarcomas, *J. Natl. Cancer Inst.* **54**, 387–393 (1975).

97. P. M. Gullino and R. H. Lanzerotti, Mammary tumor regression. II. Autophagy of neoplastic cells, *J. Natl. Cancer Inst.* **49**, 1349–1356 (1972).

98. B. A. Ehrenreich and Z. A. Cohn, The uptake and digestion of iodinated human serum albumin by macrophages *in vitro*, *J. Exp. Med.* **126**, 941–958 (1967).

99. R. T. Dean and A. J. Barrett, Lysosomes, *Essays Biochem.* **12**, 1–40 (1976).

100. P. L. Sawant, I. D. Desai, and A. L. Tappel, Digestive capacity of purified lysosomes, *Biochim. Biophys. Acta* **85**, 93–102 (1964).

101. C. de Duve, The lysosome in retrospect in: *Lysosomes in Biology and Pathology* (J. T. Dingle and H. B. Fell, eds.), Vol. 1, pp. 3–40, North-Holland Publishing Co., Amsterdam (1969).

102. D. Brandes, K. W. Sloan, E. Anton, and F. Bloedorn, The effect of X-irradiation on the lysosomes of mouse mammary gland carcinomas, *Cancer Res.* **27**, 731–746 (1967).

103. J. E. Paris, D. Brandes, and E. Anton, Distribution of properties of lysosomal enzymes in untreated and in irradiated mouse mammary-gland carcinomas, *J. Natl. Cancer Inst.* **42**, 383–398 (1969).

104. J. E. Paris and D. Brandes, Effect of X-irradiation on the functional status of lysosomal enzymes of mouse mammary gland carcinomas, *Cancer Res.* **31**, 392–401 (1971).

105. C. Clarke and E. D. Wills, Lysosomal enzyme activation in irradiated mammary tumors, *Radiat. Res.* **67**, 435–446 (1976).

106. R. J. Shamberger, Lysosomal enzyme changes in growing and regressing mammary tumours, *Biochem. J.* **111**, 375–383 (1969).

107. R. H. Lanzerotti and P. M. Gullino, Activities and quantities of lysosomal enzymes during mammary tumor regression, *Cancer Res.* **32**, 2679–2685 (1972).

108. R. H. Lanzerotti and P. M. Gullino, Immunochemical quantitation of enzymes using multispecific antisera, *Anal. Biochem.* **50**, 344–353 (1972).

109. Y. S. Cho-Chung and P. M. Gullino, Mammary tumor regression. V. Role of acid ribonuclease and cathepsin, *J. Biol. Chem.* **248**, 4743–4749 (1973).

110. Y. S. Cho-Chung and P. M. Gullino, Mammary tumor regression. VI. Synthesis and degradation of acid ribonuclease, *J. Biol. Chem.* **248**, 4750–4755 (1973).

111. J. F. Woessner, Jr., The physiology of the uterus and mammary gland, in: *Lysosomes in Biology and Pathology* (J. T. Dingle and H. B. Fell, eds.), Vol. 1, pp. 299–329, North-Holland Publishing Co., Amsterdam (1969).

112. P. Badenoch-Jones and H. Baum, Progesterone-induced permeability changes in rat liver lysosomes, *Nature (London) New Biol.* **242**, 123–124 (1973).

113. J. W. C. Bird, T. Berg, and J. H. Leathem, Cathepsin activity of liver and muscle fractions of adrenalectomized rats, *Proc. Soc. Exp. Biol. Med.* **127**, 182–188 (1968).

114. R. H. Persellin, Lysosome stabilization by leukocyte granule membrane antiserum, *J. Immunol.* **103**, 39–44 (1969).

115. M. Miyamoto and H. Terayama, Serum factors affecting cathepsin release from lysosomes, *Biochem. Biophys. Res. Commun.* **64**, 617–624 (1975).

116. K. L. Yielding and G. M. Tomkins, Structural alterations in crystalline glutamic dehydrogenase induced by steroid hormones, *Proc. Natl. Acad. Sci. U.S.A.* **46**, 1483–1488 (1960).

117. D. V. Kimberg and K. L. Yielding, Pyruvate kinase. Structural and functional changes induced by diethylstilbestrol and certain steroid hormones, *J. Biol. Chem.* **237**, 3233–3239 (1962).

118. A. W. Douville and J. C. Warren, Steroid–protein interaction at sites which influence catalytic activity, *Biochemistry* **7**, 4052–4059 (1968).

119. A. L. Goldberg and A. C. St. John, Intracellular protein degradation in mammalian and bacterial cells: Part 2, *Annu. Rev. Biochem.* **45**, 747–803 (1976).

120. R. T. Dean, Concerning a possible mechanism for selective capture of cytoplasmic proteins by lysosomes, *Biochem. Biophys. Res. Commun.* **67**, 604–609 (1975).

121. P. Bohley, H. Kirschke, J. Langner, S. Riemann, B. Wiederanders, S. Ansorge, and H. Hanson, Primary reaction of intracellular protein catabolism, in: *Intracellular Protein Catabolism II* (V. Turk and N. Marks, eds.), pp. 108–110, Plenum Press, New York (1977).

122. H. Koenig, The soluble acidic lipoproteins (SALPS) of storage granules. Matrix constituents which may bind stored molecules, in: *Advances in Cytopharmacology* (B. Ceccarelli, F. Clementi, and J. Meldolesi, eds.), Vol. 2, pp. 273–301, Raven Press, New York (1974).

123. M. R. Capecchi, N. E. Capecchi, S. H. Hughes, and G. M. Wahl, Selective degradation of abnormal proteins in mammalian tissue culture cells, *Proc. Natl. Acad. Sci. U.S.A.* **71**, 4732–4736 (1974).

124. P. J. Fritz, E. L. White, K. M. Pruitt, and E. S. Vesell, Lactate dehydrogenase isozymes. Turnover in rat heart, skeletal muscle and liver, *Biochemistry* **12**, 4034–4039 (1973).

125. A. L. Goldberg and J. F. Dice, Intracellular protein degradation in mammalian and bacterial cells, *Annu. Rev. Biochem.* **43**, 835–869 (1974).

126. M. Rouleau and P. M. Gullino, Increased susceptibility of cytosol proteins to proteolytic digestion during regression of a hormone-dependent mammary tumor, *Cancer Res.* **37**, 670–677 (1977).

127. M. Rouleau, I. Losonczy, and P. M. Gullino, Arrest of synthesis of specific proteins at the onset of mammary tumor regression, *Cancer Res.* **38**, 926–931 (1978).

128. D. Gericke and P. Chandra, Inhibition of tumor growth by nucleoside cyclic 3',5'-monophosphates, *Hoppe-Seyler's Z. Physiol. Chem.* **350**, 1469–1471 (1969).

129. R. Keller, Suppression of normal and enhanced tumor growth in rats by agents interfering with intracellular cyclic nucleotides, *Life Sci.* **11**, Part II, 485–491 (1972).

130. E. E. Smith and A. H. Handler, Apparent suppression of the tumorigenicity of human cancer cells by cyclic AMP, *Res. Commun. Chem. Pathol. Pharmacol.* **5**, 863–866 (1973).

131. Y. S. Cho-Chung, *In vivo* inhibition of tumor growth by cyclic adenosine 3',5'-monophosphate derivatives, *Cancer Res.* **34,** 3492–3496 (1974).

132. Y. S. Cho-Chung and P. M. Gullino, Effect of dibutyryl cyclic adenosine 3',5'-monophosphate on *in vivo* growth of Walker 256 carcinoma: Isolation of responsive and unresponsive cell populations, *J. Natl. Cancer Inst.* **52,** 995–996 (1974).

133. Y. S. Cho-Chung and P. M. Gullino, *In vivo* inhibition of growth of two hormone-dependent mammary tumors by dibutyryl cyclic AMP, *Science* **183,** 87–88 (1974).

134. Y. S. Cho-Chung, Cyclic AMP and tumor growth *in vivo*, in: *Influence of Hormones on Tumor Development*, Vol. 1 (J. A. Kellen and R. Hilf, eds.), pp. 55–93, CRC Press, Cleveland (1979).

135. Y. S. Cho-Chung and S. F. Newcomer: Adenylate cyclase, cyclic AMP-phosphodiesterase and regression of Walker 256 mammary carcinoma, *Cancer Res.* **37,** 4493–4499 (1977).

136. Y. S. Cho-Chung, T. Clair, and R. Porper, Cyclic AMP-binding proteins and protein kinase during regression of Walker 256 mammary carcinoma, *J. Biol. Chem.* **252,** 6342–6348 (1977).

137. E. G. Krebs, Protein kinases, *Curr. Top. Cell. Regul.* **5,** 99–133 (1972).

138. U. Eppenberger, J. Preisz, A. Salokangas, P. Huber, and K. Talmadge, Studies on the adenyl cyclase, cAMP, protein kinase system in neoplastic human breast tissue, *Experientia* **32,** 792 (1976).

139. G. C. Majumder, Protein kinase activity in mouse mammary carcinoma, *Biochem. Biophys. Res. Commun.* **74,** 1140–1145 (1977).

140. Y. S. Cho-Chung, T. Clair, P. N. Yi, and C. Parkison, Comparative studies on cyclic AMP-responsive and -unresponsive Walker 256 mammary carcinomas, *J. Biol. Chem.* **252,** 6335–6341 (1977).

141. V. Daniel, G. Litwack, and G. M. Tomkins, Induction of cytolysis of cultured lymphoma cells by adenosine 3',5'-cyclic monophosphate and the isolation of resistant variants, *Proc. Natl. Acad. Sci. U.S.A.* **70,** 76–79 (1973).

142. P. Coffino, H. R. Bourne, and G. M. Tomkins, Mechanism of lymphoma cell death induced by cyclic AMP, *Am. J. Pathol.* **81,** 199–204 (1975).

143. H. R. Bourne, P. Coffino, K. L. Melmon, G. M. Tomkins, and Y. Weinstein, Genetic analysis of cyclic AMP in a mammalian cell, in: *Advances in Cyclic Nucleotide Research* (G. I. Drummond, P. Greengard, and G. A. Robison, eds.), Vol. 5, pp. 771–786, Raven Press, New York (1975).

144. P. Coffino, H. R. Bourne, U. Friedrich, J. Hochman, P. A. Insel, I. Lamaire, K. L. Melmon, and G. M. Tomkins, Molecular mechanisms of cyclic AMP action: A genetic approach, *Recent Prog. Horm. Res.* **32,** 669–684 (1976).

145. P. Coffino and K. R. Yamamoto, Somatic genetic studies of steroid and cyclic AMP receptors, in: *Control Mechanisms in Cancer* (W. E. Criss, T. Ono, and J. R. Sabine, eds.), pp. 57–66, Raven Press, New York (1976).

146. R. A. Steinberg, P. H. O'Farrell, U. Friedrich, and P. Coffino, Mutations causing charge alterations in regulatory subunits of cAMP-dependent protein kinase of cultured S49 lymphoma cells, *Cell* **10,** 381–391 (1977).

147. M. J. Tisdale and B. J. Phillips, Alterations in adenosine 3',5'-monophosphate-binding protein in Walker carcinoma cells sensitive or resistant to alkylating agents, *Biochem. Pharmacol.* **25,** 1831–1836 (1976).

148. Y. S. Cho-Chung and T. Clair, Altered cyclic AMP-binding and db cyclic AMP-unresponsiveness *in vivo*, *Nature* **265,** 452–454 (1977).

149. Y. S. Cho-Chung and T. Clair, The role of cAMP on neoplastic cell growth and regression. III. Altered cAMP-binding in DBcAMP-unresponsive Walker 256 mammary carcinoma, *Biochem. Biophys. Res. Commun.* **64,** 768–772 (1975).

150. R. A. Jungmann, P. C. Hiestand, and J. S. Schweppe, Adenosine 3',5'-monophosphate-dependent protein kinase and the stimulation of ovarian nuclear ribonucleic acid polymerase activities, *J. Biol. Chem.* **249**, 5444–5451 (1974).

151. R. A. Jungmann, P. C. Hiestand, and J. S. Schweppe, Mechanism of action of gonadotropin. IV. Cyclic adenosine monophosphate-dependent translocation of ovarian cytoplasmic cyclic adenosine monophosphate-binding protein and protein kinase to nuclear acceptor sites, *Endocrinology* **94**, 168–183 (1974).

152. Y. S. Cho-Chung, T. Clair, and P. Huffman, Loss of nuclear cyclic AMP binding in cyclic AMP-unresponsive Walker 256 mammary carcinoma, *J. Biol. Chem.* **252**, 6349–6355 (1977).

153. Y. S. Cho-Chung and B. H. Redler, Dibutyryl cyclic AMP mimics ovariectomy: Nuclear protein phosphorylation in mammary tumor regression, *Science* **197**, 272–275 (1977).

154. Y. S. Cho-Chung, J. S. Bodwin, and T. Clair, Cyclic adenosine 3',5'-monophosphate-binding protein: Role in ovariectomy-induced regression of a hormone-dependent mammary tumor in Sprague-Dawley female rats, *J. Natl. Cancer Inst.* **60**, 1175–1178 (1978).

155. Y. S. Cho-Chung, J. S. Bodwin, and T. Clair, Cyclic AMP-binding proteins; inverse relationship with estrogen-receptors in hormone-dependent mammary tumor regression, *Eur. J. Biochem.* **86**, 51–60 (1978).

156. E. Zwilling, Controlled degeneration during development, in: *Cellular Injury* (A. V. S. de Reuck and J. Knight, eds.), pp. 352–368, Little, Brown and Co., Boston (1964).

157. F. M. Butterworth, Adipose tissue of *Drosophila melanogaster*. V. Genetic and experimental studies of an extrinsic influence on the rate of cell death in the larval fat body, *Dev. Biol.* **28**, 311–325 (1972).

158. S. Sanyal, Changes of lysosomal enzymes during hereditary degeneration and histogenesis of retina in mice. II. Localization of N-acetyl-β-glucosaminidase in macrophages, *Histochemie* **29**, 28–36 (1972).

159. R. Weber, Behaviour and properties of acid hydrolases in regressing tails of tadpoles during spontaneous and induced metamorphosis *in vitro*, in: *Lysosomes* (A. V. S. de Reuck and M. P. Cameron, eds.), pp. 282–310, Little, Brown and Co., Boston (1963).

160. E. Frieden and J. J. Just, Hormonal responses in amphibian metamorphosis, in: *Biochemical Actions of Hormones* (G. Litwack, ed.), Vol. 1, pp. 1–52, Academic Press, New York (1970).

161. M. H. I. Dodd and J. M. Dodd, The biology of metamorphosis in: *Physiology of the Amphibian* (B. Lofts, ed.), Vol. 3, pp. 467–599, Academic Press, New York (1976).

162. V. Hamburger, Regression versus peripheral control of differentiation in motor hypoplasia, *Am. J. Anat.* **102**, 365–409 (1958).

163. R. H. Angeletti, P. U. Angeletti, and R. Levi-Montalcini, The nerve growth factor, in: *Humoral Control of Growth and Differentiation* (J. Lobue and A. S. Gordon, eds.), Vol. 1, pp. 229–247, Academic Press, New York (1973).

164. J. R. Tata, Requirement for RNA and protein synthesis for induced regression of the tadpole tail in organ culture, *Dev. Biol.* **13**, 77–94 (1966).

165. K. M. Mosher, D. A. Young, and A. Munck, Evidence for irreversible, actinomycin D-sensitive, and temperature-sensitive steps following binding of cortisol to glucocorticoid receptors and preceding effects on glucose metabolism in rat thymus cells, *J. Biol. Chem.* **246**, 654–659 (1971).

166. R. A. Lockshin and J. Beaulaton, Programmed cell death, *Life Sci.* **15**, 1549–1565 (1974).

Medical Adrenalectomy for Treatment of Metastatic Breast Carcinoma

RICHARD J. SANTEN AND EUGENIUSZ SAMOJLIK

1. Introduction

Approximately one-third of unselected patients with metastatic breast carcinoma experience objective tumor regression when treated with standard surgical ablative procedures such as hypophysectomy, adrenalectomy, or ovariectomy. [1-8] By preselection of women with estrogen-receptor-positive tumors for these procedures, two thirds can be expected to respond objectively. [9] However, the appreciable morbidity and significant mortality associated with the major surgical ablative therapies, particularly in debilitated patients, has limited their use to highly selected patients with widely metastatic disease. [1,3,10] For these reasons, major investigative efforts have attempted to develop chemical methods to reduce hormone secretion or block hormone action as possible alternatives to surgical ablative techniques. The term usually utilized for techniques that attempt to suppress adrenal function in lieu of adrenalectomy is "medical adrenalectomy." In a strict sense, this term can only be validly applied to regimens that produce an identical hormonal milieu to that resulting from surgical adrenalectomy. This criterion has not been fulfilled for any of the regimens developed for medical adrenalectomy; consequently, for the purposes of this review, the term "medi-

RICHARD J. SANTEN AND EUGENIUSZ SAMOJLIK • Department of Medicine, Division of Endocrinology, and The Specialized Cancer Center, The Milton S. Hershey Medical Center, The Pennsylvania State University, Hershey, Pennsylvania 17033.

cal adrenalectomy" is applied to those therapies whose rationale is the suppression of adrenal steroidogenesis.

In this chapter, the endocrine dependence of breast carcinoma as it relates to adrenal steroid secretion will be discussed initially. The various approaches to adrenal suppression and the hormonal effects of these treatments will then be outlined. Finally, the reported clinical results of the various proposed regimens will be detailed and the relative role of medical adrenalectomy in the overall treatment of breast carcinoma will be discussed.

2. Breast Carcinoma Dependence upon Adrenal Hormones and Prehormones

The precise mechanism whereby surgical adrenalectomy produces tumor regression in women with mammary carcinoma is unknown. The most likely explanation is a reduction in estrogen production. However, an alteration in the levels of other hormones of adrenal derivation such as testosterone, dihydrotestosterone, progesterone, and cortisol could also exert important effects on breast tumor growth. Biologic actions of these steroids on normal and neoplastic breast tissue have been demonstrated both *in vivo* and *in vitro*, and receptors for them are often detected in human mammary tumors[11-20] (Fig. 1). It is possible that other adrenal steroids could also indirectly modulate the effects of the major biologically active steroids by altering their metabolism or receptor binding. Dehydroepiandrosterone (DHA), dehydroepiandrosterone sulfate (DHA-S), androstenedione, androstanediol, and the metabolic products of these compounds, could potentially produce such effects.[16,21]

Critical examination of any medical adrenalectomy regimen should then include a consideration of each adrenal steroid with potential importance in the regulation of breast cancer growth, and particularly the estrogens and androgens. To provide a background for understanding the comprehensive effects of drugs on adrenal secretion, we will initially discuss the sources and metabolism of the adrenal hormones and prehormones in postmenopausal or castrate women with breast carcinoma.

The physiology of estrogen production is of greatest importance and will be reviewed initially. Extensive studies have shown that the adrenal gland secretes little or no estrone directly in postmenopausal or castrate women.[22-24] However, a large amount of the estrogen prehormone, androstenedione, is secreted by this gland and is converted in peripheral tissues to estrone.[22-24] The series of enzymatic reactions that accomplish this conversion are called collectively aromatization, a process that occurs in fat tissue, liver, and also directly in some breast

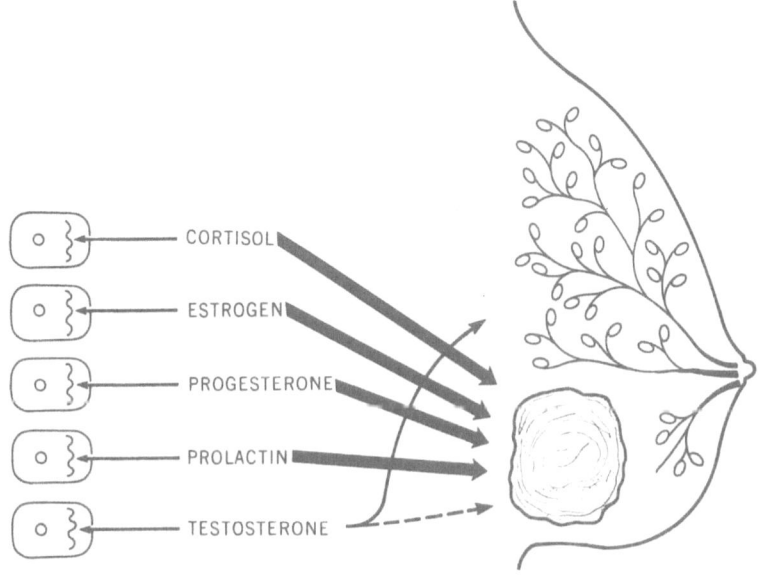

BREAST NEOPLASM

Fig. 1. Hormones for which receptor proteins have been identified in human mammary neoplasms and biologic actions on normal and neoplastic breast tissue demonstrated. The effects of all are stimulatory except testosterone (or dihydrotestosterone) which is inhibitory. Each of the steroids shown in the figure are either secreted directly by the adrenals, formed in extraglandular tissues from adrenal prehormones, or produced from both sources.

neoplasms.[25,26] Both obesity and age are known to influence the magnitude of aromatization in postmenopausal women.[27,28] Using isotopic kinetic studies, Grodin et al.[23] were able to account for all of the estrone formed in postmenopausal or castrate women by the extraglandular conversion of androstenedione to estrone. Similarly, estradiol, the most potent estrogen, is not directly secreted by the adrenal but is also formed peripherally. The synthesis of this steroid results from the enzymatic reduction of estrone in nonglandular tissues through the action of a ketoreductase. A small amount of estradiol may also result from the aromatization of testosterone.[23,29] Consequently, nearly all the estrogen produced by postmenopausal or castrate women is derived from peripherally converted steroid precursors.

Since androstenedione is such an important prehormone, it should be considered whether the postmenopausal ovary can also produce this compound and consequently contribute to the estrogen pool. Judd et al.[30] recently studied ovarian steroid secretion directly by comparing ovarian venous with peripheral venous androgen and estrogen levels in postmenopausal women. They found a negligible gradient in the estrone and estradiol levels across the ovary, suggesting that this organ does not directly secrete a significant amount of estrogen in the postmenopausal state. However, large gradients of androstenedione and testosterone were found, providing evidence of major ovarian secretion of these steroids. Since both of these compounds can be aromatized to estrogens peripherally, it is likely that the postmenopausal ovary does contribute to the estrogen pool through secretion of prehormones.[30,31]

This finding has practical relevance since it suggests the necessity of removing the ovaries at the time of surgical adrenalectomy, even in postmenopausal women. In addition, drugs used to produce medical adrenalectomy might be more effective if they were capable of suppressing the estrogens derived from ovarian as well as adrenal androstenedione.

Adrenal and ovarian prehormones are also important for the production of the androgens in postmenopausal women. Testosterone and dihydrotestosterone can be formed peripherally from androstenedione, although direct adrenal secretion of testosterone also occurs.[32-34] The weak androgens, DHA and DHA-S, on the other hand, are secreted predominantly by the adrenals.[35]

3. Approaches to Medical Adrenalectomy

3.1. ACTH Suppression with Glucocorticoids

When synthetic glucocorticoids first became widely available for clinical use, suppression of ACTH by the administration of pharmacologic doses of glucocorticoid was introduced as a method to produce medical adrenalectomy. Although this treatment suppressed cortisol production (i.e., 17-hydroxysteroids), it was not until recently that the effects of glucocorticoid administration on estrogen and androgen levels were compared to the effects produced by surgical adrenalectomy. Borkowski et al.[36] administered 3 mg of dexamethasone daily (or 4 times the physiologic replacement dose of glucocorticoid) to 6 women with metastatic breast carcinoma for 6 to 12 weeks. They found, as expected, a rapid decrease in plasma cortisol to undetectable levels. On the other hand, significant concentrations of plasma DHA, androstenedione, and testosterone persisted during dexamethasone treatment even in two surgically castrate patients. In 4 women, plasma estrone fell progressively toward undetectable levels, but in 2 patients it remained higher than the quantities observed in ovariectomized-adrenalectomized patients. Since plasma estrone results nearly exclusively from the aromatization of androstenedione in postmenopausal women, the persistence of estrone in the sera of these women may have reflected incomplete androstenedione suppression. Plasma estradiol, on the other hand, was uniformly suppressed to the levels observed in ovariectomized-adrenalectomized patients. Of interest was the fact that prolactin levels increased in all patients receiving dexamethasone and mean levels of this hormone were 3 times higher than basal after 6 to 12 weeks of treatment.

Since these studies were carried out for a maximum of only 12 weeks, the long-term adrenal-suppressive effects of pharmacologic doses of glucocortocoids on the androgens and estrogens have not been evaluated. From this study, it appears that suppression of adrenal androgens, and, to a certain extent, estrogens, to levels produced by ovariectomy and adrenalectomy, are difficult with administration of the glucocorticoids alone. These observations are likely to be a reflection of the separate regulatory mechanisms for the adrenal androgens as opposed to the glucocorticoids.[37] Data derived from studies of a number of clinical conditions such as hirsutism, puberty, and hyperprolactinemia have recently led to the concept of independently modulated adrenal androgen secretion.

What, then, are the available clinical data comparing objective response rates in women with metastatic breast carcinoma treated either with pharmacologic doses of glucocorticoid or with surgical adrenalectomy? To our knowledge, only one randomized controlled study has been performed comparing treatment with 50 mg of cortisone acetate daily to surgical adrenalectomy.[38] Because none of the patients treated with cortisone responded with objective tumor regression, the trial was terminated early and the conclusion drawn that surgical adrenalectomy is clearly superior to medical adrenalectomy with glucocorticoids. A review of the overall experience with pharmacologic doses of glucocorticoid for medical adrenalectomy revealed that 189 of 756 patients, or 25%, experienced objective tumor regression[38-54] (Table I) as we have previously discussed in detail.[55] In these studies, the response rates would appear to be less favorable than those of 30–40% reported for surgical adrenalectomy.[3-6,8] The mean duration of response also appeared shorter in patients treated with glucocorticoids alone than in women treated with surgical adrenalectomy. These conclusions are only tentative, however, since no large controlled randomized trial of these two modes of therapy has yet been conducted.

Administration of pharmacologic doses of glucocorticoids often produces clinical antitumor effects whose mechanism differs from that of surgical adrenalectomy; for example, the antiinflammatory action of the glucocorticoids may reduce measurable tumor size by decreasing the

Table I
Medical Adrenalectomy with Glucocorticoids in Advanced Breast Cancer

Author	Drug	Dose	Patients with objective remission
Segaloff et al.[39]	Cortisone	100 mg	0/12
West et al.[40]	Cortisone	300 mg	9/21
Pearson et al.[41]	Cortisone	50–75 mg	7/53
		200–400 mg	16/53
Lemon[42]	Cortisone	50–100 mg	
	Dessicated thyroid	15–120 mg	10/29[a]
Gordan et al.[43]	Hydrocortisone	30 mg	
	Triiodothyronine	50 μg	5/23
Nissen-Meyer and Vogt[44]	Cortisone	60 mg	9/18[b]
van Gilse[45]c	Cortisone or	100 mg	41/109
	prednisone	20 mg	
Bethune[46]	Cortisone	37.5 mg	6/18
Dao et al.[38]	Cortisone	50 mg	0/19
Kennedy[47]	Cortisone[d] or	300 mg	10/34
	prednisone[d]	200 mg	
Kofman et al.[48]	Prednisolone	100 mg	8/45
Lemon[49]	Prednisone and	30 mg	15/31
	triiodothyronine	15–50 μg	
Stoll[50]	Dexamethasone	6.4–9.6 mg	3/25
Gardner[51]	Prednisone and	30 mg	
	triiodothyronine	50 μg	11/46
Stoll[52]	Prednisone	80 mg	9/80
Gordan et al.[43]	Prednisone	30 mg	1/21
	Prednisone and	30 mg	
	triiodothyronine	50 μg	10/38
Farrow[53]	Prednisone	20 mg	3/18
Forrest et al.[54]	Prednisone or	30 mg	16/63
	dexamethasone	4.5 mg	
TOTAL			189/756 (25%)

[a]Remission >6 mo.
[b]Only postmenopausal patients included.
[c]Cortisone used until 1956, then prednisone.
[d]Initial dose; maintenance dose not stated.

inflammatory reaction around the neoplasm rather than by reducing tumor cell mass. Certainly, some of the short-lived responses observed with this therapy may be attributable to such an effect.

Several disadvantages of glucocorticoid-induced medical adrenalectomy have been described. These regimens frequently induce Cushing's syndrome after long-term use.[38-54] In addition, there is an alteration of the pattern of metastases in patients receiving high-dose glucocorticoids which may be attributable to diminished immunologic responses. Sherlock *et al.*[56] demonstrated that patients with breast carcinoma who had received pharmacologic amounts of glucocorticoids exhibited a much higher incidence of brain and spleen metastases at autopsy than patients given no glucocorticoid or physiologic replacement steroid. For the reasons given above, medical adrenalectomy with glucocorticoids alone has been used with decreasing frequency in recent years.

3.2. *ortho,para'*-DDD

As opposed to drugs that interfere with steroid synthesis by reversibly blocking enzymatic pathways or inhibiting ACTH secretion, *ortho, para'*-DDD [1,1-dichloro-2-(*o*-chlorophenyl) 2-(*p*-chlorophenyl) ethane] produces necrosis of adrenal cells.[57-58] A period of 3 to 6 months is usually required before this effect is complete and the degree of necrosis may be variable. This drug also alters the pattern of steroid metabolism so that the excretion of 17-hydroxyglucocorticoid metabolites, as measured by the Porter-Silber reaction, are low in relationship to actual cortisol secretion rates.[59] *ortho, para'*-DDD causes severe side effects of nausea and lethargy. Because of these limitations, only one clinical trial in breast carcinoma has been attempted with this drug and it is unlikely to find a place in the treatment of breast carcinoma.[60]

3.3. Aminoglutethimide

Aminoglutethimide is a reversible inhibitor of several enzymatic steps involved in steroid biosynthesis.[61] This compound was originally marketed in the United States in 1960 as an anticonvulsant, but was later reclassified as an investigational new drug when its adrenal-inhibitory properties were appreciated. These drug effects were exploited, then, for treatment of Cushing's syndrome and as experimental therapy for patients with mineralocorticoid hypertension.[61] In 1966, Cash *et al.* first suggested using this compound to produce adrenal suppression in patients with breast carcinoma and subsequently treated one patient with advanced disease.[62] Griffiths *et al.* reported the first series of patients treated with aminoglutethimide (1–2.5 g/day) and 0.5 mg of dexamethasone daily as glucocorticoid replacement.[63] Of 9 patients with metastatic carcinoma of the breast who were treated, 3 experienced objective tumor regression. Unexpectedly, however, it was observed that the urinary 17-hydroxysteroids and ketosteroids were suppressed only transiently with this drug.

3.3.1. Development of an Effective Method of Adrenal Blockade

a. Mechanism of Escape. To explain the apparent escape from adrenal blockade with aminoglutethimide observed by Griffiths *et al.*, and to develop an effective adrenal-inhibitory regimen with aminoglutethimide, [63] a series of systematic studies have been carried out. [55,64-72] The mechanism for escape was found to be a classical drug-drug interaction. Figure 2 reviews the pharmacologic interactions between aminoglutethimide and dexamethasone which were identified and the methods subsequently utilized for successful adrenal blockade.

1. Aminoglutethimide blocks the conversion of cholesterol to pregnenolone and initially lowers cortisol secretion. A reflex rise in ACTH results which is sufficient to overcome the blockade either partially or completely.

2. Usual replacement amounts of dexamethasone, 1 mg daily, do not prevent the reflex ACTH rise. This phenomenon suggested a drug interaction between aminoglutethimide and dexamethasone in which aminoglutethimide accelerated the metabolism and reduced the bioavailability of dexamethasone.

3. Pharmacokinetic studies confirmed this drug interaction since [^{3}H]dexamethasone half-life before aminoglutethimide therapy was 264 min and during treatment, 120 min. Further studies by Newsome[73] using a radioimmunoassay for plasma dexamethasone have extended these observations by demonstrating that aminoglutethimide administration results in a lowering of dexamethasone plasma levels as a result of accelerated metabolism.

4. An effective regimen using aminoglutethimide and larger amounts of dexamethasone (doses of 2–3 mg daily) to compensate for the reduced bioavailability and blood levels of the glucocorticoid was then developed. Careful monitoring of adrenal function during initiation of therapy was thus required. Nonetheless, once the appropriate drug dosage was determined, inhibition of plasma cortisol and urinary free cortisol excretion could be uniformly achieved for as long as 24 months without producing Cushingoid side effects[64] (Fig. 3).

b. Development of Regimen to Avoid Drug Interaction. Further studies then allowed development of a simpler fixed-drug-dosage combination of aminoglutethimide and glucocorticoid which could facilitate wide application of this method without extensive endocrine monitoring. The rationale for this regimen was to utilize as replacement glucocorticoid a steroid whose metabolism and biopotency were not altered by aminoglutethimide. Based upon data suggesting that hydrocortisone is resistant to drug-induced alterations in its metabolism, this steroid was selected for examination.[74-76] Kinetic studies then demonstrated that

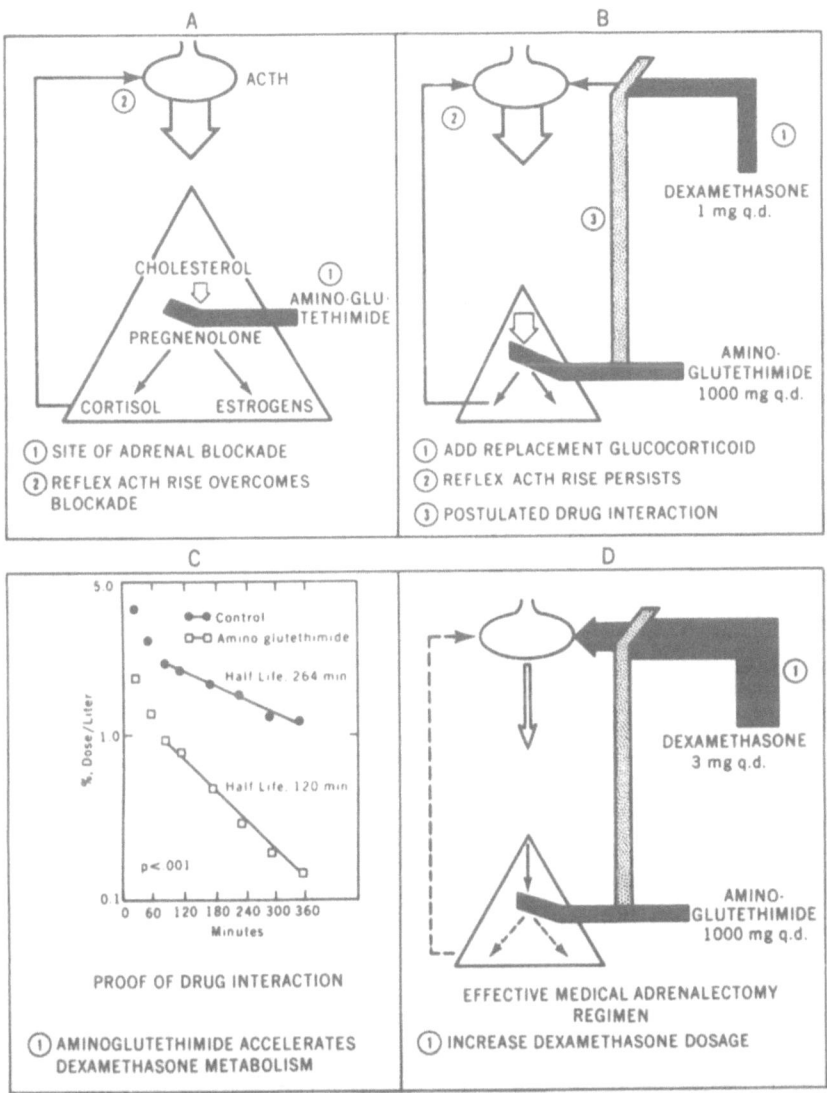

Fig. 2. Physiologic and pharmacologic principles involved in medical adrenalectomy regimen (see text for full explanation). (A) Site of action of aminoglutethimide. (B) Postulated drug interaction between aminoglutethimide and dexamethasone. (C) Kinetic studies of dexamethasone metabolism before and during treatment with aminoglutethimide. (D) Regimen developed to overcome drug interaction.

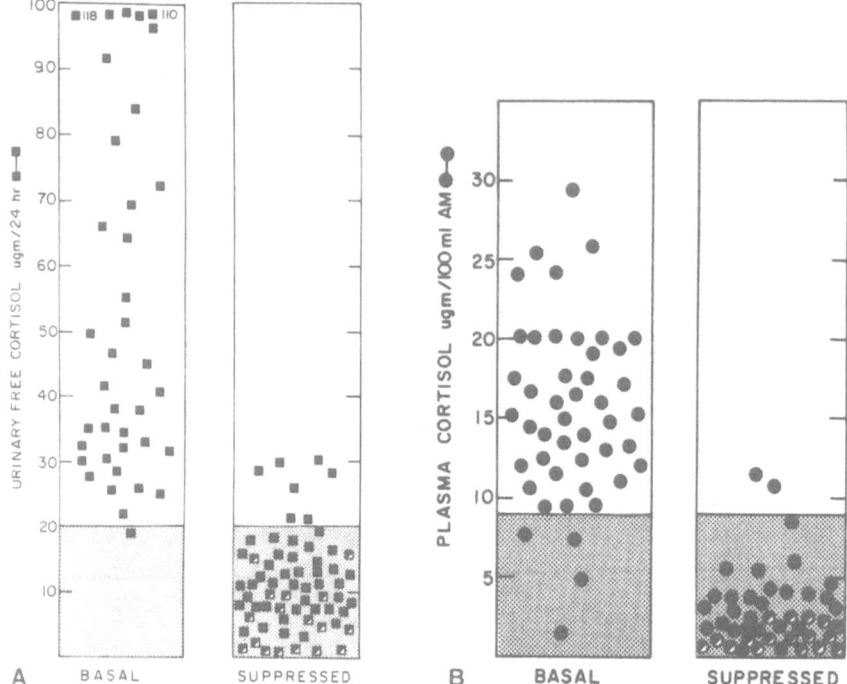

Fig. 3. (A) Urinary free cortisol levels in patients prior to (basal) and during (suppressed) aminoglutethimide therapy. The shaded area represents levels below the normal range. Partially closed squares indicate the values that were undetectable in assays with the limit of detectability of the assay represented by the position of the square. (B) Plasma cortisol levels. Design identical to that of (A).

aminoglutethimide does not cause an acceleration of the metabolism of hydrocortisone (Table II).

In the original studies with dexamethasone, 17-hydroxycorticoids or urinary free cortisol measurements were utilized to monitor adrenal function in patients receiving aminoglutethimide.[64] Since these measurements primarily reflect exogenous hormone administration in patients receiving hydrocortisone by mouth, it was necessary to develop an alternate means of assessing adrenal secretion. The assay of DHA-S was chosen for this purpose and validated by comparing the percent suppression of urinary free cortisol and DHA-S during administration of aminoglutethimide and increasing dexamethasone dosages[67] (Fig. 4). A significant correlation ($r = .79$, $p < .001$), was observed, indicating that DHA-S and urinary free cortisol provide similar information regarding adrenal suppression in patients receiving aminoglutethimide. DHA-S is convenient to assay because its plasma levels are five fold higher than

Table II
Effect of Aminoglutethimide on Cortisol Metabolism

Study period	Number of patients	Initial volume of distribution (liters)	Metabolic clearance rate (liters/24 hr)	Plasma half life (min)
Basal	10	14.5 ± 2.6	159 ± 22	73 ± 3.9
During aminoglutethimide treatment	10	14.3 ± 2.7	192 ± 37	68 ± 3.7
Significance: basal versus treatment		p = NS	p = NS	p = NS

those of cortisol and a radioimmunoassay for this hormone which does not require chromatography or plasma extraction is available. In addition, the long half life of DHA-S (approxiately 10–24 hr) in serum dampens the fluctuations resulting from episodic adrenal secretion which are so prominent for plasma cortisol. Consequently, single a.m. blood samples provide an accurate reflection of overall adrenal secretion. [77]

c. *Determination of Optimal Drug Regimen.* In patients receiving a fixed dose of 1000 mg of aminoglutethimide daily, the effects of increasing dexamethasone and hydrocortisone dosages were compared to demonstrate the feasibility of using hydrocortisone as glucocorticoid replacement in the adrenal suppression regimen (Fig. 5). DHA-S levels progressively fell from basal levels of 520 ± 90 ng/ml to a nadir of 68 ± 21 ng/ml during treatment with 1000 mg of aminoglutethimide and 3 mg of dexamethasone daily (Fig. 6). A slight increase was observed when pa-

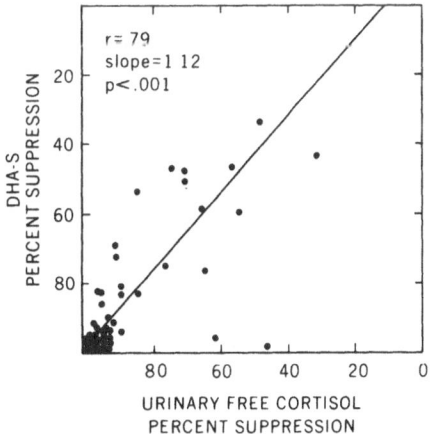

Fig. 4. Correlation of percent suppression of urinary free cortisol and plasma dehydroepiandrosterone sulfate (DHA-S) levels. Percent suppression is determined by the mean basal level of that steroid in individual patients.

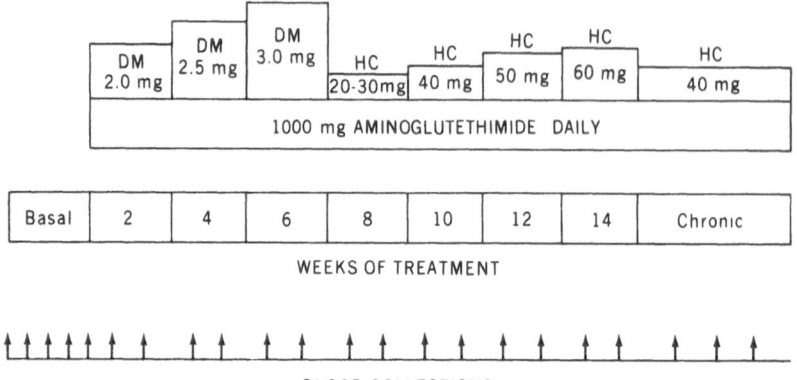

BLOOD COLLECTIONS

Fig. 5. Protocol of drug administration and blood collections. Each arrow indicates the collection of a blood sample at 0800-0900 hr. Dexamethasone (DM) and hydrocortisone (HC) are administered in divided doses with the total daily dosage given in the figure.

tients were switched to 20–30 mg of hydrocortisone daily. However, with 40–60 mg of hydrocortisone and 1000 mg of aminoglutethimide daily, a further reduction in the levels of these steroids was observed. Finally, during chronic therapy with 40 mg of hydrocortisone and 1000 mg of aminoglutethimide for up to 24 months, DHA-S remained mark-

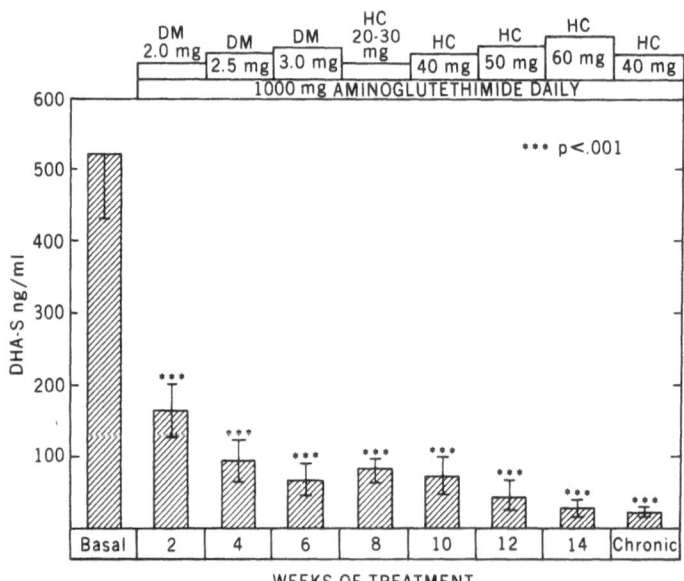

WEEKS OF TREATMENT

Fig. 6. Dehydroepiandrosterone sulfate (DHA-S) levels at various weeks of treatment in 15 patients. The height of each bar and the line above it represent the mean and S.E.M., respectively.

edly suppressed to 22.9 ± 5.0 ng/ml (p <.001). The degree of inhibition of DHA-S levels in individual patients ranged from 73% to 99.2% with a mean fall of 93%.

3.3.2. Estrogen Production during Aminoglutethimide Therapy

a. Evaluation of Estrogen Biosynthetic Pathway. To evaluate estrogen production during aminoglutethimide therapy, the androstenedione, estrone, and estradiol pathway was examined in detail. Surprisingly, the plasma levels of androstenedione measured initially, did not parallel those of other parameters of adrenal suppression such as DHA-S.[66] Androstenedione increased significantly (p < .05) from basal levels of 0.57 ± 0.07 ng/ml to 0.95 ± 0.16 ng/ml (Fig. 7) during the initial two

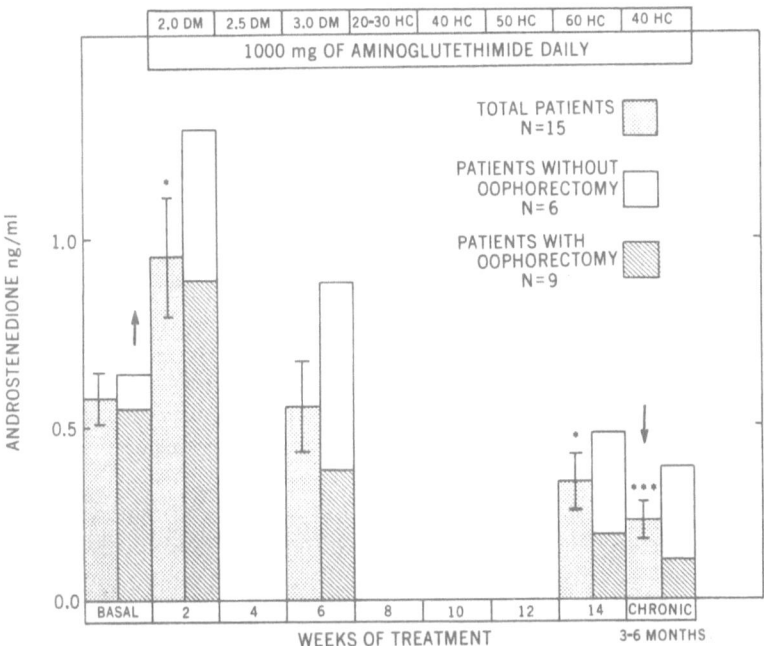

Fig. 7. Androstenedione levels during aminoglutethimide therapy. Aminoglutethimide and either dexamethasone (DM) or hydrocortisone (HC) were administered in the daily dosages indicated. Dotted areas signify mean (±S.E.M.) plasma concentrations of androstenedione in 15 postmenopausal women with breast carcinoma before (basal) and after 2, 6, and 14 weeks, and 3–6 months of treatment with aminoglutethimide. The second column represents the separate values for two subgroups: Clear portions of bars indicate mean levels in spontaneously postmenopausal women; striped areas denote surgically castrate patients. In this and subsequent similar figures, the asterisks represent significant differences between basal and treatment values in the total group of patients (*p < .05; **p < .01; ***p < .001).

weeks of the protocol when the patients received 2 mg of dexamethasone and 1000 mg of aminoglutethimide daily. Androstenedione levels then declined to baseline during administration of 3 mg of dexamethasone daily and were later suppressed to 0.34 ± 0.08 ng/ml ($p < .05$) in women receiving 60 mg of hydrocortisone daily. During chronic treatment with 40 mg of hydrocortisone and 1000 mg of aminoglutethimide, further inhibition to 0.23 ± 0.05 ng/ml ($p < .001$) was observed.

The increment in androstenedione occurring during the first two weeks of therapy could have resulted from an increase in either adrenal or ovarian secretion. To distinguish these possibilities, the data from surgically castrated women and from spontaneously postmenopausal patients were analyzed separately (Fig. 7). The greater rise in this steroid in spontaneously menopausal women (1.30 ± 0.34 ng/ml versus 0.79 ± 0.15 ng/ml) suggested that the ovary contributed to this increase. Also in support of this conclusion was the observation that the androstenedione levels were higher at each dosage level of dexamethasone plus hydrocortisone in patients with ovaries than in castrate women.

Concomitant measurements of estrone and estradiol in these patients revealed a divergent pattern from that of androstenedione. Both estrogens (Fig. 8) fell abruptly with initiation of therapy with 1000 mg of aminoglutethimide and 2 mg of dexamethasone to levels three- to fourfold lower than basal. Even during administration of large doses of dexamethasone (3 mg daily) and hydrocortisone (i.e., 60 mg daily), these steroids remained similarly suppressed. The same degree of chronic inhibition on a regimen of 1000 mg of aminoglutethimide and 40 mg of hydrocortisone was also maintained. When a separate analysis of surgically castrate versus spontaneously menopausal women was carried out, both groups exhibited a similar degree of estrogen suppression (Fig. 8).

The unexpected lack of parallel inhibition of androstenedione and the estrogens suggested that aminoglutethimide might block peripheral aromatization of androstenedione to estrone. This possibility appeared likely since aminoglutethimide is a potent aromatase inhibitor *in vitro*.[78-80] However, other explanations for the discordant pattern of suppression were possible and included an acceleration of the estrone metabolic clearance rate or reduction of the rate of androstenedione metabolism. Based upon these considerations, the effect of aminoglutethimide on aromatization and on androstenedione and estrone metabolic clearance rates were studied by direct kinetic methods *in vivo*.

Prior to aminoglutethimide therapy in 5 women with metastatic breast carcinoma, the mean transfer constant (rho value) for aromatization of androstenedione to estrone was $1.65 \pm 0.28\%$ (Fig. 9). Each subject exhibited a marked reduction in the rate of conversion of androstenedione to estrone during aminoglutethimide therapy and the mean

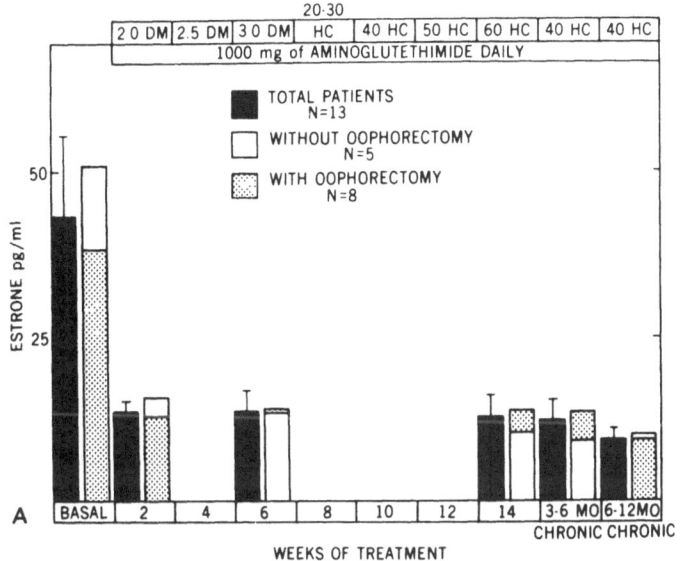

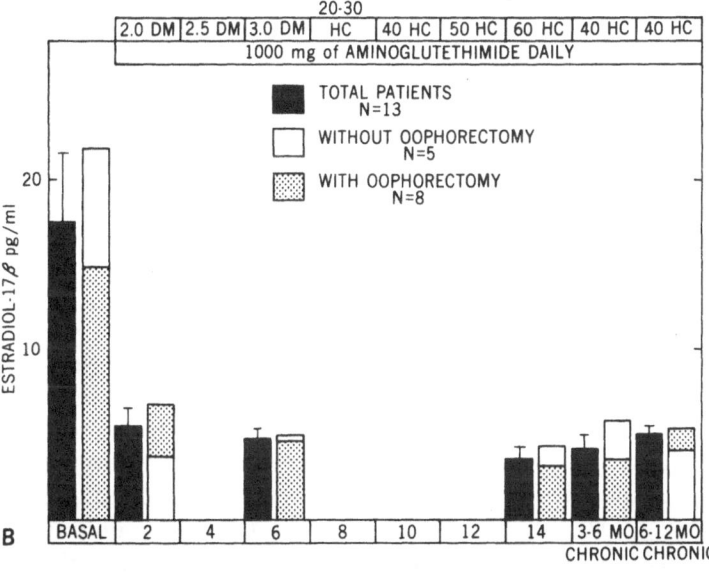

Fig. 8. (A) Estrone levels during aminoglutethimide therapy. Aminoglutethimide and either dexamethasone (DM) or hydrocortisone (HC) were administered in daily dosages indicated. Black areas indicate mean (± S.E.M.) plasma concentrations of estrone (E₁) in 13 postmenopausal women with breast carcinoma before (basal) and after 2, 6, and 14 weeks, and 3–6 months of treatment with aminoglutethimide. The second column represents the separate values for two subgroups: The clear areas show mean levels in spontaneously postmenopausal women; dotted areas indicate surgically castrate patients. (B) Estradiol levels. The format of this figure is identical to that of (A).

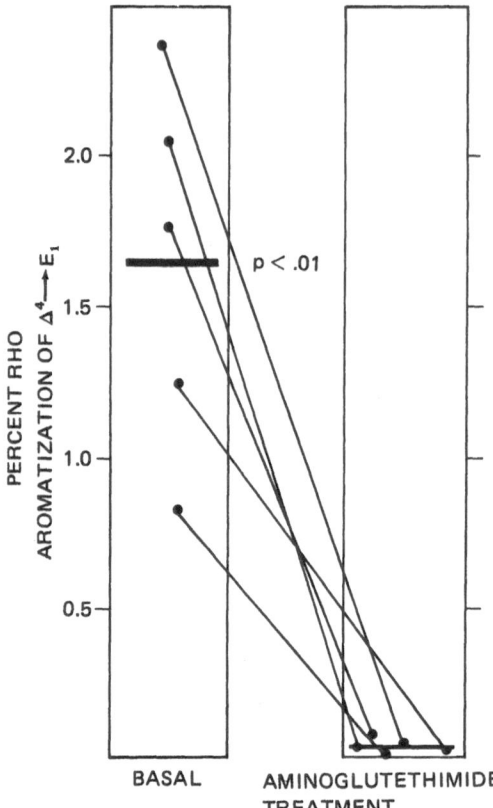

Fig. 9. Effect of aminoglutethimide on aromatization of androstenedione (Δ^4-A) to estrone (E$_1$) as measured in blood. The data points represent individual patients studied before (basal) and during treatment with 1000 mg of aminoglutethimide and 40 mg of hydrocortisone daily. The horizontal lines represent the mean value for all 5 subjects. The downward sloping lines connect individual studies before and during treatment.

value fell to $0.04 \pm 0.01\%$. This represented a highly significant ($p < .01$) 98% inhibition of aromatization. These results were confirmed by making the same measurements on 72-hr urine pools in 2 of these patients. A 95% inhibition of aromatization was demonstrated by this means.

In contrast to its effects on aromatization, no changes in androstenedione or estrone metabolic clearance rates were observed during treatment. The metabolic clearance rate of androstenedione prior to therapy was 1572 ± 241 liters/24 hr and during treatment, 1638 ± 234 liters/24-hr. The estrone metabolic clearance rate similarly did not change. Consequently, inhibition of aromatization provides the explanation for the suppression of estrone without equal inhibition of androstenedione[71] (Fig. 10).

The precise mechanism whereby aminoglutethimide blocks aromatization is unknown. This enzymatic reaction involves a series of hydroxylations of androstenedione and requires 3 mol of molecular oxygen and 3 mol of NADH for formation of 1 mol of estrone.[78,79] With elegant immunologic and chemical techniques, Thompson and Siiteri recently demonstrated that cytochrome P-450 is involved in this process, even though the reaction is not inhibited by carbon monoxide.[78,79] Aminoglutethimide blocks a number of other cytochrome P-450-mediated steroid synthetic steps including the C-20, C-21, and C-18 hydroxylations. [61,81–84] Thus, it is not surprising that aminoglutethimide also inhibits aromatization, as has now been established in post-menopausal women *in vivo* and in placental microsomes and ovarian tissues *in vitro*. [78–80]

Only one other aromatase inhibitor is available clinically. This drug, testololactone (Teslac®), was originally introduced as an impeded androgen for use in metastatic breast carcinoma but was later shown to be an aromatase inhibitor.[24,85,86] In men with gynecomastia, Teslac® produced a 50–80% inhibition of androstenedione-to-estrone conversion and reduced estradiol levels in normal men through this mechanism.[85] Teslac® also lowers the levels of estrone but, surprisingly, not those of estradiol in postmenopausal women through this mechanism.[86]

Aminoglutethimide, then, can lower estrogen production by two separate mechanisms—suppression of adrenal estrogen precursors and blockade of extraglandular aromatization (Fig. 10). Several observations suggest that the adrenal action of aminoglutethimide is not the major one in reducing estrogen synthesis. Newsome *et al.* studied patients receiving aminoglutethimide without concomitant glucocorticoid re-

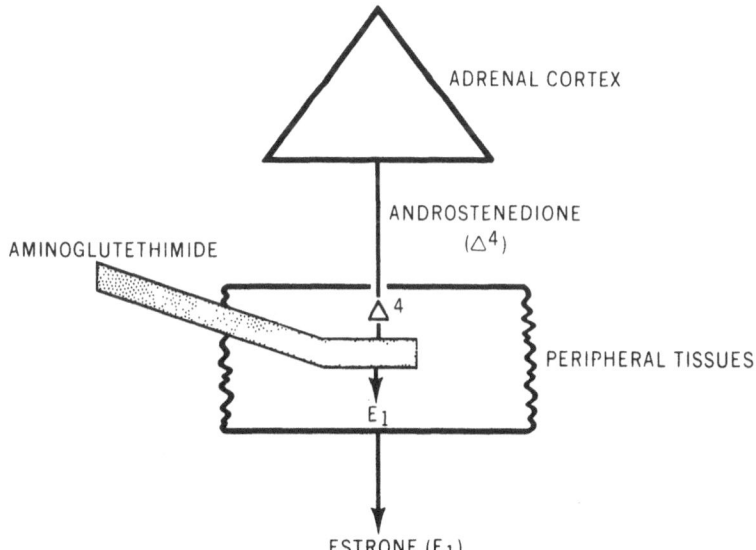

Fig. 10. Diagrammatic representation of the site of action of aminoglutethimide on the aromatization of androstenedione to estrone.

placement.[87] The lowering of cortisol induced by this regimen stimulated a reflex ACTH rise of sufficient magnitude to completely overcome the adrenal blockade and particularly the inhibition of androstenedione secretion. Even in the presence of adrenal escape, Newsome et al. observed a marked lowering of plasma estrone and estradiol concentrations with aminoglutethimide. In our studies, the estrogens were suppressed maximally prior to androstenedione inhibition. Taken together, these observations provide support for the conclusion that the estrogens can be suppressed without a concomitant adrenal blockade in patients receiving aminoglutethimide.

The effect of aminoglutethimide on aromatization is of major importance in spontaneously postmenopausal women with breast carcinoma. The postmenopausal ovary produces sufficient amounts of androstenedione to account for at least a portion of the estrogen produced after the climacteric.[30,31] Unless an ovariectomy is performed at the same time as surgical adrenalectomy in postmenopausal patients, this estrogen source will remain. On the other hand, aminoglutethimide can effectively inhibit the production of estrogens from both ovarian and adrenal androstenedione in these women.

  b. *Comparative Effects of Medical and Surgical Adrenalectomy on Estrogen Levels.* To evaluate the degree of estrogen suppression produced by aminoglutethimide, the plasma levels of estrone and estradiol were compared in one group of women treated with surgical adrenalectomy and in another receiving aminoglutethimide as medical adrenalectomy. Mean levels of these steroids fell to similar concentrations in both groups as a result of treatment[71] (Fig. 11). After surgical adrenalectomy, estrone levels were 12.0 ± 1.4 pg/ml ($n = 12$) and during aminoglutethimide, 12.3 ± 1.1 pg/ml ($n = 41$). Estradiol plasma concentrations were 5.8 ± 0.55 pg/ml ($n = 12$) in the surgically treated patients and 5.6 ± 0.65 pg/ml ($n = 42$) in the women receiving aminoglutethimide. It is of note that the basal levels of both estrone and estradiol were slightly higher in the patients given aminoglutethimide, and, consequently, the degree of suppression was greater in these patients. Therefore, aminoglutethimide induces a highly effective inhibition of estradiol production.

3.3.3. Hormonal Data during Fixed-Drug-Dosage Combination

In order to utilize the regimen of medical adrenalectomy with aminoglutethimide on a wide scale, a simple fixed-drug-dosage combination was developed as described above. Data were then collected to document the hormone levels in patients treated with this regimen exclusively. Subjects received standard drug dosages which consisted of 250 mg of aminoglutethimide 4 times daily, and hydrocortisone, 20 mg

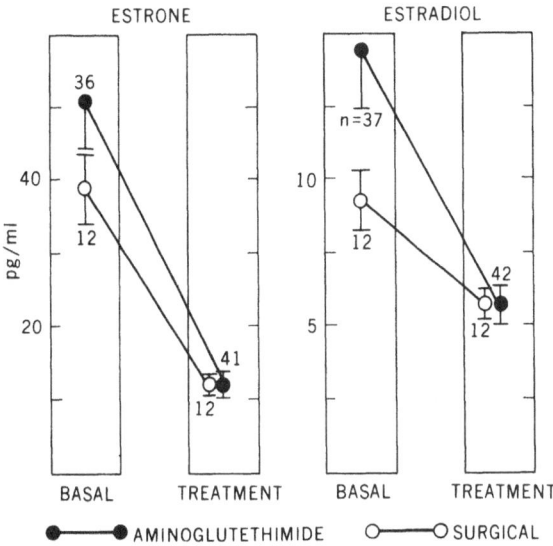

Fig. 11. Comparison of estrone and estradiol levels prior to treatment (basal) and after surgical adrenalectomy or during aminoglutethimide administration. The circles represent the mean, and the error bars the S.E.M. for each group. The numbers associated with the error bars represent the number of patients included in the particular measurement indicated.

Table III
Plasma Steroid Levels during Fixed-Dosage Regimen of
Aminoglutethimide-Hydrocortisone

HC	0	100	40					
AG	0	1000						
Weeks	Basal	2	4	6	8	10	12	Chronic
DHA-S	766	101	94.7	103	57.2	57.7	55.0	60.9
	±	±	±	±	±	±	±	±
	116	31	29	26	13	12	21	11
	$n = 29$	$n = 18$	$n = 15$	$n = 20$	$n = 17$	$n = 16$	$n = 13$	$n = 21$
Estrone	55.2	16.8	12.8	15.0	11.4	9.98	5.4	12.1
	±	±	±	±	±	±	±	±
	11.9	4.6	3.6	3.1	2.8	2.8	1.7	1.7
	$n = 17$	$n = 15$	$n = 15$	$n = 15$	$n = 13$	$n = 12$	$n = 7$	$n = 13$
Estradiol	15.3	6.08	6.02	6.4	9.7	5.2	4.2	7.9
	±	±	±	±	±	±	±	±
	2.4	1.5	1.14	1.3	2.5	1.2	1.3	1.03
	$n = 17$	$n = 14$	$n = 13$	$n = 12$	$n = 12$	$n = 9$	$n = 5$	$n = 14$

at bedtime, 10 mg in the morning, and 10 mg at 5 p.m. For the first two weeks of therapy, however, 100 mg of hydrocortisone was given to reduce the severity or prevent the drug rash that occurs in one-third of patients (see below). Hormonal data during this regimen revealed uniform suppression of DHA-S and estrogen levels (Table III), and, consequently, it can be used effectively. However, the use of mineralocorticoid therapy must be individualized. Aldosterone levels are inhibited in the majority of patients treated (Fig. 12). Only one-third of women develop symptoms of hormonal lack. In practice, standing and lying blood pressures are obtained routinely in the clinic and patients are given Florinef (0.1 mg twice a week to 0.1 mg twice a day of 9α-fluorohydrocortisone) if orthostatic hypotension develops.

3.3.4. Effects of Aminoglutethimide on Intraadrenal Enzyme Pathways

Initial studies with aminoglutethimide demonstrated a marked inhibition of DHA-S and at the same time a rise or incomplete suppression of androstenedione. A logical explanation would be that this steroid

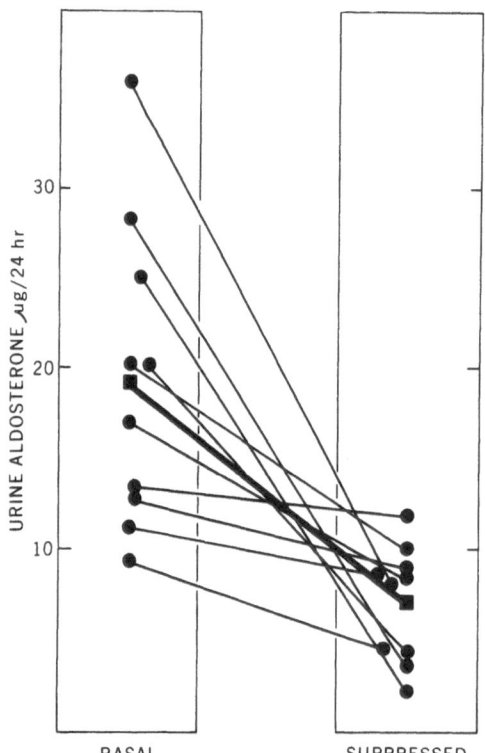

Fig. 12. Urinary aldosterone levels in patients prior to and during aminoglutethimide – dexamethasone or aminoglutethimide–hydrocortisone therapy. All values in individual subjects obtained basally or during therapy were pooled. The heavy line and squares represent mean values for each group.

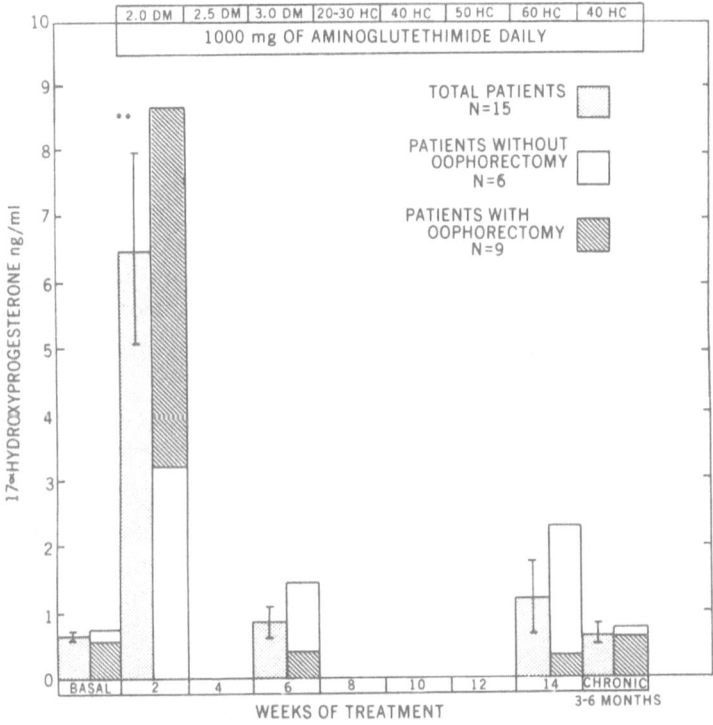

Fig. 13. 17α-Hydroxyprogesterone levels during aminoglutethimide therapy. The format of this figure is identical to that of Fig. 7.

increases as a result of the blockade of its metabolism to estrone. However, this is not the case since the metabolic clearance rate of androstenedione did not change during aminoglutethimide therapy. These findings suggest that aminoglutethimide must have an effect on other adrenal enzyme systems in addition to that proposed as its major blocking site, the conversion of cholesterol to pregnenolone. One possibility was that aminoglutethimide induces the 3β-ol-dehydrogenase-Δ^4- to Δ^5-isomerase enzyme complex in such a way as to favor secretion of Δ^4 over Δ^5 steroids. To examine this hypothesis, several Δ^4 and Δ^5 steroid pairs were examined before and during aminoglutethimide therapy.[70]

a. *Δ^4 Steroids.* The plasma levels of the Δ^4 steroids, progesterone and 17α-hydroxyprogesterone, paralleled those of androstenedione during all phases of treatment. These steroids all increased significantly over basal values during the initial two weeks of treatment with 1000 mg of aminoglutethimde and 2 mg of dexamethasone. 17α-Hydroxyprogesterone rose to the greatest extent—i.e., tenfold (Fig. 13)—from basal levels of 0.65 ± 0.07 ng/ml to 6.48 ± 1.46 ng/ml ($p < .01$). Later, all three Δ^4

steroids declined to baseline during treatment with aminoglutethimide and 3 mg of dexamethasone, and then decreased further when hydrocortisone, either 40 or 60 mg daily, was substituted for dexamathasone. Only androstenedione was significantly suppressed, however, during chronic therapy.

   b. Δ^5 *Steroids.* The patterns of the Δ^5 steroids during treatment with aminoglutethimide were strikingly different from those synthesized in the Δ^4 pathway. All Δ^5 steroids were suppressed three- to fivefold during the initial two weeks of treatment and remained inhibited throughout. (Figure 14 shows 17α-hydroxypregnenolone as an example.) As a consequence, the ratios of all Δ^5 to Δ^4 steroids were significantly altered in favor of the Δ^4 compounds during treatment.[70]

3.3.5. *Proposed Mechanisms for Hormonal Patterns Observed*

   The adrenal suppression regimen described in this chapter included coadministration of both a glucocorticoid and aminoglutethimide. It is necessary to consider whether adrenal inhibition with the current regimen might result exclusively from administration of the glucocorticoid

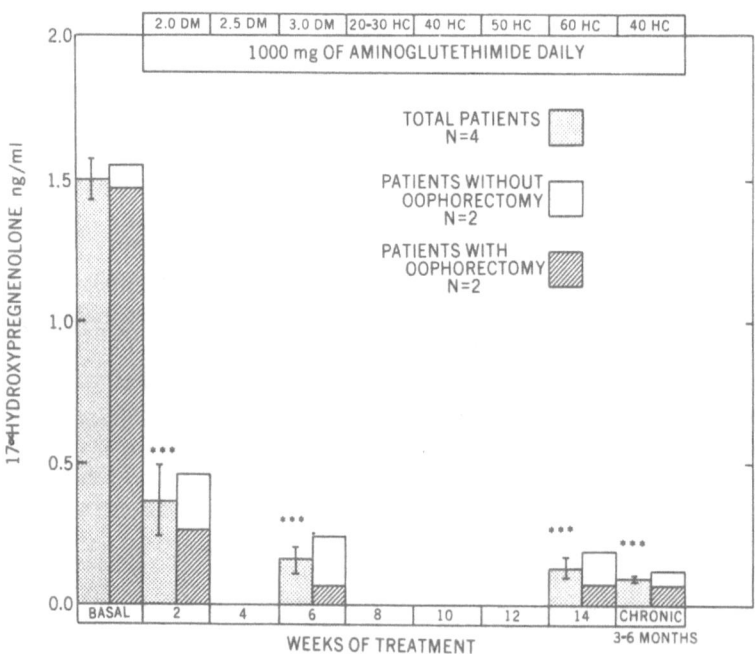

Fig. 14. 17α-Hydroxypregnenolone levels during aminoglutethimide therapy. The format of this figure is identical to that of Fig. 7.

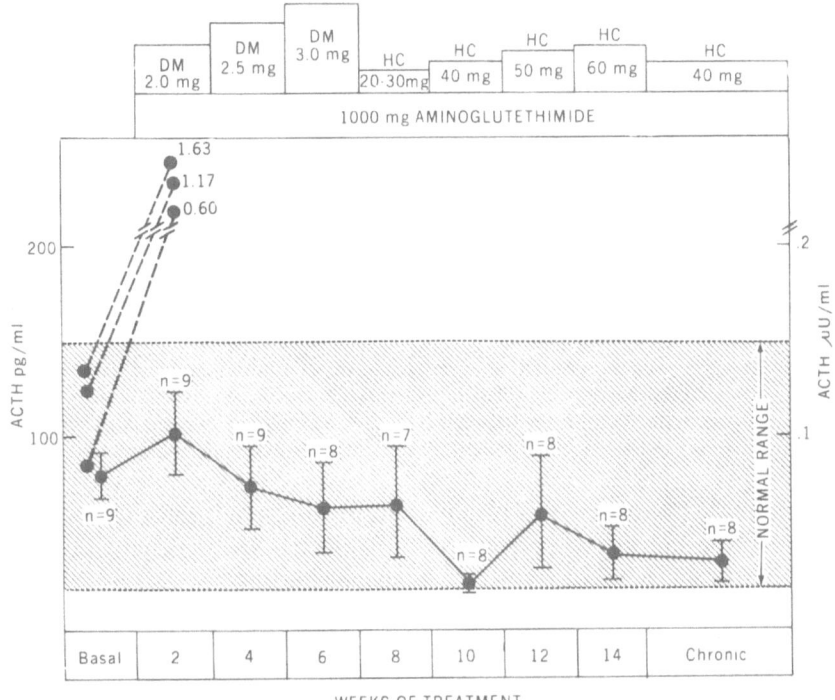

Fig. 15. Plasma ACTH levels in patients at various weeks of treatment. The data points represent mean ± S.E.M. values and the numbers of patients studied are recorded above each data point. The shaded area indicates the absolute normal range of ACTH levels of 20–150 pg/ml. For comparison, the ACTH levels measured during aminoglutethimide administration alone (i.e., with no concomitant glucocorticoid) are shown by the filled circles and dashed lines. These levels, in μU/ml, are taken from the bioassay studies of Fishman *et al.* [84]

rather than from aminoglutethimide. Examination of the ACTH data allows certain conclusions to be drawn regarding this point (Fig. 15). ACTH levels were not significantly suppressed at any time during dexamethasone administration and yet plasma DHA-S (and estrone and estradiol) concentrations were markedly lowered. These data strongly point to a predominant effect of aminoglutethimide on the inhibition of adrenal steroid synthesis. However, during chronic therapy with 40 mg of hydrocortisone and aminoglutethimide, ACTH levels, although still within the normal range of 20–150 pg/ml, were significantly suppressed below basal values. This indicates an additive effect of both ACTH suppression and direct adrenal inhibition with the latter regimen.

The observations from this and other studies also allow the formulation of a working hypothesis to explain the divergent effects of amino-

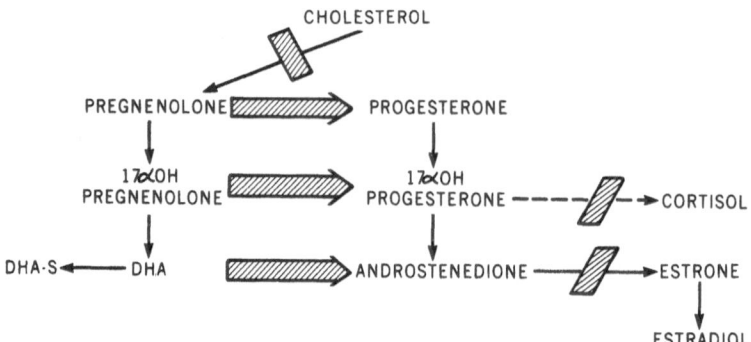

Fig. 16. Diagrammatic representation of potential sites of action of aminoglutethimide on the inhibition of pregnenolone, cortisol, and estrone synthesis (see text). The large striped arrows represent the 3β-ol-dehydrogenase-Δ⁴- to Δ⁵-isomerase enzyme system which may be enhanced in the direction shown during aminoglutethimide therapy (see text).

glutethimide on the various plasma steroids measured (Fig. 16). Aminoglutethimide blocks the conversion of cholesterol to pregnenolone and reduces the amount of substrate available for further steroid biosynthesis.[83] Enhanced conversion of the Δ^5 to Δ^4 compounds favors the secretion of progesterone, 17α-hydroxyprogesterone, and Δ^4-androstenedione. Furthermore, inhibition of the C-21 and C-11 hydroxylations reduces the formation of cortisol. In patients given aminoglutethimide, as in the C-21 and C-11 forms of congenital adrenal hyperplasia, ACTH levels rise as a result of cortisol inhibition. Absolute increments in progesterone, 17α-hydroxyprogesterone, and androstenedione then result unless sufficient amounts of glucocorticoid are given to prevent the reflex ACTH rise. In support of this proposed concept of aminoglutethimide action, Newsome studied patients receiving aminoglutethimide without any replacement glucocorticoid and demonstrated a marked increase in plasma androstenedione levels. [73]

In our studies, 2 mg of dexamethasone was given to patients as glucocorticoid replacement in the first two weeks of the aminoglutethimide regimen used. Because aminoglutethimide reduces the bioavailability of dexamethasone as previously reported, this dosage was insufficient to prevent a slight reflex rise in ACTH (Fig. 15). As a result of this and the enhanced conversion of Δ^5 and Δ^4 steroids, progesterone, 17α-hydroxyprogesterone, and androstenedione rose to levels two- to tenfold over basal values during the first two weeks of therapy. Only later when adequate amounts of replacement glucocorticoid were given did the levels of these steroids fall back to basal or suppressed values. In marked contrast, as a reflection of the altered Δ^5-toΔ^4 conversion, the Δ^5 steroids were uniformly inhibited. It should be noted that patients with a congenital absence of C-21 hydroxylase exhibit high levels of Δ^5 steroids;

consequently, aminoglutethimide cannot produce the changes observed merely by its C-21-inhibitory properties. It is apparent, then, that the diagram proposed to explain the effects of aminoglutethimide is consistent with most observed data.

3.3.6. Side Effects of Aminoglutethimide

A major side effect of aminoglutethimide, a derivative of the soporific drug glutethimide, is transient lethargy.[69] This symptom appeared early in therapy (Table IV) and was nearly uniformly resolved after three to six weeks of treatment. One explanation for the transient nature of this side effect is the fact that aminoglutethimide induces an acceleration of its own metabolism (Fig. 17). The mean half life of aminoglutethimide prior to therapy in 6 patients was 13.3 ± 2.6 (S.E.) hr and during chronic treatment, 7.3 ± 2.1 hr ($p < .01$). In recognition of this fact, patients may be advised to start on one-half the aminoglutethimide dosage for the first two to three weeks of therapy until the rate of metabolic clearance of this drug stabilizes at a more rapid rate. A total dosage of 1000 mg/day is the maximum required to inhibit estrogen secretion and aromatization. Doses that have been previously recommended for treatment of Cushing's syndrome, i.e., 1500–2500 mg per day, are not necessary and may produce an unacceptable incidence of side effects.

Skin rash also occurs commonly in response to aminoglutethimide and is moribiliform in type.[69] The rash is occasionally associated with fever and usually begins approximately ten days after the start of therapy. However, aminoglutethimide may be continued and the rash resolves spontaneously within four to five days. Higher steroid doses are highly effective in reducing the fever and diminishing the severity of the rash and are required only for five to seven days. For this reason, it has been found practical to routinely administer 100 mg of hydrocor-

Table IV
Acute and Chronic Aminoglutethimide Toxicity

	Lethargy	Skin rash	Ataxia	Other
Acute	22/53 (41.5%)	19/53 (35.8%)	6/53 (11.3%)	5/53 (9.4%)[a]
Chronic	0/49	0/49	0/49	9/49 (18.5%)[b]

[a]Dizziness.
[b]Weight gain,[5] facial fullness,[3] leg cramps.[2]

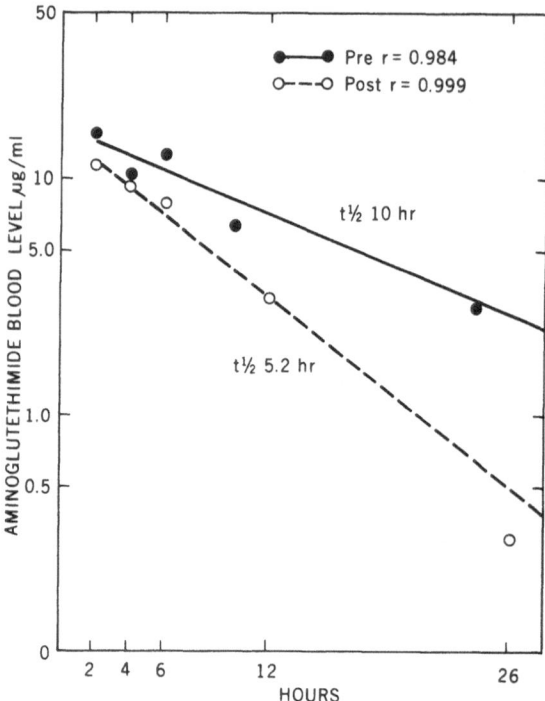

Fig. 17. Example of the half life of aminoglutethimide before and after 6 weeks of treatment with aminoglutethimide and hydrocortisone in a single patient.

tisone daily for the first two weeks of therapy to all patients to prevent or diminish the severity of the rash.

During chronic treatment with aminoglutethimide, the medical adrenalectomy regimen is well tolerated with only minor side effects such as weight gain, facial fullness, and leg cramps in about 18% of patients. In susceptible individuals, hypothyroidism may occur as a result of the effects of aminoglutethimide on thyroxine synthesis [68,88-90]; however, in the majority of patients, TSH levels rise by an average of threefold[68] to overcome the antithyroid effects of the drug (Fig. 18). To detect incipient hypothyroidism, thyroxine levels should be monitored periodically. Although TSH and prolactin secretion are tightly interrelated in some patients with chronic hypothyroidism, [91,92] serially measured levels of prolactin did not increase in patients receiving the aminoglutethimide medical adrenalectomy regimen (Fig. 19).

3.3.7. Clinical Studies

Medical adrenalectomy with aminoglutethimide was first utilized in a series of patients with breast carcinoma by Griffiths *et al.* in 1969 and these authors subsequently reported that 3 of 9 women responded objectively.[63] The degree of adrenal suppression in these patients was highly variable since a recognition of the effects of aminoglutethimide on synthetic glucocorticoid metabolism had not been identified. A joint study carried out at Duke University and The Pennsylvania State University was recently reported, in which 55 patients were treated with aminoglutethimide and adrenal blockade achieved. All of these women had previously undergone mastectomy for carcinoma of the breast and subsequently developed recurrent disease. Exclusions included lym-

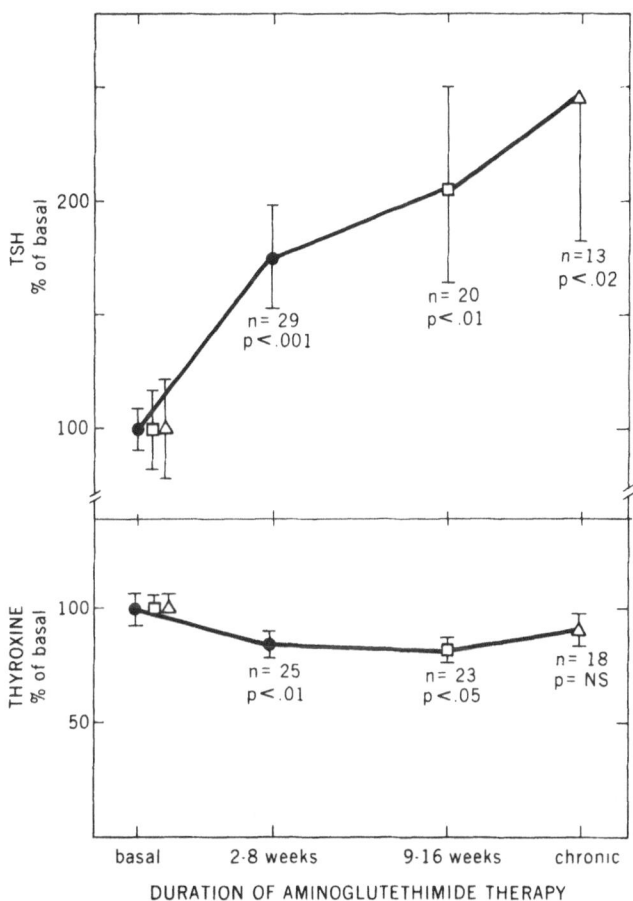

Fig. 18. TSH and thyroxine levels expressed as mean percent of basal values (± S.E.M.) during treatment with aminoglutethimide and either hydrocortisone or dexamethasone. Paired t tests were used to determine the statistical significance of the differences between values observed during treatment and basal levels. Each symbol indicates the group of subjects available for analysis at each time point with the number (n) of subjects in that group indicated.

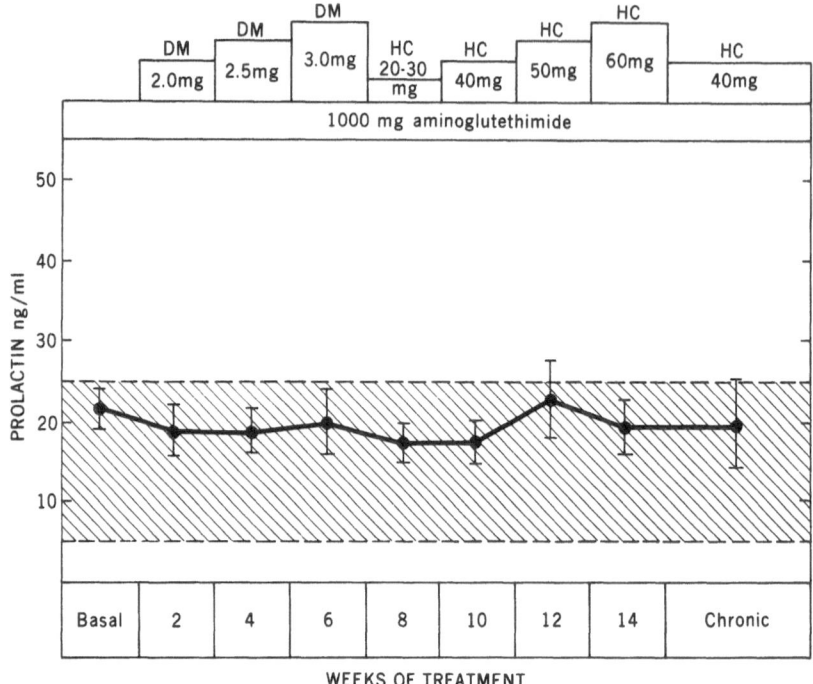

Fig. 19. Prolactin levels during aminoglutethimide and either dexamethasone (DM) or hydrocortisone (HC) in women with breast carcinoma. The shaded area represents the normal range of prolactin levels. After collection of basal samples, all subjects received 1000 mg of aminoglutethimide daily. At the same time, these women received DM at an initial dosage of 2 mg daily for 2 weeks and then were given increasing amounts at 2-week intervals. Later, women were switched to HC in increasing amounts as shown.

phangitic metastases to lung or central nervous system and patient age over 80. Two women were lost to follow-up and 3 withdrew from the study because of toxic reactions to aminoglutethimide. The relevant clinical data from these patients have been reported.[69] Estrogen receptor values were available in only 5 patients. Classification of a response as an objective complete remission required that all metastatic lesions disappear for at least 3 months. A partial remission was defined as a decrease of 50% or greater in the sums of the products of the two largest perpendicular diameters of all measurable lesions and/or partial recalcification of osteolytic lesions for a period of 3 months. Regression of osteoblastic lesions or stability with regression of other lesions were also considered objective responses. Stable disease was defined as a decrease of less than 50% or an increase of less than 25% in metastatic lesions for at least 3 months. Progressive disease required an increase of 25% or greater over original measurements.

Of the 50 evaluable patients, 16% underwent complete tumor regression and 22% partial objective remission. Twenty percent had stabilization of disease and 40% demonstrated disease progression. The duration of complete remissions was 25.2 ± 6.3 months and 12.8 ± 2.0 months for partial objective responses. Soft-tissue and osseous metastases responded more frequently than metastatic lesions in lung or liver. Of the 5 estrogen-receptor-positive patients, 3 exhibited objective tumor regression. A previous response to other endocrine therapy also predicted a favorable effect of medical adrenalectomy with aminoglutethimide.

Gale *et al.* reported the use of an aminoglutethimide medical adrenalectomy regimen consisting of 1000 mg of aminoglutethimide daily and variable doses of dexamethasone.[93] They obtained a 33% objective remission rate in 65 patients unselected by estrogen receptor testing. Newsome *et al.* observed a similar rate of response to treatment with 1000 mg of aminoglutethimide and 3 mg of dexamethasone daily.[94] These results suggest that medical adrenalectomy with aminoglutethimide may produce tumor regression with a frequency and duration similar to that achieved by surgical adrenalectomy.

A comparative randomized trial of aminoglutethimide medical adrenalectomy with surgical adrenalectomy in patients stratified by clinical parameters and estrogen receptor status is now being undertaken. Preliminary data in 65 patients entered suggest an equal rate of response to these two treatments, but patient entry and duration of follow-up are still limited. Such a study is necessary to provide a valid direct comparison of these two treatment modalities.

Newsome and associates have been conducting additional studies to determine whether an initial response to aminoglutethimide medical adrenalectomy is predictive for a later response to surgical adrenalectomy. As of January, 1978 (personal communication), 41 of 48 patients entering the trial were evaluable. Twenty experienced a subjective or objective response to a 12-week course of aminoglutethimide. Eighteen of these women had persistence of these effects for at least six months following surgical adrenalectomy. Six nonresponders to aminoglutethimide medical adrenalectomy were later subjected to surgical adrenalectomy. None of these women benefited from surgery. These data provide support for the concept that individual patients respond identically to medical or surgical adrenalectomy.

A further study has compared medical adrenalectomy with aminoglutethimide to surgical hypophysectomy. The rationale for this comparison is the following[95]: Carcinoma of the breast regresses as frequently following surgical hypophysectomy as with surgical adrenalectomy.[1–8] While the precise mechanistic effect of pituitary ablation is unclear, ad-

renal function and estrogen levels are suppressed following this procedure and recent data suggest that reduction of prolactin levels are probably not important in mediating the responses to hypophysectomy.
Based upon the concept that in postmenopausal women, hypophysectomy acts through suppression of adrenal-related estrogen production,
it is reasonable to compare medical adrenalectomy with aminoglutethimide to hypophysectomy.

Thirty-three patients were randomly selected for hypophysectomy
or medical adrenalectomy with aminoglutethimide and two patients
were crossed over to medical adrenalectomy after initial therapy with
hypophysectomy. Three of 14 patients experienced partial objective
tumor regression with a median duration of 4 to 6 months following
hypophysectomy, whereas 10 of 21 women receiving aminoglutethimide objectively responded (2 complete, 8 partial) with a median duration of 11.5 months (Table V). Side effects in the medical group were
minimal, while surgical complications included two cases of cerebro-
spinal fluid rhinorrhea, one leading to meningitis and death. Also reported in this study were the hormonal data from 2 patients crossed
over to medical adrenalectomy after a surgical hypophysectomy and 3
additional patients treated with both modalities. The levels of DHA-S,
estrone, and estradiol were all suppressed further by aminoglutethimide
in patients previously treated with hypophysectomy (Table VI). Careful
endocrine evaluation following hypophysectomy revealed residual
pituitary function in each of the 5 patients studied. It is not clear whether

Table V
Response Rates to Hypophysectomy and Estrogen Suppression

	Hypophysectomy	Estrogen suppression	
Number of patients	14	21	
Overall responses			
Stable	1	0	
Complete regression (CR)	0	2	
Partial regression (PR)	3	8	
CR and PR	3 (21%)	10 (47%)	p = NS
Responses by site of lesion[a]			
Soft tissue	3/7 (1 CR)	4/9	
Pleura	1/4	2/6 (1 CR)	
Lung	0/5	2/6 (1 CR)	
Bone	2/5 (1 CR)	5/10 (2 CR)	
Liver	0/3	0/7	
Median duration of response	4.6 mo	11.5 mo	

[a]Number of patients responding/number of patients with lesion.

Table VI
Hormonal Data in Hypophysectomized Patients before and after
Aminoglutethimide Treatment

	DHA-S (ng/ml)		Estrone (pg/ml)		Estradiol (pg/ml)	
	Basal	Treated	Basal	Treated	Basal	Treated
Patient						
1	732	194	177	9.6	5.2	4.3
2	1119	28	26	15.4	9.2	3.1
3	100	12	48	5.1	15.1	3.3
4	254	45	58	13.2	6.0	<.5
5	94	4.8	22	2.3	6.1	1.4
Mean ± S.E.M.	459 ± 202	57 ± 35	66 ± 28	9.1 + 2.4	8.3 ± 1.8	2.5 ± 0.69

	Urine			
	Estrone (μg/24 hr)		Estradiol (μg/24 hr)	
	Basal	Treated	Basal	Treated
Patient				
1	3.4	.086	.60	.11
2	1.11	.056	.34	.14
Mean	2.25	.071	.47	.125

further hormonal suppression could be produced in all hypophysectomized patients by the addition of aminoglutethimide.

The observations of Manni et al. in this regard are of interest.[96] They observed frequent responses to antiestrogens in patients following hypophysectomy. It may be, then, that the degree of residual estrogen secretion following hypophysectomy is important[97,98] and amenable to reduction with medical adrenalectomy or antiestrogens.

Clinical data regarding the rate of response to aminoglutethimide in patients selected on the basis of estrogen receptor positivity are limited. Three of five estrogen-receptor-positive patients treated by Wells et al. had objective tumor regression after treatment with aminoglutethimide. [69] More recent data from our group which correlate the response rates in estrogen-receptor-positive and estrogen-receptor-negative patients are available. In the group of 35 patients with ER < 10 fm/mg cytosol protein, 72% experienced either complete or partial objective responses or stabilization for greater than 6 months. Of these, 50% were noted to have objective responses. Three of 7 patients with estrogen-receptor levels between 3 and 10 fmol/mg cytosol protein also responded objectively. All 4 patients with both estrogen-receptor and progesterone-receptor positively experienced objective tumor regression.

4. Role of Medical Adrenalectomy in the Treatment of Breast Carcinoma

The development of an effective fixed-dosage regimen to suppress adrenal estrogens with aminoglutethimide circumvents problems inherent in the use of high-dose glucocorticoids to produce a medical adrenalectomy. Consequently, the role of medical adrenalectomy as a therapeutic strategy must now be reconsidered. Firstly, it should be emphasized that estrogen-receptor-negative patients would not be expected to benefit from this medical adrenalectomy regimen.[9] Certainly aminoglutethimide treatment would be useful for postmenopausal patients with breast carcinoma who would otherwise be candidates for surgical adrenalectomy or hypophysectomy but are too debilitated for surgery. Although present data suggest that medical adrenalectomy with aminoglutethimide is as effective as surgical adrenalectomy, a conclusive recommendation that medical is preferable to surgical adrenalectomy awaits the results of controlled clinical trials. Patients who fail to respond to hypophysectomy or have an initial response with later relapse should also be considered for aminoglutethimide. Finally, earlier use of aminoglutethimide as adjuvant therapy in estrogen-receptor-positive postmenopausal or surgically castrate patients warrants a clinical trial. A more difficult question relates to the relative roles of aminoglutethimide medical adrenalectomy and antiestrogens in the treatment of women with metastatic breast carcinoma. Controlled trials of the relative efficacy of each and perhaps combination therapy are required before any answer to this question can be forthcoming.

ACKNOWLEDGMENTS: The authors wish to thank Mrs. Marlene Thompson for invaluable help in the preparation of this manuscript. Appreciation is expressed to Dr. C. Wayne Bardin for encouragement in the performance of these studies, and to Drs. Allan Lipton, Harold Harvey, Samuel Wells, Edward Ruby, John Kendall, Robert Misbin, Laurence Demers, Elwood Foltz, Chhanda Gupta, Slobodan Runic, and Darrow Haagensen, who made major contributions to the work from our laboratory reviewed in this chapter. This work was sponsored in part by NIH Contract No. N01-CB-13851 and Specialized Cancer Grant No. 1 P30 CA18450 from the National Cancer Institute, Department of Health, Education, and Welfare.

5. References

1. O. H. Pearson and B. S. Ray, Results of hypophysectomy in the treatment of metastatic mammary carcinoma, *Cancer* **12**, 85–92 (1959).
2. B. S. Ray, Carcinoma of the breast—hypophysectomy as palliative treatment, *J. Am. Med. Assoc.* **200**, 974–975 (1967).
3. A. A. Fracchia, H. T. Randall, and J. H. Farrow, The results of adrenalectomy in advanced breast cancer in 500 consecutive patients, *Surg. Gynecol. Obstet.* **125**, 747–756 (1967).
4. A. A. Fracchia, Indications for castration and adrenalectomy for advanced breast cancer, *Cancer* **28**, 1699–1701 (1971).
5. A. A. Fracchia, J. H. Farrow, T. R. Miller, R. H. Tofflefsen, E. J. Greenberg, and W. H. Knapper, Hypophysectomy as compared with adrenalectomy in the treatment of advanced carcinoma of the breast, *Surg. Gynecol. Obstet.* **133**, 241–246 (1971).
6. B. A. Stoll (ed.), The basis of endocrine therapy, in: *Endocrine Therapy in Malignant Disease*, Chapter 6, pp. 111–137, W. B. Saunders, Philadelphia, (1972).
7. P. Juret and M. Hayem, Pituitary ablation in the treatment of breast cancer, in: *Mammary Cancer and Neuroendocrine Therapy* (B. A. Stoll, ed.), pp. 283–311, Butterworths, London (1974).
8. M. J. Silverstein, R. L. Byron, Jr., R. H. Yonemoto, D. U. Riihimaki, and G. Schuster, Bilateral adrenalectomy for advanced breast cancer. A 21-year experience, *Surgery* **77**, 825–832 (1975).
9. W. L. McGuire, P. P. Carbone, and E. P. Vollmer (eds.), *Estrogen Receptors in Human Breast Cancer*, Raven Press, New York (1975).
10. J. S. Spratt, and W. L. Donegan (eds.), Adrenalectomy, in: *Cancer of the Breast*, Chapter 5, pp. 107–108, W. B. Saunders, Philadelphia (1967).
11. A. T. Cowie, Hormone factors in mammary development and lactation, in: *Mammary Cancer and Neuroendocrine Therapy* (B. A. Stoll, ed.), pp. 3–24, Butterworths, London (1974).
12. J. C. Porter, Hormonal regulation of breast development and activity, *J. Invest. Dermatol.* **63**, 85–92 (1974).
13. R. K. Wagner, L. Gorlick, and P. W. Jungblut, Dihydrotestosterone receptors in human mammary cancer, *Acta Endocrinol. (Copenhagen) Suppl.* **173**, 65 (Abst.) (1973).
14. K. B. Horwitz, and W. L. McGuire, Specific progesterone receptors in human breast cancer, *Steroids* **25**, 497–505 (1975).
15. R. P. Persijn, C. B. Korsten, and E. Engelsman, Oestrogen and androgen receptors in breast cancer and response to endocrine therapy, *Br. Med. J.* **4**, 503 (1975).
16. J. Poortman, J. A. C. Prenen, F. Schwarz, and J. H. H. Thijssen, Interaction of Δ^5-androstene-$3\beta,17\beta$-diol with estradiol and dihydrotestosterone receptors in human myometrial and mammary cancer tissue. *J. Clin. Endocrinol. Metab.* **40**, 373–379 (1975).
17. F. A. G. Teulings, and H. A. van Gilse, Demonstration of glucocorticoid receptors in human mammary carcinomas, *Horm. Res.* **8**, 107–116 (1977).
18. D. G. Gardner and J. L. Wittliff, Demonstration of a glucocorticoid hormone-receptor complex in the cytoplasm of a hormone-responsive tumour, *Br. J. Cancer* **27**, 441–444 (1975).
19. G. Shyamala, Glucocorticoid receptors in mouse mammary tumors, *J. Biol. Chem.* **249**, 2160–2163 (1974).
20. J. E. Goral, and J. L. Wittliff, Comparison of glucocorticoid-binding proteins in normal and neoplastic mammary tissues of the rat, *Biochemistry* **14**, 2944–2952 (1975).
21. J. H. H. Thijssen, Androgens in human postmenopausal breast cancer, *Horm. Res.* **6**, 289–309 (1975).

22. P. C. MacDonald, R. P. Rombaut, and P. K. Siiteri, Plasma precursors of estrogen. I. Extent of conversion of plasma Δ^4-androstenedione to estrone in normal males and nonpregnant, normal, castrate and adrenalectomized females, *J. Clin. Endocrinol. Metab.* **27**, 1103–1111 (1967).

23. J. M. Grodin, P. K. Siiteri, and P. C. MacDonald, Source of estrogen production in postmenopausal women, *J. Clin. Endocrinol. Metab.* **36**, 207–214 (1973).

24. P. K. Siiteri, J. E. Williams, and N. K. Takaki, Steroid abnormalities in endometrial and breast carcinoma: A unifying hypothesis, *J. Steroid Biochem.* **7**, 897–903 (1976).

25. J. B. Adams, and K. Li, Biosynthesis of 17β-oestradiol in human breast carcinoma tissue and a novel method for its characterization, *Br. J. Cancer* **31**, 429–433 (1975).

26. D. Jones, E. H. D. Cameron, K. Griffiths, E. N. Gleare, and A. P. M. Forrest, Steroid metabolism by human breast tumours, *Biochem. J.* **116**, 919–921 (1970).

27. P. C. MacDonald, J. M. Grodin, and P. K. Siiteri, The utilization of plasma androstenedione for estrone production in women, in: *Progress in Endocrinology* (C. Gual, ed.), pp. 770–776, Excerpta Medica International Congress Series, No. 184 (1969).

28. C. Longcope, Metabolic clearance and blood production rates of estrogens in postmenopausal women, *Am. J. Obstet. Gynecol.* **111**, 778–781 (1971).

29. C. E. Bird, W. Finnis, and A. F. Clark, Kinetics of testosterone metabolism in postmenopausal women with and without breast cancer, *Proceedings of the 60th Annual Meeting of The Endocrine Society*, Abstract No. 905 (1978).

30. H. L. Judd, G. E. Judd, W. E. Lucas, and S. S. C. Yen, Endocrine function of the postmenopausal ovary: Concentration of androgens and estrogens in ovarian and peripheral vein blood, *J. Clin. Endocrinol. Metabol.* **39**, 1029–1024 (1974).

31. H. L. Judd, W. E. Lucas, and S. S. C. Yen, Effect of oophorectomy on circulating testosterone and androstenedione levels in patients with endometrial cancer, *Am. J. Obstet. Gynecol.* **118**, 793–798 (1974).

32. R. Horton, and J. F. Tait, Androstenedione production and interconversion rates measured in peripheral blood and studies on the possible site of its conversion to testosterone, *J. Clin. Invest.* **45**, 301–313 (1966).

33. C. W. Bardin, and M. B. Lipsett, Testosterone and androstenedione blood production rates in normal women and women with idiopathic hirsutism or polycystic ovaries, *J. Clin. Invest.* **46**, 891–901 (1967).

34. M. A. Kirschner and C. W. Bardin, Androgen production and metabolism in normal and virilized women, *Metabolism* **21**, 667–688 (1972).

35. E. Nieschlag, D. L. Loriaux, H. J. Ruder, I. R. Zucker, M. A. Kirschner, and M. B. Lipsett, The secretion of dehydroepiandrosterone and dehydroepiandrosterone-sulfate in man, *J. Endocrinol.* **57**, 123–134 (1973).

36. A. Borkowski, M. L. L'Hermite, P. Dor, E. Longeval, M. Rozencweig, C. Muquardt, and E. van Cauter, Steroid sex hormones and prolactin in postmenopausal women with generalized mammary carcinoma during prolonged dexamethasone treatment, *J. Endocrinol.* **73**, 235–246 (1977).

37. N. Deshpande, Regulation of androgen synthesis in the human adrenal gland *in vivo* and *in vitro*, *Horm. Res.* **6**, 289–309 (1975).

38. T. L. Dao, E. Tan, and V. Brooks, A comparative evaluation of adrenalectomy and cortisone in the treatment of advanced mammary carcinoma, *Cancer* **14**, 1259–1265 (1961).

39. A. Segaloff, R. Carabasi, B. N. Horwitt, J. V. Schlosser, and P. J. Murison, Hormonal therapy in cancer of the breast, *Cancer* **7**, 331–334 (1954).

40. C. D. West, M. C. Li, J. P. Maclean, G. C. Escher, and O. H. Pearson, Cortisone-induced remissions in women with metastatic mammary cancer, *Proc. Am. Assoc. Cancer Res.* **1**, 51–52 (1954).

41. O. H. Pearson, M. C. Li, J. P. Maclean, M. B. Lipsett, and C. D. West, The use of hydrocortisone in cancer, *Ann. N. Y. Acad. Sci.* **61**, 393–396 (1955).
42. H. M. Lemon, Cortisone–thyroid therapy of metastatic mammary cancer, *Ann. Int. Med.* **46**, 457–484 (1957).
43. G. S. Gordan, W. P. Graham, III, L. Goldman, R. Papac, G. E. Sheline, J. Vaeth, and J. Witt, Hormonal treatment of disseminated cancer of the female breast, *Calif. Med.* **98**, 189–194 (1963).
44. R. Nissen-Meyer and J. H. Vogt, Cortisone treatment of metastatic breast cancer, *Acta Unio Int. Contra Cancrum* **15**, 1140–1144 (1959).
45. H. A. van Gilse, Long-term treatment with corticosteroids of patients with metastatic breast cancer, *Cancer Chemother. Rep.* **16**, 293–298 (1962).
46. G. W. Bethune, Cortisone in palliative treatment of breast cancer, *Can. J. Surg.* **7**, 289–291 (1964).
47. B. J. Kennedy, The present status of hormone therapy in advanced breast cancer, *Radiology* **69**, 330–340 (1967).
48. S. Kofman, D. Nagamani, R. E. Buenger, and S. G. Taylor, III, The use of prednisolone in the treatment of disseminated breast carcinoma, *Cancer* **11**, 226–232 (1958).
49. H. M. Lemon, Prednisone therapy of advanced mammary cancer, *Cancer* **12**, 93–107 (1959).
50. B. A. Stoll, Dexamethasone in advanced breast cancer, *Cancer* **13**, 1074–1080 (1960).
51. B. Gardner, A. N. Thomas, and G. S. Gordan, Antitumor efficacy of prednisone and sodium liothyronine in advanced breast cancer, *Cancer* **15**, 334–337 (1962).
52. B. A. Stoll, Corticosteroids in therapy of advanced mammary cancer, *Br. Med. J.* **1**, 210–214 (1963).
53. J. H. Farrow, The management of metastatic breast cancer by hormone manipulation, *Bull N. Y. Acad. Med.* **38**, 151–196 (1962).
54. A. P. M. Forrest, H. J. Stewart, E. A. Benson, H. Ker, V. Jones, P. B. Kunkler, and H. Campbell, Controlled studies in advanced breast cancer, in: *Proceedings of First Tenovus Symposium* (A. P. M. Forrest and P. B. Kunkler, eds.), pp. 186–196, E. & S. Livingstone, Edinburgh and London (1968).
55. A. Lipton and R. J. Santen, Medical adrenalectomy using aminoglutethimide and dexamethasone in advanced breast cancer, *Cancer* **33**, 503–512 (1974).
56. P. Sherlock, and W. H. Hartmann, Adrenal steroids and the pattern of metastases of breast cancer, *J. Am. Med. Assoc.* **181**, 313–317 (1962).
57. A. A. Nelson and G. Woodard, Severe adrenal cortical atrophy (cytotoxic) and hepatic damage produced in dogs by feeding 2,2-Bis(Parachlorophenyl)-1,1-dichloroethane (DDD or TDE), *Arch. Pathol.* **48**, 387–394 (1949).
58. J. Nichols and H. L. Sheehan, Effect of partial adrenal cortical atrophy on the course of alloxan diabetes, *Endocrinology* **51**, 362–377 (1952).
59. T. Bledsoe, D. P. Island, R. L. Ney, and G. W. Liddle, An effect of o,p'-DDD on the extra-adrenal metabolism of cortisol in man, *J. Clin. Endocrinol Metab.* **24**, 1303–1311 (1964).
60. S. Weisenfeld, A. Hecht, D. Leighter, and M. Goldner, o,p'DDD in the treatment of advanced mammary carcinoma, *Cancer* **17**, 1258–1266 (1964).
61. D. B. Gower, Modifiers of steroid-hormone metabolism: A review of their chemistry, biochemistry and clinical applications, *J. Steroid Biochem.* **5**, 501–523 (1974).
62. R. Cash, A. J. Brough, M. N. P. Cohen, and P. S. Satoh, Aminoglutethimide (Elipten–Ciba) as an inhibitor of adrenal steroidogenesis: Mechanism of action and therapeutic trial, *J. Clin. Endocrinol. Metab.* **27**, 1239–1248 (1967).
63. C. T. Griffiths, T. C. Hall, Z. Saba, J. J. Barlow, and H. B. Nevinny, Preliminary trial of aminoglutethimide in breast cancer, *Cancer* **32**, 31–37 (1973).

64. R. J. Santen, A. Lipton, and J. Kendall, Successful medical adrenalectomy with aminoglutethimide: Role of altered drug metabolism. *J. Am. Med. Assoc.* **230**, 1661–1665 (1974).

65. R. J. Santen, E. Samojlik, A. Lipton, H. Harvey, E. B. Ruby, S. A. Wells, and J. Kendall, Kinetic, hormonal and clinical studies with aminoglutethimide in breast cancer, *Cancer* **39**, 2948–2958 (1977).

66. E. Samojlik, R. J. Santen, and S. A. Wells, Adrenal suppression with aminoglutethimide. II. Differential effects of aminoglutethimide on plasma androstenedione and estrogen levels, *J. Clin. Endocrinol. Metab.* **45**, 480–487 (1977).

67. R. J. Santen, S. A. Wells, S. Runic, C. Gupta, J. Kendall, E. B. Ruby, and E. Samojlik, Adrenal suppression with aminoglutethimide. I. Differential effects of aminoglutethimide on glucocorticoid metabolism as a rationale for use of hydrocortisone, *J. Clin. Endocrinol. Metab.* **45**, 469–479 (1977).

68. R. J. Santen, S. A. Wells, N. Cohn, L. M. Demers, R. I. Misbin, and E. L. Foltz, Compensatory increase in TSH secretion without effect on prolactin secretion in patients treated with aminoglutethimide. *J. Clin. Endocrinol. Metab.* **45**, 739–746 (1977).

69. S. A. Wells, R. J. Santen, A. Lipton, D. E. Haagensen, E. B. Ruby, H. Harvey, and W. G. Dilley, Medical adrenalectomy with aminoglutethimide: Clinical studies in postmenopausal patients with metastatic breast carcinoma, *Ann. Surg.* **187**, 475–484 (1978).

70. E. Samojlik and R. J. Santen, Adrenal suppression with aminoglutethimide III. Comparison of plasma Δ^4 and Δ^5-steroids in postmenopausal women treated for breast carcinoma, *J. Clin. Endocrinol. Metab.* **47**, 717–724 (1978).

71. R. J. Santen, S. Santner, B. Davis, J. Veldhuis, E. Samojlik, and E. Ruby, Aminoglutethimide inhibits extraglandular estrogen production in postmenopausal women with breast carcinoma, *J. Clin. Endocrinol. Metab.* **47**, 1257–1265 (1978).

72. F. T. Murray, S. Santner, E. A. Samojlik, and R. J. Santen, Serum aminoglutethimide levels: Studies of serum half life, clearance, and patient compliance, *J. Clin. Pharmacol.* (1979) (in press).

73. H. H. Newsome, Jr., Some actions of aminoglutethimide on steroid metabolism, secretion, and pituitary feedback control, in: *Proceedings of the Vth International Congress of Endocrinology*, Hamburg, Germany, p. 1 (1976).

74. E. E. Werk, Jr., J. MacGee, and L. S. Sholiton, Effect of diphenylhydantoin on cortisol metabolism in man, *J. Clin. Invest.* **43**, 1824–1835 (1964).

75. Y. Choi, K. Thrasher, E. E. Werk, Jr., L. J. Sholiton, and C. Olinger, Effect of diphenylhydantoin on cortisol kinetics in humans, *J. Pharmacol. Exp. Ther.* **176**, 27–34 (1971).

76. M. Philbert, M. H. Laudat and L. H. Bricaire, Etude clinique et biologique d'un inhibiteur de l'hormonosynthèse corticosurrénale: l'aminoglutethimide, *Ann. Endocrinol.* **29**, 189–209 (1966).

77. R. S. Rosenfeld, B. J. Rosenberg, D. K. Fukushima, and L. Hellman, 24-Hour secretory pattern of dehydroisoandrosterone and dehydroisoandrosterone sulfate, *J. Clin. Endocrinol. Metab.* **40**, 850–855 (1975).

78. E. A. Thompson, Jr. and P. K. Siiteri, The involvement of human placental microsomal cytochrome P-450 in aromatization, *J. Biol. Chem.* **249**, 5373–5378 (1974).

79. E. A. Thompson, Jr. and P. K. Siiteri, Utilization of oxygen and reduced nicotinamide adenine dinucleotide phosphate by human placental microsomes during aromatization of androstenedione, *J. Biol. Chem.* **249**, 5364–5372 (1974).

80. Y. Katz, The inhibitory effects of aminoglutethimide phosphate (AGP) on estradiol-17β production in the ovaries of prepubertal, PMS-treated rats, *Proceedings of the Tenth Annual Meeting of the Society for the Study of Reproduction*, p. 40 (1977).

81. F. W. Kahnt and R. Neher, Uber die adrenale steroid-biosynthese *in vitro*. III. Selektive hemmung der nebennierenrinden-funktion. *Helv. Chim. Acta* **49**, 725–732 (1966).

82. R. N. Dexter, L. M. Fishman, R. L. Ney, and G. W. Liddle, Inhibition of adrenal corticosteroid synthesis by aminoglutethimide: Studies of the mechanism of action, *J. Clin. Endocrinol Metab.* **27**, 473–480 (1967).

83. M. P. Cohen and P. P. Foa, Aminoglutethimide inhibition of adrenal desmolase activity, *Proc. Soc. Exp. Biol. Med.* **127**, 1086–1090 (1969).

84. L. M. Fishman, G. W. Liddle, D. P. Island, N. Fleischer, and O. Kuchel, Effects of aminoglutethimide on adrenal function in man, *J. Clin. Endocrinol. Metab.* **27**, 481–490 (1967).

85. S. P. Marynick, R. J. Sherins, J. C. Pita, Jr., and M. B. Lipsett, Evidence for direct testosterone suppression of pituitary luteinizing hormone secretion in men, *Proceedings of the 59th Annual Meeting of The Endocrine Society*, Abstract No. 148, p. 130 (1977).

86. I. M. Shamonki, R. M. Barone, P. K. Siiteri, and H. L. Judd, Inhibition of peripheral aromatization in postmenopausal women, *Proceedings of the 60th Annual Meeting of The Endocrine Society*, Abstract No. 587, p. 368 (1978).

87. H. H. Newsome, Jr., P. W. Brown, J. J. Terz, and W. Lawrence, Jr., Medical adrenalectomy and plasma steroids in advanced breast carcinoma, *Surgery* **83**, 83–89 (1978).

88. M. L. Rallison, F. H. Tyler, and L. F. Kumagai, Goitrous hypothyroidism induced by an anticonvulsant drug, *J. Pediatr.* **65**, 1095–95 (1964).

89. J. A. Pittman and R. W. Brown, Antithyroid and antiadrenocortical activity of aminoglutethimide, *J. Clin. Endocrinol. Metab.* **26**, 1014–1016 (1966).

90. M. L. Rallison, L. F. Kumagai, and F. H. Tyler, Goitrous hypothyroidism induced by aminoglutethimide, anticonvulsant drug. *J. Clin. Endocrinol. Metab.* **27**, 265–272 (1967).

91. C. R. W. Edwards, I. A. Forsyth, and G. M. Besser, Amenorrhea, galactorrhea, and primary hypothyroidism with high circulating levels of prolactin, *Br. Med. J.* **3**, 462–464 (1971).

92. K. Miyai, T. Onishi, M. Hosokawa, K. Ishibashi, and Y. Kumahara, Inhibition of thyrotropin and prolactin secretions in primary hypothyroidism by 2-Br-α-ergocryptine, *J. Clin. Endocrinol. Metab.* **39**, 391–394 (1974).

93. K. E. Gale, P. R. Sheehe, L. V. Gould, and R. Rohner, Treatment of advanced breast cancer with aminoglutethimide, *Clin. Res.* **24**, 376A (1976).

94. H. H. Newsome, P. W. Brown, J. J. Terz, and W. Lawrence, Jr., Medical and surgical adrenalectomy in patients with advanced breast carcinoma, *Cancer* **39**, 542–546 (1977).

95. H. A. Harvey, R. J. Santen, J. Osterman, E. Samojlik, D. S. White, and A. Lipton, A comparative trial of transsphenoidal hypophysectomy and estrogen suppression with aminoglutethimide in advanced breast cancer, *Cancer* (1979) (in press).

96. A. Manni, J. Trujillo, J. S. Marshall, and O. H. Pearson, Treatment of breast cancer with antiestrogen: Approach to medical hypophysectomy? *Clin. Res.* **25**, 524A (1977).

97. G. C. L. Lachelin, S. S. C. Yen, and J. F. Alksne, Hormonal changes following hypophysectomy in humans, *J. Obstet. Gynecol.* **50**, 333–338 (1977).

98. J. T. LaRossa and J. C. Melby, Endocrinologic completeness of transsphenoidal hypophysectomy in postmenopausal patients with metastatic breast cancer, *Clin. Res.* **25**, 409A (1977).

4

Actions and Metabolism of Intracellular Mediators in Neoplastic Mammary Cells

JAMES A. RILLEMA

1. Introduction

The division of cells is a complex process which is required for both the development of multicellular organisms and the maintenance of certain of their tissues. At the present time we are just beginning to understand some of the intricate control mechanisms which regulate the rates of cell division and the differentiation of cells. Our understanding of the molecular basis for the regulation of these processes in normal and neoplastic cells may be of fundamental importance to our understanding of why neoplastic cells continue to divide under conditions where normal cells do not divide.

There are several primary processes associated with neoplastic cells. These include (1) the induction or transformation of normal to neoplastic cells, (2) the promotion of neoplastic cell growth, (3) the regression of neoplastic tissues, and (4) the metastasis of neoplastic tissues. Under specific experimental conditions, certain hormones have been shown to either inhibit or promote each of these processes in certain mammary carcinomas. Several authors have recently reviewed specific aspects of the actions of hormones on neoplastic mammary cells.[1-11] In this chap-

JAMES A. RILLEMA • Department of Physiology, Wayne State University School of Medicine, Detroit, Michigan 48201.

ter I shall review the literature concerning the possible relationship of several intracellular regulatory agents to the mammary carcinoma problem; the regulatory agents to be discussed will include the cyclic nucleotides, the prostaglandins, the polyamines, and calcium ions. The actions of hormones on the regulation of the metabolism of these intracellular mediators will be discussed. Finally, an attempt will be made to relate these observations to the primary processes associated with neoplastic mammary cells.

2. Cyclic Nucleotides

The literature contains a plethora of information suggesting that cyclic AMP (cAMP) and cyclic GMP (cGMP) regulate the rates of proliferation and differentiation of a variety of normal and neoplastic cells and tissues. In view of the large number of publications that are available relative to this topic, only those that are relevant to our discussion of the mammary carcinoma problem will be referenced. In the early 1970s the bulk of the experimental studies with cultured cells and tissues suggested that the division of normal and neoplastic cells might be stimulated by cGMP but inhibited by cAMP. This conclusion was based primarily on two types of observations. First, the proliferation of several cell lines is inhibited by the addition of phosphodiesterase inhibitors or cAMP to the medium bathing the cultured cells. And second, cAMP levels are decreased while cGMP levels are increased in these cell lines during periods of rapid growth. [12-18] In contrast to these types of cells, however, there are a few other cell types which behave in a seemingly reciprocal fashion, i.e., cAMP stimulates their rates of proliferation and cAMP levels are elevated in the cells during periods of rapid growth. An example of this latter type of cell is the thymocyte.[19-21] The cyclic nucleotides have also been shown to affect processes associated with the differentiation of certain types of cells. [22-24] It is thus clear that the cyclic nucleotides have a number of actions on processes associated with the proliferation and differentiation of cells. However, no consistent pattern has yet emerged.

2.1. Actions of cAMP on the Proliferation of Neoplastic Mammary Cells

Two laboratories have studied the effect of $N^6,O^{2'}$-dibutyryl cAMP (DBcAMP) injections on the rate of growth of mammary tumors. Different types of tumors had differing responses to the DBcAMP. In 1974 Cho-Chung and Gullino[25-27] reported that a Walker 256 hormone-dependent tumor, most DMBA [7,12-dimethylbenz(α)anthracene]-induced tumors, and a MTW9 tumor regressed when the tumor-bearing rats were injected with DBcAMP. In contrast, DBcAMP had little or no effect on the growth rates of a CSETB fibrosarcoma, a nitrosomethylurea-induced mammary carcinoma, or a non-hormone-dependent Walker 256 tumor. More recently, Klein and Loizzi[28] observed that the growth rate of the R3230AC rat mammary tumor, which is hormonally independent, was stimulated by DBcAMP injections. Thus it is clear that DBcAMP can either stimulate, inhibit, or have no effect on the rates of growth of specific experimental mammary tumors when the drug is administered *in vivo*. Even if a consistent effect had been observed in these types of experiments, however, it would be exceedingly difficult to properly interpret the results. One simply does not know whether the action of DBcAMP is direct, or whether a secondary action of DBcAMP, such as an altered rate of secretion of a certain hormone, is responsible for the observed effects. In this regard, Cho-Chung and Gullino[26] observed no change in the plasma estrogen levels in their tumor-bearing, DBcAMP-treated rats, suggesting that altered estrogen availability is probably not responsible for the altered rates of growth of the tumors. Nevertheless, other secondary actions of DBcAMP may be responsible for the differential actions of DBcAMP on the growth rates of various experimental mammary tumors. In subsequent studies carried out in the laboratory of Cho-Chung[29-36] a number of actions of *in vivo* administered DBcAMP on the biochemical processes of rat mammary tumors were investigated; the details of these studies will be discussed below in Section 2.4. In any case, although the studies in which DBcAMP was administered to tumor-bearing animals have provided some very interesting data, they have provided little definitive insight into the primary processes associated with the mammary carcinoma problem.

The effect of DBcAMP has also been tested on a mammary cell line (BT-20) of human origin.[37] The authors of this work found that DBcAMP, cAMP and theophylline, an inhibitor of cyclic nucleotide phosphodiesterases, inhibit the aggregation of these cells in culture. Since it has been proposed that factors intrinsic to the formation of cellular aggregates may be involved in the spread of cancer cells, the authors propose that cAMP may have a role in the propagation of cancer. However, since the action of DBcAMP on the aggregation of nonneoplastic mammary cells was not reported, it is not known if this action of DBcAMP is specific for neoplastic cells.

Recently, Yang and Nandi[38] have shown that DBcAMP potentiates the stimulatory actions of the glucocorticoids on mammary tumor virus (MTV) production in primary cultures derived from mammary tumors that developed in MTV-infected female BALB/cfCH3 mice. Isoproterenol and epinephrine, agents that stimulate adenylate cyclase activity in most cells and thus enhance the rate of cAMP production, similarly potentiated the action of hydrocortisone on MTV production in the cultured tumor cells. These observations may be of great importance if it becomes apparent that viruses are involved in mammary carcinoma cell induction in humans.

2.2. Cyclic Nucleotide Levels in Mammary Gland Neoplasms

cAMP and cGMP levels have been determined in several experimental rat tumors and in human breast neoplasms. In 1974 Minton et al. reported that cAMP levels were fifteenfold higher in human breast cancer tissues than in adjacent normal breast tissues[39]; cAMP content was expressed on the basis of wet tissue weight. In contrast to these results, Oertel et al.[40] reported that neoplastic human mammary tissues had 70% less cAMP than did adjacent normal mammary tissues; again the cAMP content was expressed on the basis of wet tissue weights. More recently two other laboratories have reported cyclic nucleotide levels in normal and neoplastic human breast tissues. Both Guerinot et al.[41] and Küng et al.[42] observed that cAMP levels were sevenfold higher and cGMP levels were twofold higher in neoplastic tissues than in normal adjacent tissues when calculated on the basis of the wet weight of the tissues. Küng et al.,[42] however, also expressed their results on the basis of the numbers of cells; then the levels of both cAMP and cGMP were significantly lower in the neoplastic tissues. Thus, most of the above studies indicate that cyclic nucleotide levels are elevated in neoplastic mammary cells when levels are expressed on the basis of the wet weight of the tissues, but the reciprocal is the case when the cyclic nucleotide levels are expressed on the basis of the numbers of cells. The proper way to express the results is difficult to assess in view of a number of conditions which differ in normal and neoplastic tissues. Some of these factors include differences in the densities of the cells, differences in the intracellular volumes of the cells, and, finally, differences in the relative abundance of different types of cells.

Cyclic nucleotide levels have also been measured in several types of mammary tumors from experimental animals. Cohen and Chan[43] reported a four- to fivefold higher level of cAMP in DMBA-induced mammary tumors of rats than in mammary glands from nonpregnant rats; the data were expressed on the basis of the wet tissue weight. Cohen and Chan also measured cAMP levels in a neoplastic cell line derived from DMBA-induced rat tumors and in normal mammary epithelial cells growing in monolayer cultures. In this case, they found that cAMP levels were more than 50% lower in the neoplastic cells, but the results of the culture studies were expressed on the basis of the protein content of the tissues. As was clearly pointed out by Cohen and Chan, the types of cells in the DMBA-induced tumors are quite different from those in the mammary glands from nonpregnant rats, and it is difficult to assess the significance of these cAMP measurements. Studies have recently been carried out in my laboratory in which the levels of both cAMP and cGMP were measured in DMBA-induced mammary tumors of rats.[44] The results were then compared with cyclic nucleotide levels present in mammary glands obtained from virgin and midpregnant (12–14 days) rats. A comparison of cyclic nucleotide levels in the tumors with the levels in glands from midpregnant rats would appear to be better than a comparison with the glands from the virgin animals in view of the significantly higher percentage of epithelial cells in the glands of pregnant animals. Our results were expressed on the basis of wet tissue weight, DNA content, RNA content, and protein content. Based on all of these parameters, cAMP levels were significantly higher in the tumor tissues than in the glands from the midpregnant rats. In contrast, cGMP levels were not different in the tumors and glands from midpregnant rats based on the wet weight of the tissues, but based on DNA, RNA, and protein contents, cGMP levels were in all cases significantly lower in the tumor tissues. It is also of interest that the ratio of cAMP to cGMP was about twofold higher in the tumor tissues than in the mammary glands from either the virgin or midpregnant animals. We do not currently know the significance of this latter observation.

Several studies have been carried out in which cyclic nucleotide levels were measured and compared in growing and regressing rat mammary tumors. Matusik and Hilf[45] and Hilf et al.[46] reported cAMP and cGMP levels in DMBA-induced rat tumors that were induced to regress by a number of endocrine manipulations, including ovariectomy, streptozotocin-induced diabetes, and inhibition of prolactin secretion with lergotrile mesylate. Based on wet tissue weights or protein content, they found that cAMP levels were lower in growing tumors than in regressing tumors; in contrast, no differences in cGMP levels were observed. When the cAMP levels were expressed on the basis of the tissue DNA content, however, the cAMP levels were not different in the growing and regressing tumors. These investigators also reported that the ratio of cAMP to cGMP was not different in the growing and regressing tumors. Again, these studies from Hilf's laboratory point out the critical importance of the manner in which cyclic nucleotide levels are calculated.

More recently, Cho-Chung et al.[47,48] confirmed the results from Hilf's laboratory, in that the regression of DMBA-induced mammary tumors in rats in response to ovariectomy was found to occur in concert with an elevated tissue content of cAMP based on the wet weight of the tissues; estrogen administration returned the cAMP levels to those observed in the nonovariectomized animals.

Chatterjee and Kim[49] measured cAMP levels and cAMP phosphodiesterase activities in a series of metastasizing and nonmetastasizing rat mammary tumors. They found that cAMP levels were 1.3–2.0 times higher in the highly metastatic carcinomas, whereas the cAMP phosphodiesterase activity was inversely proportional to the metastatic capacity of the carcinoma tissue. Whether elevated cAMP levels were directly or indirectly responsible for the metastatic processes was not demonstrated.

Tisdale and Philips[50] tested the ability of a number of antitumor agents to alter the level of cAMP in Walker carcinoma cells. They found that only the alkylating drugs elevated cAMP levels in the neoplastic cells. These authors suggest that the alkylating agents may act by inhibiting the activity of a cAMP phosphodiesterase.

A variety of processes associated with mammary carcinogenesis are therefore clearly accompanied by significant changes in cyclic nucleotide levels. In many cases, however, the magnitude and direction of the changes depended on the nature of the tissues being compared and on whether cyclic nucleotide levels were expressed on the basis of wet tissue weight, cell number, or some other macromolecular parameter. The possible implications of the observations cited above to our understanding of the mammary carcinoma problem will be further discussed later in this chapter.

2.3. Enzymes of Cyclic Nucleotide Metabolism

cAMP and cGMP are formed from ATP and GTP, respectively; the formation of cAMP is catalyzed by the enzyme adenylate cyclase and the formation of cGMP gy guanylate cyclase. The catabolism of the cyclic nucleotides occurs by their conversions to their respective 5'-monophosphate derivatives; there are at least four cyclic nucleotide phosphodiesterases which catalyze these reactions. There have been several studies carried out in which the activities of these enzymes have been measured in normal and neoplastic mammary tissues.

Cohen et al.[51] studied cyclic nucleotide phosphodiesterase activities in monolayer cultures of epithelial cells derived from virgin rat mammary glands and in cells from DMBA-induced rat mammary tumors. Total cAMP phosphodiesterase activity was severalfold higher in the normal cells than in the neoplastic cells. In contrast, the activity of a low-K_m cAMP phosphodiesterase was higher in the tumor-derived cells; the authors feel that the low-K_m cAMP phosphodiesterase may be the dominant cAMP catabolic enzyme and that the elevated activity of this enzyme in the neoplastic cells may be responsible for the lower levels of cAMP present in these cells.[43] Since these investigators did not measure adenylate cyclase activity in the cultured cells, however, it is not possible to evaluate the possible contribution of the rate of synthesis of cAMP to the levels of cAMP which were reported earlier.[43] We have compared the activities of both the low-K_m and high-K_m cyclic nucleotide phosphodiesterases in DMBA-induced rat mammary tumors with those in mammary glands from virgin and midpregnant rats.[44] Both the low-K_m and high-K_m cAMP and cGMP phosphodiesterase activities were generally higher in the mammary glands from the midpregnant rats than in the tumor tissues when the results were expressed on the basis of the DNA contents of the tissues; when the enzyme activities were expressed on the basis of wet tissue weight, however, the activity of the low-K_m cyclic nucleotide phosphodiesterase of the neoplastic tissues was elevated, whereas no difference was detected in the high-K_m phosphodiesterase activity. Küng et al.[42] and Singer et al.[52] have measured cyclic nucleotide phosphodiesterase activities in normal and neoplastic human mammary tissues. In both studies, the activities of the low-K_m cAMP[42,52] and cGMP[52] phosphodiesterases were significantly higher in the neoplastic tissues when the results were expressed on the basis of wet tissue weight or protein content. Küng et al.,[42] however, found no detectable differences when the results were expressed on the basis of the number of cells. Singer et al.[52] observed that the neoplastic human mammary tissue had a 60–70% higher content of a protein activator of cGMP phosphodiesterase. As mentioned above, Chatterjee and Kim[49] found higher levels of cAMP phosphodiesterase activities in several highly metastatic rat mammary tumors than in low metastatic tumors.

Guanylate and adenylate cyclase activities have been compared in several normal and neoplastic mammary cells and tissues. Sheth et al.[53] reported that based on the tissue protein contents, adenylate cyclase activity is three- to fourfold higher in mouse mammary tumors than in normal mouse mammary tissues. Schorr and Russell[54] similarly found measurable levels of adenylate cyclase activities in murine mammary carcinomas, but undetectable levels in mammary glands from lactating mice. Several years ago Brown et al.[55] reported that adenylate cyclase activities are severalfold higher in chemically induced rat mammary carcinomas than in normal rat mammary gland tissue; their data were expressed on the basis of the wet weights of the tissues. We[44] found that the adenylate cyclase activity of DMBA-induced rat mammary tumors was significantly higher than that of mammary glands from either virgin or midpregnant rats when the data were expressed on the basis of wet

tissue weight, DNA content, protein content, or RNA content. Guanylate cyclase activities, in contrast, were the same in the DMBA-induced
tumors and normal mammary tissues unless the data were expressed on
the basis of the DNA content, in which case guanylate cyclase activity
was significantly less in the neoplastic tissues. Recently, Cho-Chung *et
al.*[48] have reported that both adenylate cyclase and cAMP phosphodiesterase activities were elevated in DMBA-induced rat mammary tumors
that were regressing in response to ovariectomy; their results, however,
were expressed only on the basis of the wet weight of the tissues. Cho-
Chung and Newcomer[33] have also measured adenylate cyclase and
cAMP phosphodiesterase activities in two Walker 256 mammary carcinomas, one of which is hormone responsive; basal enzyme activities
were the same in the two types of cells, but the fluoride-stimulated
adenylate cyclase activity was twice as high in the hormone-responsive
cells. Küng *et al.*[42] have measured adenylate cyclase activities in human
neoplastic breast tissues. They observed elevated activities of adenylate
cyclase in the carcinoma tissues when the results were expressed on the
basis of wet tissue weight or tissue protein content; however, enzyme
activities were significantly lower in the neoplastic tissues when expressed on the basis of cell number.

The interpretation of the results of studies in which the activities of
enzymes associated with cyclic nucleotide metabolism are compared in
normal and neoplastic mammary tissues is complicated by the same
factors that were described above for studies in which cyclic nucleotide
levels were compared in these tissues. In addition, the enzyme studies
are further complicated by the fact that the enzyme activities were all
determined in broken cell preparations, and whether the measured activities reflect the relative activities of these enzymes in the whole cells is
not known.

2.4. Cyclic-Nucleotide-Binding Proteins and
Cyclic-Nucleotide-Dependent Protein Kinases

In general, the cyclic nucleotides are believed to exert their actions
on the metabolism of cells by stimulating the activity of cyclic-
nucleotide-dependent protein kinases. Accordingly, several laboratories
have measured cAMP-binding and/or protein kinase activities in normal
and neoplastic mammary cells. Eppenberger *et al.*[56] reported that
cAMP-binding activity and the activity of cAMP-dependent protein
kinases are higher in human primary mammary carcinomas when expressed on the basis of wet tissue weight or tissue protein content, but
lower when expressed on the basis of cell number. Based on the DNA
content of tissues, Majumder[57] observed significantly lower activities of

cAMP-dependent and -independent protein kinases in C3H mouse mammary carcinoma cells than in normal mouse mammary tissues; Majumder also found smaller amounts of a specific cAMP-binding protein in the neoplastic cells. Anderson and Mendelson[58] observed different binding patterns of cAMP and cGMP to nuclear extracts from mammary glands of normal rats and a transplantable R-35 mammary tumor. These investigators observed a similar distribution of three DNA-dependent RNA polymerases (I, II, and III) in the normal and neoplastic tissues, but polymerase II was inhibited by cAMP more in the nuclear extracts from the normal tissues than in those from the tumors. The authors concluded that the altered cyclic nucleotide binding pattern may be a fundamental defect associated with mammary carcinogenesis.

Recently, Cho-Chung and his colleagues have published a number of studies in which cAMP-binding and protein kinase activities were measured in several rat mammary tumor models.[30,34-36,47,48] In two Walker 256 mammary carcinomas,[30,34-36] one of which regresses in response to DBcAMP, they showed several differences in cAMP binding and the activities of cAMP-dependent protein kinases. The authors concluded that the failure of one type of Walker 256 carcinoma to regress in response to DBcAMP may be related to the inability of DBcAMP to stimulate the production of a nuclear cAMP binding protein in that type of Walker 256 tumor. In further studies Cho-Chung et al.[47,48] reported that cAMP binding was increased twofold in the cytoplasm and fivefold in the nucleus of DMBA-induced rat tumors that were regressing in response to ovariectomy; estrogen administration to the ovariectomized animals reversed these effects. Most of the data from Cho-Chung's laboratory, however, were expressed on the basis of tissue protein content or wet weight of the tissues; perhaps if they had expressed their data on the basis of the number of cells and/or the tissue DNA content, their conclusions might have been different. The experiments by Cho-Chung et al. may provide some insight into the primary processes whereby estrogen promotes the growth of certain tumors, but they do not help us understand the primary biochemical differences between normal and neoplastic cells.

2.5. Hormones and Cyclic Nucleotides in Mammary Neoplasms

Few studies have been carried out with regard to the hormonal regulation of cyclic nucleotide metabolism in neoplastic mammary cells. As discussed above, Matusik and Hilf[45] found that cAMP levels were reduced (based on wet tissue weight or protein content) in DMBA-induced rat tumors in response to ovariectomy, chemically induced diabetes, and inhibition of prolactin secretion. These results suggest that estrogen, insulin, and prolactin may be needed to suppress cAMP levels in growing DMBA-induced tumors. Cho-Chung et al.[47,48] confirmed the observation that ovariectomy of rats bearing DMBA-induced tumors results in elevated cAMP levels based on the wet weights of the tissues; they further observed that ovariectomy increased the activities of adenylate cyclase and cAMP phosphodiesterase in the tumors. Estrogen administration to the ovariectomized animals returned cAMP levels to those observed in the tumors of nonovariectomized animals. Cho-Chung et al. further observed that ovariectomy of rats bearing DMBA-induced tumors resulted in an increased level of cAMP binding; this effect again was reversed by the administration of estrogen. In contrast to the behavior of adenylate cyclase in DMBA-induced mammary tumors of rats, Sheth et al. [53] reported that the activity of this enzyme was elevated about threefold in mammary tumors of mice that were injected with estrogen. Whether any or all of these observations are related to the primary processes associated with mammary carcinogenesis is not known.

Stimulatory effects of the prostaglandins on adenylate cyclase activity has been observed in Walker 256 mammary carcinoma cells[33,36] and in a murine mammary carcinoma.[54] These observations will be discussed later with regard to the possible relationship of the prostaglandins to mammary carcinogenesis.

2.6. Cyclic Nucleotides and the Cell Cycle

The cyclic nucleotides have been implicated as regulators of various stages of the cell cycles of a number of synchronized cell populations.[59-62] Accordingly, peaks and nadirs of cAMP and cGMP levels have been observed, while elevated levels of cAMP have been shown to arrest the proliferation of specific types of cells at specific stages of their cycles. Howard et al.[63] have recently compared cyclic nucleotide levels in high- and low-tumorigenic mouse mammary epithelial cells in monolayer cultures. In cells whose growth had been arrested by culturing with 1% serum, cGMP levels were about threefold higher in the tumorigenic cells, whereas cAMP levels were about threefold higher in the nontumorigenic cells. When the growth-arrested cells were stimulated to proliferate by a 5% serum medium, both cell lines responded within five to ten minutes with a four- to fivefold increase in cGMP levels and a 50% decrease in cAMP levels. The significance that these observations have to the differential regulation of proliferative processes in normal and neoplastic mammary cells is not presently known. The studies by Howard et al., however, do show that peaks and nadirs of cAMP and cGMP levels probably do occur during the cell cycles of mammary cells as they do in other types of cells.[59-62] The determination of the role of the cyclic nucleotides in the cell cycles of normal and neoplastic mammary cells may be of fundamental importance to our understanding of the mammary carcinoma problem.

2.7. Assessment of the Current Status of the Cyclic Nucleotides and Mammary Neoplasms

The studies described above clearly show that there are a number of significant differences between processes associated with cyclic nucleotide metabolism in normal and neoplastic mammary cells. Certain of these studies suggest that cAMP may be involved in the promotional aspects of certain types of neoplastic mammary cells; other studies suggest that cAMP may be involved in the metastases of other types of mammary cells. However, in most cases, the data are difficult to interpret. One critical concern is the nature of the control tissues to which the neoplastic tissues are compared. Normal and neoplastic mammary tissues are heterogeneous with regard to their cellular composition and may differ in cell density and cellular content of macromolecules (protein and DNA). Thus, the magnitude and direction of changes in various aspects of cyclic nucleotide metabolism often depend on whether comparisons are made on the basis of wet tissue weights or on the basis of the tissue protein or DNA content. It is not possible at present to state which is the proper method of expressing data.

Studies have recently shown that the cyclic nucleotides are involved in the cell cycles of a number of types of cells. The studies by Howard *et al.*[63] are compatible with the idea that the cyclic nucleotides may also be involved in the regulation of the cell cycles of normal and neoplastic mammary cells. If this is the case, then cyclic nucleotide levels and other processes associated with cyclic nucleotide metabolism in a population of cells, such as in tumor or normal mammary tissues, would depend on the number and types of cells in the various phases of the cell cycle; the duration of time that individual cells spend in each phase of the cell cycle would also be of critical importance. In retrospect, then, the studies in which events associated with cyclic nucleotide metabolism were compared in normal and neoplastic tissues would appear to provide very little insight into our understanding of the primary processes associated with mammary tumorigenesis. In order to determine whether an altered event(s) associated with cyclic nucleotide metabolism is of critical importance with regard to the primary processes associated with mammary carcinogenesis, it would first appear to be essential to understand how the cyclic nucleotides and related processes are involved in the regulation of the cell cycles of normal and neoplastic mammary cells. It may

then be possible to assess whether important differences in cyclic nucleotide metabolism do in fact exist between the normal and neoplastic
mammary cells. Finally, it may then be possible to determine the precise
locus at which hormones[64] affect the promotion, induction, and/or regression of specific neoplasms.

3. Prostaglandins

In recent studies it has been suggested that the prostaglandins may
have a role in the regulation of cellular proliferation and differentiation.[65-69] Furthermore, most if not all of the actions of the prostaglandins
in cells appear to be mediated through some aspect of cyclic nucleotide
metabolism. Thus, many of the observations discussed above concerning altered cyclic nucleotide metabolism in neoplastic cells may be associated with possible alterations in the metabolism of the prostaglandins.

3.1. Prostaglandin Levels and Rates of Production of Prostaglandins

Elevated levels of prostaglandins have been found in a number of
neoplastic tissues, including DMBA-induced mammary tumors of rats[70]
and human breast tumors.[71-73] Tan et al.[70] reported that the levels of
radioimmunoassayable prostaglandin E_2 were about threefold higher in
DMBA-induced mammary tumors of rats than in normal rat mammary
tissues; their results were expressed on the basis of dry tissue weights.
Had they expressed their data on the basis of cell numbers or tissue
DNA contents, their conclusions might have been different. Tan et al.
also measured the rates of prostaglandin production when a variety of
precursors were added to the media bathing explants from DMBA-
induced tumors of rats and mammary glands from normal rats. They
found that the neoplastic cells produced three- to fourfold more prostaglandins than did the cells of the normal tissues. More recently, Carpenter et al.[74] reported observations similar to those from Tan's laboratory; they found that explants from DMBA-induced rat tumors produced five- to twentyfold more prostaglandins from arachidonic acid
than did explants from virgin rats.

Several studies concerning the prostaglandins have been carried
out. Bennett et al.[71-73] reported severalfold higher levels of prostaglandin E_2 in malignant human breast carcinomas than in either benign
breast tumors or normal breast tissue. They also reported a significantly
higher rate of synthesis of the prostaglandins in the malignant tissues.
All the data of Bennett et al., however, were expressed on the basis of
the wet weight. Nevertheless, Bennett et al. further observed a positive

correlation between the rate of bone destruction in tumor-bearing women and the rate of prostaglandin production. Since certain of the prostaglandins are known to stimulate the catabolism of bone, Bennett *et al.* have suggested that in certain mammary-tumor-bearing patients, an elevated rate of production of the prostaglandins from metastatic mammary cells may be responsible for the coexisting osteolysis. In this regard, Powles *et al.*[75] have reported that the osteolytic effect of Walker carcinoma cells in rats can be abolished by administration of inhibitors of prostaglandin biosynthesis such as aspirin and indomethacin. Powles *et al.*[76] have further observed that 15-keto-13,14-dihydroprostaglandin E_2 levels are elevated in the sera of patients with metastatic breast carcinomas. Finally, Dowsett *et al.*[77] have reported that the osteolysis of bone *in vitro* by breast carcinomas can be inhibited by aspirin. They concluded, however, that the osteolytic principle from breast carcinomas is probably something other than the prostaglandins, since the media from cultured breast carcinomas had no action on cultured bone tissues when aspirin was added to the incubation media. Most studies, therefore, suggest that neoplastic mammary tissues, both animal and human, have either a higher rate of production of the prostaglandins or a higher output of a substance that enhances the rate of production of the prostaglandins.

Kibbey *et al.*[78] have recently studied the rates of production of prostaglandin E_2 from a highly metastatic rat mammary tumor and from three nonmetastatic tumors. Prostaglandin E_2 production was more than an order of magnitude higher in the nonmetastatic tumors. These results are therefore in apparent opposition to those of Bennett *et al.*,[71–73] in which malignant human breast tumors were found to produce prostaglandins at a higher rate than benign tumors.

Jacobson[79] has studied the effects of the *in vivo* administration of prostaglandin $F_{2\alpha}$ to rats bearing the DMBA-induced tumors. He observed a significant regression of the tumors with prostaglandin administration; tumor growth was resumed following withdrawal of the prostaglandin injection regimen. Although it could be argued that the prostaglandin $F_{2\alpha}$ could be affecting the rates of growth of the tumors by an indirect mechanism, experiments by Thomas *et al.*[80] suggest that this may not be the case. They reported that the growth rate of a human adenocarcinoma cell line (HT-29) was inhibited by the addition of prostaglandin E_1 to the incubation medium, while the addition of indomethacin, an inhibitor of prostaglandin biosynthesis, stimulated the rate of proliferation of these cells. Similar observations have been reported for cell lines of nonmammary origin.[65,81] In contrast to the studies discussed above, the prostaglandins have been reported to stimulate the rates of DNA synthesis in several other types of cells of nonmammary origins.[82-84] It is therefore not possible at present to make a conclusive statement concerning a general relationship of the prostaglandins to the rates of proliferation of neoplastic and normal cells.

3.2. Regulation of Prostaglandin Biosynthesis

The prostaglandins are synthesized from long-chained polyunsaturated free fatty acids that are derived from essential free fatty acids. The rate-limiting process for the regulation of the intracellular levels of prostaglandins could involve (1) the activities of the enzymes that catalyze the rate of degradation of the prostaglandins, (2) the activities of the enzymes (prostaglandin synthetase complex) that catalyze the synthesis of the prostaglandins, and/or (3) the availability of the precursor free fatty acids. The latter is believed to be rate limiting under most circumstances. It is therefore of great interest that a number of studies have shown that the incidence of mammary carcinogenesis is markedly increased when a high-polyunsaturated diet is ingested. It is of further interest that the distribution of fatty acids is markedly different in various lipid fractions of normal and neoplastic mammary cells.

3.2.1. Dietary Studies

High-fat diets, and especially those high in polyunsaturated lipids, have been correlated with higher incidences of mammary tumors in both animals and humans.[85-91] Several years ago, Carroll and Khor[91] tested the effects on mammary tumor incidence of a variety of lipids added to the diets of DMBA-fed rats; they observed a positive correlation between tumor incidence and the degree of polyunsaturation of the lipids in the diets. More recently, Hopkins et al.[92] have confirmed these results. In addition, Hopkins et al.[93] tested the effect of feeding a high-polyunsaturated diet before or after the administration of DMBA to rats. They observed that only when the high-polyunsaturated diet was fed after DMBA administration was the incidence of mammary tumors increased. These authors concluded that the high-polyunsaturated diet was probably involved in the promotional aspects of mammary tumorigenesis rather than in the induction process. Dayton et al.[94] have compared the effects of diets containing high-oleate and high-linoleate safflower oils on the incidence of mammary tumors in DMBA-fed rats; no differences in tumor incidence were detected in the groups of animals fed these diets or in animals fed a diet containing coconut oil. However, coconut oil contains 2% linoleate and the high-oleate safflower oil contained 13% linoleate; thus, it is possible that this quantity of linoleate may have been adequate to stimulate mammary tumorigenesis. This idea is supported by the data of Abraham and Rao.[95,96] They found that a diet containing as little as 1% corn oil was adequate to enhance the rate of mammary tumor growth in C3H mice. They further observed that the administration to their experimental mice of a substance (5,8,11,14-eicosatetranoic acid) that inhibits arachidonic acid conversion to the prostaglandins inhibits the promotion of tumor growth in the C3H mice. The probable involvement of the prostaglandins in some aspect of the promotion of the tumor growth in the C3H mice is thus apparent. Most of the dietary studies, therefore, appear to support the idea that high-polyunsaturated-fat diets tend to promote the growth of mammary tumors. In addition, the effects of the polyunsaturated fatty acids may be carried out via an enhanced rate of prostaglandin biosynthesis. In this regard, it is of relevance that inhibitors of prostaglandin synthesis have been shown to inhibit the growth rate of mammary tumors[95] and certain other tumors.[97] Also, Tisdale has shown that a variety of antitumor agents inhibit prostaglandin biosynthesis.[98]

Although a high-polyunsaturated-fat diet has been shown to promote mammary tumorigenesis and inhibitors of prostaglandin synthesis have been shown to inhibit mammary tumor growth, it is not known if these agents act directly on the neoplastic cells. Relative to this problem, Chan et al.[88,99] have observed that plasma levels of estrogen and prolactin are elevated in rats fed high-fat diets. Moreover, Hill et al.[89] and Chan and Cohen[100] found that the high incidence of tumors in DMBA-fed rats that were on a high-fat diet was significantly reduced[89] or completely suppressed[100] by administration of bromoergocryptine, an inhibitor of prolactin secretion. In addition, the administration of an antiestrogen partially reduced the extent and progression of tumor development in DMBA-injected rats. The modulation of the hormonal milieu in the plasma of the DMBA-treated rats may thus explain, at least in part, how the incidence of mammary carcinomas is enhanced in response to the high-polyunsaturated-fat diets. Many additional laboratory studies, however, need to be carried out in order to clarify the precise mechanism whereby dietary lipids affect mammary carcinogenesis.

3.2.2. Fatty Acid Distribution in Mammary Tumors

Many investigators feel that the rate-limiting step for the synthesis of the prostaglandins may be the rate of release of unsaturated free fatty acids from the phospholipids present in cellular membranes.[101] Accordingly, the rate of availability of the prostaglandin precursors could depend on both the fatty acid composition of the cell lipids and the activities of phospholipases. Recently, we have found that phospholipase A_2

activity in DMBA-induced rat mammary tumors is more than an order of magnitude higher than that in mammary glands from either virgin or midpregnant rats (unpublished observations).

There are several studies in which the lipid constituents of normal and neoplastic mammary tissues have been compared.[95,102-107] Although a number of significant differences have been measured, we will consider only those differences which may be related to the regulation of prostaglandin metabolism. Tan et al.[105] found a significantly higher content of polyunsaturated free fatty acids, including arachidonic acid, in the phospholipids from DMBA-induced mammary tumors of rats than in normal rat mammary tissues. In contrast, Leung and Sun[104] reported little or no difference in the arachidonic acid content of the phospholipids from DMBA-induced rat mammary tumors and normal tissues; their normal tissues, however, were tissues adjacent to the tumors in the DMBA-injected rats. In similar studies, we measured the arachidonic acid levels in the phospholipids from DMBA-induced rat tumors; we then compared these results with the arachidonic acid distribution in mammary glands from virgin and midpregnant rats.[107] The phospholipids from the DMBA-induced tumors and mammary glands of midpregnant rats contained a severalfold higher percentage of arachidonic acid than the phospholipids from the mammary glands of virgin rats. Like Leung and Sun,[104] however, we found no difference in the arachidonic acid content of the phospholipids from the DMBA-induced tumors and normal mammary tissue from the tumor-bearing animals (unpublished observations). It is thus possible that the high proportion of arachidonic acid in the phospholipids of DMBA-induced tumors and/or the elevated phospholipase A_2 activity may contribute to the elevated content and rate of production of prostaglandins in the DMBA-induced tumors as demonstrated by Tan et al.[70] It is of further interest that Abraham and Rao[95] found no arachidonic acid in the fatty acids from preneoplastic or normal mammary tissues from either virgin or lactating C3H mice, but about 10% of the fatty acids in neoplastic tissue from these mice were arachidonic acid.

3.3. Prostaglandins and the Cyclic Nucleotides

In a variety of biological systems there is an interrelationship between the prostaglandins and cyclic nucleotides.[65-67] Many of the actions of the E prostaglandins are known to occur via stimulation of adenylate cyclase and a consequent increase in the rate of synthesis of cAMP. Several years ago Bär[108] reported that prostaglandin E_1 stimulates adenylate cyclase activity in mammary tissues from mice and rabbits. More recently, Burstein et al.[109] have shown that the prostaglandins of the E series stimulate the accumulation of cAMP in monolayer cultures of epithelial cells from midpregnant mice. Prostaglandin E_1 has also been shown to stimulate adenylate cyclase activity in Walker 256 mammary carcinoma cells[33,36] and in a murine mammary carcinoma.[54] In primary epithelial cell cultures of tumors from C3H mice, Burstein *et al.*[110] have shown that arachidonic acid enhances the rates of synthesis of both cAMP and the prostaglandins of the E and F series. Although these studies clearly demonstrate that the prostaglandins and archidonic acid can elevate the rate of production of cAMP in a variety of mammary tissues, the relevance that these observations have to the regulation of the metabolism of normal and neoplastic mammary cells has not been established. Moreover, it has been shown in certain cells of nonmammary origin that the cyclic nucleotides can regulate the rate of prostaglandin biosynthesis[80]; such a relationship has not been reported for mammary cells.

3.4. Hormones and the Prostaglandins

Only a limited number of studies have been carried out with regard to the hormonal regulation of prostaglandin metabolism in normal and neoplastic mammary cells. In our studies concerning the regulation of metabolism in normal mammary cells, we have observed several actions of the prostaglandins.[111–113] We have also shown that prolactin stimulates the activity of phospholipase A_2 in microsomal preparations from mouse mammary glands[114] and that phospholipase A_2 has actions similar to those of prolactin.[115] In more recent studies, we have found that the rate of prostaglandin E production from mouse mammary gland explants is enhanced more than twofold by the addition of prolactin to the medium bathing the explants (unpublished observations). In this regard, it is also of interest that Horrobin *et al.*[116] found that prolactin causes about a 50-fold increase in the rate of prostaglandin output from the perfused rat mesenteric bed. It remains to be established whether other hormones have actions on prostaglandin metabolism in normal and neoplastic mammary cells. It also remains to be established whether the hormonal actions on the primary processes associated with mammary carcinogenesis are carried out via the regulation of prostaglandin metabolism.

3.5. Prostaglandins and the Cell Cycle

Since certain of the prostaglandins are known to affect cyclic nucleotide levels in normal and neoplastic cells, and since the cyclic nucleotides may participate in the regulation of the cell cycle, it is possible that the prostaglandins may contribute to the regulation of the latter. Although Bayer and Beaven[117] reported that indomethacin inhibits the growth of both transformed and nontransformed fibroblasts in the G_1 phase of the cell cycle, we do not know if the prostaglandins may participate in the regulation of the cell cycles of normal and neoplastic mammary cells; nor do we know if alterations in specific aspects of prostaglandin metabolism are responsible for primary processes associated with mammary tumorigenesis.

3.6. Assessment of the Current Status of the Prostaglandins and Mammary Neoplasms

Although the levels of prostaglandins and their rates of production appear to be elevated in a number of mammary tumor cells, we have little knowledge at present of how these substances are functioning in either normal or neoplastic mammary cells. It is indeed possible that the prostaglandins may be of critical importance for the regulation of the cell cycles of mammary cells. It is accordingly possible that a defect associated with the regulation of prostaglandin metabolism may be responsible for one or more of the primary processes associated with mammary tumorigenesis. Finally, it is possible that the actions of hormones on normal and neoplastic mammary cells may be related to their actions on prostaglandin metabolism.

4. Polyamines

Putrescine and the polyamines spermidine and spermine are thought to be of importance for both normal proliferative processes and the growth of many neoplastic cells.[118-123] Elevated levels of these substances have been measured in a number of neoplastic and growing tissues. In addition, elevated levels of these substances have been found in the sera and urine of tumor-bearing patients. Although precise functions for the polyamines have not been established in all cells, they have been shown to affect the rate of synthesis of several macromolecules in various types of cells.

4.1. Polyamine Levels in Mammary Tumors and in the Sera and Urine of Tumor-Bearing Females

Several years ago Russell and colleagues[124,125] reported that cancer patients, including mammary cancer patients, excreted many more polyamines into the urine than did normal individuals. The removal of the neoplastic tissues tended to reduce the rate of excretion of the polyamines. Subsequently, it was reported in several additional studies that a large percentage of breast cancer patients excrete elevated levels of the polyamines.[126-130] Serum levels of the polyamines, however, were found to be elevated only in a small percentage of human breast cancer cases.[131]

Polyamine metabolism also has been studied in several types of mammary tumor models in experimental animals. In 1974 Russell *et al.*[132] studied polyamine levels in rats bearing MTW9 tumors. They found that regression of the tumors in response to the withdrawal of lactogenic hormone from the tumor-bearing animals resulted in a rise in the concentrations of spermidine in the sera, but a reduced content of spermidine in the tumors. Andersson *et al.*[133] studied polyamine metabolism in DMBA-induced mammary tumors of rats. They reported that spermidine and spermine levels were about threefold higher in the tumor tissues than in mammary glands from nonpregnant rats; their results were expressed on the basis of the wet weight of the tissues. Andersson *et al.* further reported that the excretion rates of spermidine and putrescine are generally elevated in the tumor-bearing animals. Most of the studies cited above, therefore, clearly show that mammary tumors of both human and animal origin have elevated levels of certain of the polyamines. The importance of these observations, however, is not immediately apparent since the functions of the polyamines in neoplastic mammary cells have not yet been established.

4.2. The Enzymes of Polyamine Metabolism

Enzymes involved in the synthesis of the polyamines include arginase, ornithine decarboxylase (ODC), *S*-adenosyl-methionine decarboxylase (SAMD), spermidine synthase, and spermine synthase. Of these enzymes, only arginase and ODC have been studied in neoplastic mammary cells. Rao *et al.*[134] have recently shown that hydrocortisone *in vitro* induces a threefold increase in arginase activity in mammary tumors of ICRC mice. Andersson *et al.*[133] observed an eightfold higher activity of ODC in DMBA-induced mammary tumors of rats than in mammary glands of nonpregnant rats. Since ODC under most circumstances is believed to be the rate-limiting enzyme for the synthesis of the polyamines, the enhanced activity of ODC as shown by Andersson *et al.* may explain why polyamine levels are generally elevated in neoplastic mammary cells. Further information concerning the enzymes of polyamine metabolism in neoplastic mammary cells is not presently available.

4.3. Hormones and Polyamine Metabolism

In normal mammary gland tissues, it has been shown that insulin, hydrocortisone, and prolactin have actions on the rates of polyamine formation and the activities of the enzymes that catalyze the synthesis of the polyamines.[135-144] In addition, the binding of prolactin to its receptor sites in mouse mammary cells is enhanced by putrescine and the polyamines.[145] The only study presently available concerning hormones and their actions on polyamine metabolism in neoplastic mammary cells is that by Rao et al.,[134] in which they showed that hydorcortisone elevates arginase activity in cultured mammary tumor tissues from ICR mice. Clearly, much further work needs to be carried out to clarify the actions of hormones on polyamine metabolism in neoplastic mammary tissues.

4.4. Polyamines and the Cell Cycle

Evidence suggests that the polyamines, like the cyclic nucleotides and perhaps also the prostaglandins, may be involved in the regulation of the cell cycles of certain cells.[146-149] For example, Gerner and Russell[150] and Fuller et al.[151] have shown that in Chinese hamster ovarian cells, spermidine and spermine accumulate during the S phase of the cell cycle; this corresponds to the time at which DNA synthesis is occurring. Fuller et al. have further reported that SAMD activity is increased during the G_1 to S phase transition. Polyamine accumulation has also been associated with an enhanced ODC activity in synchronized cells.[152,153] Of further interest is the observation that MGAG [methylglyoxal bis(guanylhydrazone)], an inhibitor of SAMD and hence polyamine synthesis, inhibits the proliferation of several types of cells; cells inhibited with MGAG accumulate in the G_1 phase of the cell cycle.[154-160] The inhibition of MGAG is reversible by the addition of spermidine to the media bathing the cultured cells; thus, the specific locus of action of MGAG which is responsible for its inhibition of cellular proliferation would appear to be its inhibition of polyamine synthesis. Studies have not yet been published concerning the possible participation of the polyamines in the regulation of the cell cycles in normal and/or neoplastic mammary cells.

4.5. Assessment of the Current Status of the Polyamines and Mammary Neoplasms

Although levels of the polyamines are clearly elevated in certain neoplastic cells, we know very little at present of how the polyamines may participate in the proliferative processes of normal and neoplastic mammary cells. If the polyamines are involved in the S phase of the cell cycles of mammary cells, as appears to be the case in other types of cells, then it is indeed possible that hormonal actions on polyamine metabolism, as have been clearly demonstrated in normal cells, may be causally related to their actions on cellular proliferation. For example, the effect of antiestrogens on the inhibition of growth of some mammary tumors may be related to their inhibition of the estrogen stimulation of ODC activity.[152]

Further studies have suggested that the polyamines may have actions on cyclic nucleotide metabolism and, reciprocally, the cyclic nucleotides may have effects on polyamine metabolism.[161–164] Such possible relationships have not yet been studied in mammary tissues, nor has the possible significance of these interrelationships been established for any types of cells. It is also possible that prostaglandin metabolism may be regulated by the polyamines or that the prostaglandins may have effects on polyamine metabolism.

5. Calcium Ions

Berridge[165] has advocated the idea that the division of cells may be regulated by the intracellular concentration of calcium ions. He and other authors[166,167] have recently reviewed the literature with regard to the complex interrelationship of calcium ions and cyclic nucleotide metabolism. In addition, certain steps in the biosynthesis of the prostaglandins also require calcium ions; these include the activation of phospholipase A_2 by calcium ions and the stimulation of thromboxane synthesis by calcium.[168] It is thus possible that a modulation of the intracellular calcium ion concentration may have effects of specific biochemical events whereby the processes of cell division are regulated. It is further possible that an aberrant regulation of calcium ion levels in cells may be of primary importance with regard to the uncontrolled growth rates of neoplastic cells. At the present time our knowledge concerning the actions of calcium ions in the regulation of the division of normal and neoplastic mammary cells is nil, and future work in this area may be of great importance.

6. Summary

Alterations in the metabolism of the cyclic nucleotides, prostaglandins, and polyamines have been demonstrated in mammary cancer cells from both humans and experimental animals. Since each of these agents as well as calcium ions may be of critical importance to the regulation of the cell cycles of both normal and neoplastic mammary cells, it is indeed possible that an altered metabolism of one or more of these intracellular mediators may be of fundamental importance to the primary processes associated with mammary carcinogenesis. At the present time, however, our knowledge concerning the precise mechanisms whereby these intracellular mediators may regulate the cell cycles of normal and/or neoplastic mammary cells is quite limited. Future research activities focusing on this issue would appear to be of great importance in furthering our understanding of the mammary carcinoma problem.

The actions of hormones on the primary processes associated with mammary tumorigenesis may also be carried out via an alteration of the metabolism of one or more of the intracellular mediators. In this regard, considerable progress has already been made relative to the mechanism by which estrogen may act as a promoter for neoplastic mammary cells; i.e., estrogen may act by altering the tissue levels of a cAMP-binding protein. Clearly, further studies concerning the actions of hormones on the metabolism of intracellular mediators may enhance our understanding of how mammary tumor cells are regulated.

ACKNOWLEDGMENT: Observations from the author's laboratory were supported by U.S.P.H.S. Grant No. CA 18296.

7. References

1. W. L. McGuire, Physiological principles underlying endocrine therapy of breast cancer, in: *Breast Cancer: Advances in Research and Treatment* (W. L. McGuire, ed.), Vol. 1, pp. 217–262, Plenum Press, New York (1977).
2. W. L. McGuire, Prolactin and breast cancer, *Prolactin and Human Reproduction* (P. G. Crosignani and C. Robyn, eds.), pp. 143–151, Academic Press, New York (1977).
3. A. Segaloff, Hormones and mammary carcinogenesis, in: *Breast Cancer: Advances in Research and Treatment* (W. L. McGuire, ed.), Vol. 2, Plenum Press, New York (1978).
4. C. W. Welsch and J. Meites, in: *Endocrine Control in Neoplasia* (R. K. Sharma and W. E. Criss, eds.), Vol. 9, pp. 71–92, Raven Press, New York (1978).
5. V. P. Hollander and E. J. Diamond, Hormonal control in animal breast cancer, in: *Endocrine Control in Neoplasia* (R. K. Sharma and W. E. Criss, eds.), Vol. 9, pp. 93–120, Raven Press, New York (1978).
6. M. E. Costlow and W. E. McGuire, Prolactin receptors and hormone dependence in mammary carcinoma, in: *Endocrine Control in Neoplasia* (R. K. Sharma and W. E. Criss, eds.), Vol. 9, pp. 121–152, Raven Press, New York (1978).
7. R. Hilf, J. T. Harmon, and S. M. Shafie, Insulin and insulin receptors in mammary cancer, in: *Endocrine Control in Neoplasia* (R. K. Sharma and W. E. Criss, eds.), Vol. 9, pp. 153–168, Raven Press, New York (1978).

8. N. Legros and J. C. Heuson, Hormone action in breast cancer explants, in: *Endocrine Control in Neoplasia* (R. K. Sharma and W. E. Criss, eds.), Vol. 9, pp. 169–190, Raven Press, New York (1978).

9. M. Monaco and M. E. Lippman, Interaction between hormones and human breast cancer in long-term tissue culture, in: *Endocrine Control in Neoplasia* (R. K. Sharma and W. E. Criss, eds.), Vol. 9, pp. 233–248, Raven Press, New York (1978).

10. S. Mohla and W. A. Anderson, Role of steroid hormones in mammary cancer, in: *Endocrine Control in Neoplasia* (R. K. Sharma and W. E. Criss, eds.), Vol. 9, pp. 315–334, Raven Press, New York (1978).

11. Y. S. Cho-Chung, Interaction of cyclic AMP and estrogen in tumor growth controls, in: *Endocrine Control in Neoplasia* (R. K. Sharma, and W. E. Criss, eds.), Vol. 9, pp. 335–348, Raven Press, New York (1978).

12. F. J. Chlapowski, L. A. Kelly, and R. W. Butcher, Cyclic nucleotides in cultured cells, in: *Advances in Cyclic Nucleotide Research* (P. Greengard and G. A. Robison, eds.), Vol. 6, pp. 245–338, Raven Press, New York (1975).

13. W. L. Ryan and M. L. Heidrick, Role of cyclic nucleotides in cancer, in: *Advances in Cyclic Nucleotide Research* (P. Greengard and G. A. Robison, eds.), Vol. 4, pp. 81–116, Raven Press, New York (1974).

14. G. S. Johnson, Regulation of cell functions in fibroblasts by cyclic AMP, in: *The Role of Cyclic Nucleotides in Carcinogenesis* (J. Schultz and H. G. Gratzner, eds.), pp. 39–46, Academic Press, New York (1973).

15. I. Pastan, M. Willingham, R. Carchman, and W. B. Anderson, Cyclic AMP metabolism in normal and transformed fibroblasts, in: *The Role of Cyclic Nucleotides in Carcinogenesis* (J. Schultz and H. G. Gratzner, eds.), pp. 47–56, Academic Press, New York (1973).

16. W. D. Wicks, R. Van Wijk, K. Clay, and C. Beavy, Regulation of growth rate, DNA synthesis and specific protein synthesis by derivatives of cyclic AMP in cultured hepatoma cells, in: *The Role of Cyclic Nucleotides in Carcinogenesis* (J. Schultz and H. G. Gratzner, eds.), pp. 103–126, Academic Press, New York (1973).

17. P. Furmanski and M. Lublin, Cyclic AMP and the expression of differentiated properties *in vitro*, in: *The Role of Cyclic Nucleotides in Carcinogenesis* (J. Schultz and H. G. Gratzner, eds.), pp. 239–262, Academic Press, New York (1973).

18. J. Voorhees, W. Kelsey, M. Stawiski, E. Smith, and E. Duell, Increased cyclic GMP and decreased cyclic AMP levels in the rapidly proliferating epithelium of psoriasis, in: *The Role of Cyclic Nucleotides in Carcinogenesis* (J. Schultz and H. G. Gratzner, eds.), pp. 325–373, Academic Press, New York (1973).

19. K. N. Prasad, Role of cyclic AMP in the differentiation of neuroblastoma cell culture, in: *The Role of Cyclic Nucleotides in Carcinogenesis* (J. Schultz and H. G. Gratzner, eds.), pp. 207–238, Academic Press, New York (1973).

20. D. McMahon, Chemical messengers in development: A hypothesis, *Science* **185**, 1012–1021 (1974).

21. K. N. Prasad, S. K. Sahu, and P. K. Sinha, Cyclic nucleotides in the regulation of expression of differentiated functions in neuroblastoma cells, *J. Natl. Cancer Inst.* **57**, 619–629 (1976).

22. C. W. Abell and T. M. Monahan, The role of adenosine 3′,5′-cyclic monophosphate in the regulation of mammalian cell division, *J. Cell Biol.* **59**, 549–558 (1973).

23. W. E. Seifert and P. S. Rudland, Possible involvement of cyclic GMP in growth control of cultured mouse cells, *Nature* **248**, 138–140 (1973).

24. I. Pastan, Regulation of cellular growth, *Adv. Metab. Disord.* **8**, 7–16 (1975).

25. Y. S. Cho-Chung, *In vivo* inhibition of tumor growth by cyclic adenosine 3′,5′-monophosphate derivatives, *Cancer Res.* **34**, 3492–3496 (1974).

26. Y. S. Cho-Chung and P. M. Gullino, *In vivo* inhibition of growth of two hormone-dependent mammary tumors by dibutyryl cyclic AMP, *Science* **183**, 87–88 (1974).
27. Y. S. Cho-Chung and P. M. Gullino, Effect of dibutyryl cyclic adenosine 3′,5′-monophosphate on *in vivo* growth of Walker 256 carcinoma: Isolation of responsive and unresponsive cell populations, *J. Natl. Cancer Inst.* **52**, 995–996 (1974).
28. D. M. Klein and R. F. Loizzi, Enhancement of R3230AC rat mammary tumor growth and cellular differentiation by dibutyryl cyclic adenosine monophosphate, *J. Natl. Cancer Inst.* **58**, 813–818 (1977).
29. Y. S. Cho-Chung and B. Berghoffer, The role of cyclic AMP in neoplastic cell growth and regression II. Growth arrest and glucose-6-phosphate dehydrogenase isozyme shift by dibutyryl cyclic AMP, *Biochem. Biophys. Res. Commun.* **60**, 528–534 (1972).
30. Y. S. Cho-Chung and T. Clair, The role of cAMP on neoplastic cell growth and regression. III. Altered cAMP-binding in DBcAMP-unresponsive Walter 256 mammary carcinoma, *Biochem. Biophys. Res. Commun.* **64**, 768–772 (1975).
31. J. S. Bodwin and Y. S. Cho-Chung, Decreased estrogen binding in hormone-dependent mammary carcinoma following ovariectomy of dibutyryl cyclic AMP treatment, *Cancer Lett.* **3**, 289–294 (1977).
32. Y. S. Cho-Chung and B. H. Redler, Dibutyryl cyclic AMP mimics ovariectomy: Nuclear protein phosphorylation in mammary tumor regression, *Science* **197**, 272–275 (1977).
33. Y. S. Cho-Chung and S. F. Newcomer, Adenylate cyclase, cyclic adenosine 3′:5′-monophosphate phosphodiesterase, and regression of Walker 256 mammary carcinoma, *Cancer Res.* **37**, 4493–4499 (1977).
34. Y. S. Cho-Chung, T. Clair, P. N. Yi, and C. Parkinson, Comparative studies on cyclic AMP binding and protein kinase in cyclic AMP-responsive and unresponsive Walker 256 mammary carcinomas, *J. Biol. Chem.* **252**, 6335–6341 (1977).
35. Y. S. Cho-Chung, T. Clair, and R. Porper, Cyclic AMP-binding proteins and protein kinase during regression of Walker 256 mammary carcinoma, *J. Biol. Chem.* **252**, 6342–6348 (1977).
36. Y. S. Cho-Chung, T. Clair, and P. Huffman, Loss of nuclear cyclic AMP binding in cyclic AMP-unresponsive Walker 256 mammary carcinoma, *J. Biol. Chem.* **252**, 6349–6355 (1977).
37. R. Tchao and J. Leighton, Inhibitory effect of dibutyryl cyclic AMP and theophylline on the aggregation of human breast tumour cell line BT-20, *Nature* **259**, 220–222 (1976).
38. J. Yang and S. Nandi, Cyclic AMP regulation of mammary tumor virus production, *J. Virol.* **21**, 815–819 (1977).
39. J. P. Minton, T. Wisenbaugh, and R. H. Matthews, Elevated cyclic AMP levels in human breast-cancer tissue, *J. Natl. Cancer Inst.* **53**, 283–284 (1974).
40. G. W. Oertel, P. Benes, G. Hoffman, and E. Shuy, Interaction between dehydroepiandrosterone, glucose-6-phosphate dehydrogenase, and cyclic adenosine 3′,5′-monophosphate in neoplastic and normal human mammary tissue, *Experientia* **31**, 1124–1125 (1975).
41. F. Guerinot, J. C. Delarue, G. Contesso, and C. Bohoun, Adenosine 3′,5′-cyclic monophosphate and guanosine 3′,5′-cyclic monophosphate levels in human breast cancer tissue, *Oncology* **34**, 261–263 (1977).
42. W. Küng, E. Bechtel, E. Guyer, A. Salokangas, J. Preisz, P. Huber, J. Torhorst, R. A. Jungmann, K. Talmadge, and U. Eppenberger, Altered levels of cyclic nucleotides, cyclic AMP phosphodiesterase and adenylyl cyclase activities in normal, dysplastic and neoplastic human mammary tissue, *FEBS Lett.* **82**, 102–106 (1977).

43. L. A. Cohen and P. C. Chan, Intracellular cAMP levels in normal rat mammary gland and adenocarcinoma. *In vivo* vs. *in vitro, Life Sci.* **16**, 107–115 (1975).

44. J. A. Rillema, J. A. Mulder, and L. D. Anderson, Cyclic nucleotides and their associated enzymes in 9,10-dimethyl-1,2-benzanthracene-induced mammary tumors of rats, *Cancer Res.* **38**, 741–744 (1978).

45. R. J. Matusik and R. Hilf, Relationship of adenosine 3′,5′-cyclic monophosphate and guanosine 3′,5′-cyclic monophosphate to growth of dimethylbenz[a]anthracene-induced mammary tumors in rats, *J. Natl. Cancer Inst.* **56**, 659–661 (1976).

46. R. Hilf, J. T. Harmon, R. J. Matusik, and M. B. Ringler, Hormonal control of mammary cancer, in: *Control Mechanisms in Cancer* (W. E. Criss, T. Ono, and J. R. Sabine, eds.), pp. 1–24, Raven Press, New York (1976).

47. Y. S. Cho-Chung, J. S. Bodwin, and T. Clair, Cyclic adenosine 3′,5′-monophosphate-binding protein: Role in ovariectomy-induced regression of hormone-dependent mammary tumor in Sprague–Dawley female rats, *J. Natl. Cancer Inst.* **60**, 1175–1178 (1978).

48. Y. S. Cho-Chung, J. S. Bodwin, and T. Clair, Cyclic AMP-binding proteins: Inverse relationship with estrogen-receptors in hormone dependent mammary tumor regression, *Eur. J. Biochem.* **86**, 51–60 (1978).

49. S. K. Chatterjee and U. Kim, Adenosine-3′,5′-cyclic monophosphate levels and adenosine-3′,5′-cyclic monophosphate phosphodiesterase activity in metastasizing and nonmetastasizing rat mammary carcinomas, *J. Natl. Cancer Inst.* **54**, 181–186 (1975).

50. M. J. Tisdale and B. J. Phillips, Comparative effects of alkylating agents and other anti-tumour agents on the intracellular level of adenosine 3′,5′-monophosphate in Walker carcinoma, *Biochem. Pharmacol.* **24**, 1271–1276 (1975).

51. L. A. Cohen, D. Straka, and P. C. Chan, Cyclic nucleotide phosphodiesterase activity in normal and neoplastic rat mammary cells grown in monolayer culture, *Cancer Res.* **36**, 2007–2012 (1976).

52. A. L. Singer, R. P. Sherwin, A. S. Dunn, and M. M. Appleman, Cyclic nucleotide phosphodiesterases in neoplastic and nonneoplastic human mammary tissues, *Cancer Res.* **36**, 60–66 (1976).

53. N. A. Sheth, S. V. Bhide, and K. J. Ranadive, Behavior of adenyl cyclase in mammary gland of mice subsceptible and resistant to breast cancer, *Indian J. Cancer* **11**, 177–182 (1974).

54. I. Schorr and A. Russell, Properties of adenylate cyclase of murine mammary carcinoma, *Biochim. Biophys. Acta* **364**, 173–180 (1974).

55. H. D. Brown, S. K. Chattopadhyay, H. J. Spjut, J. S. Spratt, Jr., and S. N. Pennington, Adenyl cyclase activity in dimethylaminobiphenyl-induced breast carcinoma, *Biochim. Biophys. Acta* **192**, 372–375 (1969).

56. U. Eppenberger, K. Talmadge, W. Küng, E. Bechtel, J. Preisz, P. Huber, R. A. Jungmann, and A. Salokangas, Adenosine 3′,5′-cyclic-monophosphate dependent protein kinase and cyclic-AMP-binding in human mammary tumors, *FEBS Lett.* **80**, 229–234 (1977).

57. G. C. Majumder, Protein kinase activity in mouse mammary carcinoma, *Biochem. Biophys. Res. Commun.* **74**, 1140–1145 (1977).

58. K. M. Anderson and I. S. Mendelson, Solubilized nuclear DNA-dependent RNA polymerases from normal rat mammary glands and from transplantable R-35 rat mammary tumors, *Oncology* **31**, 338–356 (1975).

59. M. J. Berridge, Control of cell division: A unifying hypothesis, *J. Cyclic Nucleotide Res.* **1**, 305–320 (1975).

60. J. F. Whitfield, J. P. MacManus, R. H. Rixon, A. L. Boynton, T. Youdale, and S. Swierenga, The positive control of cell proliferation by the interplay of calcium ions and cyclic nucleotides. A review, *In Vitro* **12**, 1–18 (1976).
61. K. M. Halprin, Cyclic nucleotides and epidermal cell proliferation, *J. Invest. Dermatol.* **66**, 339–343 (1976).
62. D. A. Chambers, Molecular mediators of cell proliferation, *J. Invest. Dermatol.* **67**, 661–664 (1976).
63. E. F. Howard, D. F. Scott, and J. O. Manter, Cyclic nucleotide levels in mouse mammary epithelial cells during growth arrest and growth initiation in culture, *J. Natl. Cancer Inst.* **59**, 145–149 (1977).
64. F. K. Lin, M. R. Banerjee, and L. R. Crump, Cell cycle-related hormone carcinogen interaction during chemical carcinogen induction of nodule-like mammary lesions in organ culture, *Cancer Res.* **36**, 1607–1614 (1976).
65. B. M. Jaffe and M. G. Santoro, Prostaglandins and cancer, in: *The Prostaglandins* (P. W. Ramwell, ed.), Vol. 3, pp. 329–351, Plenum Press, New York (1977).
66. J. J. Voorhees, D. A. Chambers, E. A. Duell, C. L. Marcelo, and G. G. Krueger, Molecular mechanisms in proliferative skin disease, *J. Invest. Dermatol.* **67**, 442–450 (1976).
67. B. M. Jaffe, Prostaglandins and cancer: An update, *Prostaglandins* **6**, 453–461 (1974).
68. S. M. M. Karim and B. Rao, Prostaglandins and tumors, in: *Prostaglandins: Physiological, Pharmacological and Pathological Aspects* (S. M. M. Karim, ed.), pp. 303–325, University Park Press, Baltimore (1976).
69. A. M. Neville and E. H. Cooper, Biochemical monitoring of cancer. A review, *Ann Clin. Biochem.* **13**, 283–305 (1976).
70. W. C. Tan, O. S. Privett, and M. E. Goldyne, Studies of prostaglandins in rat mammary tumors induced by 7,12-dimethylbenz(a)anthracene, *Cancer Res.* **34**, 3229–3231 (1974).
71. A. Bennett, A. M. McDonald, J. S. Simpson, and I. F. Stamford, Breast cancer, prostaglandins and bone metastases, *Lancet* **1**, 1218–1220 (1975).
72. A. Bennett, E. M. Charlier, A. M. McDonald, J. S. Simpson, I. F. Stamford, and T. Zebro, Prostaglandins and breast cancer, *Lancet* **2**, 624–625 (1977).
73. A. Bennett, M. Charlier, A. M. McDonald, J. S. Simpson, and I. F. Stamford, Bone destruction by breast tumours, *Prostaglandins* **11**, 461–463 (1976).
74. M. P. Carpenter, R. O. Robinson, and L. P. Thuy, Prostaglandin synthesis and prostaglandin E-9-ketoreductase in normal and neoplastic rat mammary gland, *Fed. Proc. Fed. Am. Soc. Exp. Biol.* **36**, 767, Abstract No. 2612 (1977).
75. T. J. Powles, S. A. Clark, D. M. Easty, and A. M. Neville, The inhibition by aspirin and indomethacin of osteolytic tumour deposits and hypercalcaemia in rats with Walker tumour, and its possible application to human breast cancer, *Br. J. Cancer* **28**, 316–321 (1973).
76. T. J. Powles, R. C. Coombes, A. M. Neville, H. T. Ford, J. C. Gazet, and L. Levine, 15-Keto-13,14-dihydroprostaglandin E_2 concentrations in serum of patients with breast cancer, *Lancet* **2**, 138 (1977).
77. M. Dowsett, G. C. Easty, T. J. Powles, D. M. Easty, and A. M. Neville, Human breast tumour-induced osteolysis and prostaglandins, *Prostaglandins* **11**, 447–455 (1976).
78. W. E. Kibbey, D. G. Bronn and J. P. Minton, Prostaglandins and metastasis, *Lancet* **1**, 101 (1978).
79. H. I. Jacobson, Oncolytic action of prostaglandins, *Cancer Chemother. Rep. Part 1*, **58**, 503–511 (1974).
80. D. R. Thomas, G. W. Philpott, and B. M. Jaffe, Prostaglandin E (PGE) control of cell proliferation *in vitro*: Characteristics of HT-29, *J. Surg. Res.* **16**, 463–465 (1974).

81. D. R. Thomas, G. W. Philpott, and B. M. Jaffe, The relationship between concentration of prostaglandin E and rates of cell replication, *Exp. Cell Res.* **84,** 40–46 (1974).

82. O. J. Franks, J. P. MacManus, and J. F. Whitfield, The effect of prostaglandins on cyclic AMP production and cell proliferation in thymic lymphocytes, *Biochem. Biophys. Res. Commun.* **44,** 1177–1183 (1971).

83. I. Feher and J. Gidali, Prostaglandin E_2 as stimulator of haemopoietic stem cell proliferation, *Nature* **247,** 550–551 (1974).

84. L. J. DeAsua, D. Clingan, and P. S. Rudland, Initiation of cell proliferation in culture mouse fibroblasts by prostaglandin $F_{2\alpha}$, *Proc. Natl. Acad. Sci. U.S.A.* **72,** 2724–2728 (1975).

85. A. B. Miller, Role of nutrition in the etiology of breast cancer, *Cancer* **39,** 2704–2708 (1977).

86. E. L. Wynder, Nutrition and cancer, *Fed. Proc. Fed. Am. Soc. Exp. Biol.* **35,** 1309–1315 (1976).

87. K. K. Carroll, Experimental evidence of dietary factors and hormone-dependent cancers, *Cancer Res.* **35,** 3374–3383 (1975).

88. P. C. Chan, J. F. Head, L. A. Cohen, and E. L. Wynder, Influence of dietary fat on the induction of mammary tumors by N-nitrosomethylurea: Associated hormone changes and differences between Sprague–Dawley and F344 rats, *J. Natl. Cancer Inst.* **59,** 1279–1283 (1977).

89. P. Hill, P. Chan, L. Cohen, E. Wynder, and K. Kuno, Diet and endocrine-related cancer, *Cancer* **39,** 1820–1826 (1977).

90. K. K. Carroll, Dietary factors in hormone-dependent cancers, in: *Nutrition and Cancer* (M. Winick, ed.), pp. 25–40, John Wiley and Sons, New York (1977).

91. K. K. Carroll and H. T. Khor, Effects of level and type of dietary fat on incidence of mammary tumors in female Sprague–Dawley rats by 7,12-dimethylbenz(α)anthracene, *Lipids* **6,** 415–420 (1971).

92. G. J. Hopkins, C. E. West, and G. C. Hard, Effect of dietary fats on the incidence of 7,12-dimethylbenz(α)anthracene-induced tumors in rats, *Lipids* **11,** 328–333 (1976).

93. G. J. Hopkins, G. C. Hard, and C. E. West, Carcinogenesis induced by 7,12-dimethylbenz(α)anthracene in C3H-A ^{vy}fB mice: Influence of different dietary fats, *J. Natl. Cancer Inst.* **60,** 849 (1978).

94. S. Dayton, S. Hashimoto, and J. Wollman, Effect of high-oleic and high-linoleic safflower oils on mammary tumors induced in rats by 7,12-dimethylbenz(α)anthracene, *J. Nutr.* **107,** 1353–1360 (1977).

95. S. Abraham and G. A. Rao, Lipids and lipogenesis in a murine mammary neoplastic system, in: *Control Mechanisms in Cancer* (W. E. Criss, T. Ono, and J. R. Sabine, eds.), pp. 363–378, Raven Press, New York (1976).

96. G. A. Rao and S. Abraham, Enhanced growth rate of transplanted mammary adenocarcinoma induced in C3H mice by dietary linoleate, *J. Natl. Cancer Inst.* **56,** 431–432 (1976).

97. V. Hial, Z. Horakova, R. E. Shaff, and M. A. Beaven, Alteration of tumor growth by aspirin and indomethacin: Studies with two transplantable tumors in mouse, *Eur. J. Pharmacol.* **37,** 367–376 (1976).

98. M. J. Tisdale, Inhibition of prostaglandin synthetase by anti-tumour agents, *Chem. Biol. Interact.* **18,** 91–100 (1977).

99. P. Chan, F. Didato, and L. A. Cohen, High dietary fat, elevation of rat serum prolactin and mammary cancer, *Proc. Soc. Exp. Biol. Med.* **149,** 133–135 (1975).

100. P. Chan and L. A. Cohen, Effect of dietary fat, antiestrogen and antiprolactin on the development of mammary tumors in rats, *J. Natl. Cancer Inst.* **52,** 25–30, (1974).

101. N. W. Schoene and J. M. Iacono, The influence of phospholipase A_2 on prostaglandin

production in platelets, in: *Advances in Prostaglandin and Thromboxane Research* (B. Samuelsson and R. Paoletti, eds.), Vol. 2, 763–766, Raven Press, New York (1976).

102. V. F. Lindlar and H. Wagener, Zur lipid-und fettsaurenzusammensetzung experimenteller tumoren, *Schweiz. Med. Wochenschr.* **7**, 243–250 (1964).

103. R. Wood, Oleic and vaccinec acid levels in lipid classes of tumors, *Lipids* **11**, 578–580 (1976).

104. B. S. Leung and G. Y. Sun, Acyl group composition of membrane phospholipids in mammary tissues and carcinoma induced by dimethylbenz(α)anthracene, *Proc. Soc. Exp. Biol. Med.* **152**, 671–676 (1976).

105. W. C. Tan, C. Chapman, T. Takatori, and O. S. Privett, Studies of lipid class and fatty acid profiles of rat mammary tumors induced by 7,12-dimethylbenz(α)anthracene, *Lipids*, **10**, 70–74 (1975).

106. E. D. Rees, A. E. Shuck, and H. Ackerman, Lipid composition of rat mammary carcinomas, mammary glands and related tissues: Endocrine influences, *J. Lipid Res.* **7**, 396–402 (1966).

107. J. A. Rillema and J. A. Mulder, Arachidonic acid distribution in lipids of mammary glands and DMBA-induced tumors of rats, *Prostagl. Med.* **1**, 31–38 (1978).

108. H. P. Bär, Epinephrine- and prostaglandin-sensitive adenyl cyclase in mammary gland, *Biochim. Biophys. Acta* **321**, 397–406 (1973).

109. S. Burstein, G. Gagnon, S. A. Hunter, and D. V. Maudsley, Prostaglandin biosynthesis and stimulation of cyclic AMP in primary monolayer cultures of epithelial cells from mouse mammary gland, *Prostaglandins* **11**, 85–99 (1976).

110. S. Burstein, G. Gagnon, S. A. Hunter, and D. A. Maudsley, Elevation of prostaglandin and cyclic AMP levels by arachidonic acid in primary epithelial cell cultures of C3H mouse mammary tumors, *Prostaglandins* **13**, 41–53 (1977).

111. J. A. Rillema, Effects of prostaglandin on RNA and casein synthesis in mammary gland explants of mice, *Endocrinology* **99**, 490–495 (1976).

112. J. A. Rillema, Activation of casein synthesis by prostaglandins plus spermidine in mammary gland explants of mice, *Biochem. Biophys. Res. Commun.* **70**, 45–49 (1976).

113. J. A. Rillema, Possible role of prostaglandin $F_{2\alpha}$ in mediating effect of prolactin on RNA synthesis in mammary gland explants of mice, *Nature* **253**, 466–467 (1975).

114. J. A. Rillema and E. A. Wild, Prolactin activation of phospholipase A activity in membrane preparations from mammary glands, *Endocrinology* **100**, 1219–1222 (1977).

115. J. A. Rillema and L. D. Anderson, Phospholipases and the effect of prolactin on uridine incorporation into RNA in mammary gland explants of mice, *Biochim. Biophys. Acta* **428**, 819–824 (1976).

116. D. F. Horrobin, M. S. Manku, R. A. Karmali, B. A. Nassar, and M. W. Greaves, Prolactin and prostaglandin synthesis, *Lancet* **2**, 1154 (1974).

117. B. M. Bayer and M. A. Beaven, Evidence that indomethacin inhibits growth of cells in the G_1 phase of the cell cycle, *Fed. Proc. Fed. Am. Soc. Exp. Biol.* **37**, 896 (1978).

118. D. H. Russell, The roles of the polyamines, putrescine, spermidine and spermine in normal and malignant tissues, *Life Sci.* **13**, 1635–1647 (1973).

119. D. C. Tormey and T. P. Waalkes, Biochemical markers in cancer of the breast, *Recent Results Cancer Res.* **57**, 78–94 (1976).

120. C. W. Tabor and H. Tabor, 1,4-Diaminobutane (putrescene), spermidine and spermine, *Annu. Rev. Biochem.* **45**, 285–306 (1976).

121. D. H. Russell, Clinical relevance of polyamines as biochemical markers of tumor kinetics, *Clin. Chem.* **23**, 22–27 (1977).

122. U. Bachrach, Polyamines as chemical markers of malignancy, *Ital. J. Biochem.* **25**, 77–93 (1976).

123. D. Russell, *Polyamines in Normal and Neoplastic Growth*, Raven Press, New York (1973).

124. D. H. Russell, Increased polyamine concentration in the urine of human cancer patients, *Nature (London) New Biol.* **233**, 144–145 (1971).

125. D. H. Russell, C. C. Levy, S. C. Schimpff, and I. A. Hawk, Urinary polyamines in cancer patients, *Cancer Res.* **31**, 1555–1558 (1971).

126. A. Lipton, L. M. Sheehan, and G. F. Kessler, Jr., Urinary polyamine levels in human cancer, *Cancer* **35**, 464–468 (1975).

127. J. H. Fleisher and D. H. Russell, Estimation of urinary diamines and polyamines by thin-layer chromatography, *J. Chromatogr.* **110**, 335–340 (1975).

128. B. G. M. Durie, S. E. Salmon, and D. H. Russell, Polyamines as markers of response and disease activity in cancer chemotherapy, *Cancer Res.* **37**, 214–221 (1977).

129. K. Fujita, T. Nagatsu, K. Maruta, M. Ito, H. Senba, and K. Miki, Urinary putrescine, spermidine and spermine in human blood and solid cancers and in an experimental gastric tumor of rats, *Cancer Res.* **36**, 1320–1324 (1976).

130. O. Heby and G. Andersson, Simplified micro-method for the quantitative analysis of putrescine, spermidine and spermine in urine, *J. Chromatogr.* **145**, 73–80 (1978).

131. D. C. Tormey, T. P. Waalkes, D. Ahmann, C. W. Gehrke, R. W. Zumwalt, J Snyder, and H. Hansen, Biological markers in breast carcinoma, *Cancer* **35**, 1095–1100 (1975).

132. D. H. Russell, P. M. Gullino, L. J. Marton, and S. M. LeGendre, Polyamine depletion of the MTW9 mammary tumor and subsequent elevation of spermidine in the sera of tumor-bearing rats as a biochemical marker of tumor regression, *Cancer Res.* **34**, 2378–2381 (1974).

133. A. C. Andersson, S. Heningsson, L. Lundell, E. Rosengren, and F. Sundler, Diamines and polyamines in DMBA-induced breast carcinoma containing mast cells resistant to compound 48/80, *Agents Actions* **6**, 577–583 (1976).

134. K. V. K. Rao, A. V. Bhat, and C. B. Bapat, Effect of hydrocortisone on arginase activity in ICRC mouse mammary tumors *in vitro, Indian J. Physiol. Pharmacol.* **21**, 145–146 (1977).

135. R. P. G. Aisbitt and J. M. Barry, Stimulation by insulin of ornithine decarboxylase activity in cultured mammary tissue, *Biochim. Biophys. Acta* **320**, 610–616 (1973).

136. T. Oka and J. W. Perry, Arginase affects lactogenesis through its influence on the biosynthesis of spermidine, *Nature* **250**, 660–661 (1974).

137. T. Oka and J. W. Perry, Studies on the function of glucocorticoid in mouse mammary epithelial cell differentiation *in vitro, J. Biol. Chem.* **249**, 3586–3591 (1974).

138. J. A. Rillema, Action of prolactin on ornithine decarboxylase activity in mammary gland explants of mice, *Endocr. Res. Commun.* **3**, 297–305 (1976).

139. T. Oka and J. W. Perry, Studies on regulatory factors of ornithine decarboxylase activity during development of mouse mammary gland epithelium *in vitro, J. Biol. Chem.* **251**, 1738–1744 (1976).

140. T. Oka and J. W. Perry, Spermidine as a possible mediator of glucocorticoid effect on milk protein synthesis in mouse mammary epithelium *in vitro, J. Biol. Chem.* **249**, 7647–7652 (1974).

141. T. Oka, Spermidine in hormone-dependent differentiation of mammary gland *in vitro, Science* **184**, 78–80 (1974).

142. K. Kano and T. Oka, Polyamine transport and metabolism in mouse mammary gland, *J. Biol. Chem.* **251**, 2795–2800 (1976).

143. J. A. Rillema, B. E. Linebaugh, and J. A. Mulder, Regulation of casein synthesis by polyamines in mammary gland explants in mice, *Endocrinology* **100**, 529–536 (1977).

144. T. Oka, J. W. Perry, and K. Kano, Hormone regulation of spermidine synthase during the development of mouse mammary epithelium *in vitro, Biochem. Biophys. Res. Commun.* **79**, 979–986 (1977).

145. N. A. Sheth, S. S. Tikekar, K. J. Ranadive, and A. R. Sheth, Enhancement of *in vitro*

binding of rat prolactin to murine mammary gland by polyamines, *IRCS Med. Sci. Biochem. Cancer Cell Membr. Biol. Endocr. Syst. Reprod. Obstet. Gynecol.* **4**, 323 (1976).

146. M. Winther and L. Stevens, Polyamine stimulation of *in vivo* rates of macromolecular synthesis in a putrescine auxotroph of *Aspergillus nidulans*, *FEBS Lett.* **85**, 229–231 (1978).

147. O. Heby, G. Andersson and J. W. Gray, Interference with S and G_2 phase progression by polyamine synthesis inhibitors, *Exp. Cell Res.* **111**, 461–464 (1978).

148. C. Lafarge-Frayssinet, O. Bertaux, R. Valencia, and C. Frayssinet, Evolution of ornithine decarboxylase activity during the cell cycle of *Euglena gracilis Z* in synchronous culture, *Biochim. Biophys. Acta* **539**, 435–444 (1978).

149. H. Hibasami, M. Tanaka, J. Nagai, and T. Ikeda, Changes in ornithine decarboxylase activity and cyclic adenosine-3′,5′-monophosphate concentrations during the cell cycle of synchronized BHK cells, *Aust. J. Exp. Biol. Med. Sci.* **55**, 379–383 (1977).

150. E. W. Gerner and D. H. Russell, The relationship between polyamine accumulation and DNA replication in synchronized chinese hamster ovary cells after heat shock, *Cancer Res.* **37**, 482–489 (1977).

151. D. J. M. Fuller, E. W. Gerner, and D. H. Russell, Polyamine biosynthesis and accumulation during the G_1 to S phase transition, *J. Cell. Physiol.* **93**, 81–88 (1977).

152. W. H. Bulger and D. Kupfer, Induction of uterine ornithine decarboxylase (ODC) by antiestrogens. Inhibition of estradiol-mediated induction of ODC: A possible mechanism of action of antiestrogens, *Endocr. Res. Commun.* **3**, 209–218 (1976).

153. U. Bachrach, Polyamines and neoplastic growth: Stabilization of ornithine decarboxylase during transformation, *Biochem. Biophys. Res. Commun.* **72**, 1008–1013 (1976).

154. E. Mihick, Current studies with methylglyoxylbis(guanylhydrazone), *Cancer Res.* **23**, 1375 (1963).

155. D. H. Russell and P. J. Strambrook, Cell cycle specific fluctuations in adenosine-3′,5′-cyclic monophosphate and polyamines of chinese hamster ovary cells, *Proc. Natl. Acad. Sci. U.S.A.* **72**, 1482–1486 (1975).

156. O. D. Helby, J. W. Gray, P. A. Lindl, L. J. Marton, and C. B. Wilson, Changes in L-ornithine decarboxylase activity during the cell cycle, *Biochem. Biophys. Res. Commun.* **71**, 99–105 (1976).

157. J. C. Knutson, L. Graham, and D. R. Mouris, DNA synthesis in nuclei from activated lymphocytes inhibited in polyamine accumulation, *Fed. Proc. Fed. Am. Soc. Exp. Biol.* **35**, 1488 (1976).

158. O. Heby, L. J. Marton, C. Wilson, and J. W. Gray, Effect of methylglyoxal-bis(guanylhydrazone), an inhibitor of spermidine and spermine synthesis on cell cycle traverse, *Eur. J. Cancer* **13**, 1009–1017 (1977).

159. H. T. Rupniak and D. Paul, Regulation of the cell cycle by polyamines in normal and transformed fibroblasts, in: *Advances in Polyamine Research* (R. A. Campbell, D. R. Morris, D. Bartos, G. D. Daves, Jr., and F. Bartos, eds.), Vol. 1, pp. 117–126, Raven Press, New York (1978).

160. H. T. Rupniak and D. Paul, Inhibition of spermidine and spermine synthesis leads to growth arrest of rat embryo fibroblasts in G_1, *J. Cell. Physiol.* **94**, 161–170 (1978).

161. C. V. Byus and D. H. Russell, Effects of methyl xanthine derivatives on cyclic AMP levels and ornithine decarboxylase activity of rat tissues, *Life Sci.* **15**, 1991–1997 (1974).

162. B. Hogan, R. Shields, and D. Curtis, Effect of cyclic nucleotides on the induction of ornithine decarboxylase in BHK cells by serum and insulin, *Cell* **2**, 229–233 (1974).

163. V. J. Atmar and G. D. Kuehn, Effects of polyamines on adenylate cyclase activity and acidic nuclear protein phosphorylation in *Physarum polycephalum*, *Fed. Proc. Fed. Am. Soc. Exp. Biol.* **36**, 686 (1977).

164. J. H. Levine, A. B. Leaming, and P. Ruskin, On the mechanism of activation of

hepatic ornithine decarboxylase by cyclic AMP, in: *Advances in Polyamine Research* (R. A. Campbell, D. R. Morris, D. Bartos, G. D. Daves, Jr., and F. Bartos, eds.), Vol. 1, pp. 51–58, Raven Press, New York (1978).

165. M. J. Berridge, The interaction of cyclic nucleotides and calcium in the control of cellular activity, *Adv. Cyclic Nucleotide Res.* **6**, 1–98 (1975).

166. J. F. Whitfield, R. H. Rixon, J. P. MacManus, and S. D. Balk, Calcium, cyclic adenosine 3',5'-monophosphate and the control of cell proliferation: A review, *In Vitro* **8**, 257–278 (1973).

167. H. Rasmussen and D. B. P. Goodman, Relationship between calcium and cyclic nucleotides in all activation, *Physiol. Rev.* **57**, 421–509 (1977).

168. O. Oelz, H. R. Knapp, L. J. Roberts, R. Oelz, B. J. Sweetman, J. A. Oats, and P. W. Reed, Calcium-dependent stimulation of thromboxane and prostaglandin biosynthesis by ionophores, in: *Advances in Prostaglandin and Thromboxane Research* (C. Galli, G. Galli, and G. Porcellati, eds.), Vol. 3, pp. 147–158, Raven Press, New York (1978).

5

Methods for Analyzing Steroid Receptors in Human Breast Cancer

GARY C. CHAMNESS AND WILLIAM L. McGUIRE

1. Introduction

For almost a century, it has been known that human breast cancer may respond favorably to ovariectomy[1] or other ablative endocrine treatments such as adrenalectomy.[2] Further understanding of this phenomenon, however, awaited the synthesis in about 1960 of high-specific-activity radioactive estrogens, [³H]hexestrol by Glascock and Hoekstra[3] and [³H]estradiol by Jensen and Jacobson.[4,5] Almost immediately, it was reported by Folca *et al.* that four patients whose tumors contained excess [³H]hexestrol after *in vivo* injection responded to later ablative treatment, while six others whose tumors did not concentrate [³H]hexestrol did not respond.[6] *In vivo* concentration of labeled estrogens by human breast tumors was also reported by others,[7–12] but the technique has obvious limitations.

In 1965, Toft and Gorski first used an *in vitro* approach to demonstrate the estrogen receptor protein in uterine tissue.[13] Cytoplasmic estrogen receptor was then found in human breast cancer tissues by Jensen and associates,[14,15] who speculated that its presence might signal hormone dependence of the tumors. The present decade has seen a proliferation of estrogen receptor assay methods and reports of clinical correlations in breast cancer, many of which were summarized at

GARY C. CHAMNESS AND WILLIAM L. McGUIRE • Department of Medicine, University of Texas Health Science Center, San Antonio, Texas 78284.

an international workshop in 1974.[16] It was concluded that the absence of cytoplasmic estrogen receptor in a breast tumor makes a favorable response to any endocrine therapy very unlikely. Unfortunately, the converse correlation is much less striking; only 55–60% of receptor-positive tumors respond. In an effort to improve the ability to predict the hormone responsiveness of a breast tumor, a number of further approaches are being investigated.

First, the mechanism by which estrogen receptor affects target cell growth and function is being examined to discover steps at which a defect in neoplastic tissues might render them insensitive to estrogen, even when the cytoplasmic receptor itself is present. Current information on this mechanism has been extensively reviewed.[17–20] In particular, shortly after the discovery of estrogen receptor in the cytoplasm of target cells it was found that binding of estradiol *in vivo* causes a very rapid translocation of the receptor into cell nuclei.[21,22] Thus, the presence of receptor in cell nuclei of human breast tumor biopsies would presumably indicate that the translocation step was intact and also that the patient was producing sufficient estrogen to stimulate the tumor.[23,24] Methods for determining estrogen receptor in nuclei of human breast tumor specimens are therefore being developed.

Second, the presence of other steroid receptors may give further information about the state of hormone responsiveness in a human breast cancer. Progesterone receptor, for example, is induced by estrogen in many normal tissues, and might therefore serve as a marker of estrogen stimulation in a tumor.[25] Both glucocorticoids and androgens sometimes induce breast cancer regression, so that it seems possible that presence of receptors for these two classes of hormones in breast tumors may be correlated with the effectiveness of these treatments. Assays for all of these receptors in human breast cancer have been reported, though the data relating these to the results of therapy are as yet very sparse.

It is the purpose of this chapter to review the methods available for determining the presence and amount of steroid receptors in human breast cancers. We will first describe those methods used for the cytoplasmic estrogen receptor, since these have been in use longest and have provided the foundation for all of the other assay methods. The list will include both well-established procedures and newer techniques that seem promising. We will then discuss methods for evaluating estrogen receptor in tumor cell nuclei, followed by procedures for studying progesterone, glucocorticoid, and androgen receptors. Finally, we will comment briefly on the choice of receptor assay methods and on their use and interpretation. Some of these topics have been reviewed recently,[16,26-28] while more general coverage of hormones and their receptors in the control of breast cancer is found elsewhere in these volumes and in a number of other recent publications (see, for example, References 29–35).

2. General Considerations

2.1. Approaches to Assay and Analysis

Almost all existing methods are based on measurement of the binding of a radiolabeled steroid, either to tissue slices or, more usually, to the soluble proteins contained in the supernatant (cytosol) of a tissue homogenate. These methods differ primarily in the procedure used to separate hormone bound to the receptor protein from that which remains unbound. This problem is complicated by the fact that steroids may bind to a number of proteins in addition to the receptor, including albumin, α_1-acidic glycoprotein, corticosteroid-binding globulin (CBG), and sex-hormone-binding globulin (SHBG).[33] These are plasma proteins, but since human tumor specimens nearly always contain substantial amounts of plasma protein contamination,[36] the ability of a method to distinguish these from true receptor is critical. Each method offers certain advantages and disadvantages, and a number of variations are possible within each.

Methods for separating bound from free ligand are inherently nonequilibrium procedures—for at least a brief period, hormone must remain bound to receptor in the absence of any free hormone while the separation is being effected. True equilibrium methods, such as either equilibrium dialysis or steady-state electrophoresis or gel filtration, have not been useful for receptor assay primarily because the very small amounts of receptor that must be measured do not perturb the equilibrium distribution of ligand enough for accurate measurement. But there is another advantage besides sensitivity in nonequilibrium separations. Many of the nonreceptor proteins bind steroids with relatively low affinity, so that dissociation is rapid and frequently complete during the time required for separation, whereas the receptor–steroid complex barely dissociates at all. Indeed, some of the methods to be discussed below purposely increase the time or temperature of the separation step in an attempt to optimize the dissociation of nonspecifically bound steroid. Although clearly useful, this feature of nonequilibrium procedures does make it difficult to determine the true affinity constant of receptors for their ligands, since the equilibrium is established between receptor and *free* ligand, not including that ligand which may be even temporarily bound to other proteins. The effects of serum proteins in particular on determinations of receptor affinity have been examined.[37-39]

In spite of the problem just noted, the affinity constant is frequently used to distinguish receptor and nonreceptor binding. This takes advantage of the fact that receptors have a higher affinity for their ligands than even the high-affinity plasma-binding globulins, and insures that the binding measured has the appropriate affinity. The amount of steroid bound at (approximate) equilibrium with a number of different free-steroid concentrations is plotted and extrapolated to reveal the amount of high-affinity binding at saturation (and therefore the number of receptor sites present) as well as the affinity constant. This is done using the double reciprocal plot of Lineweaver and Burk or the plot suggested by Scatchard[40]; the Scatchard plot is probably better suited to receptor binding analysis since it does not falsely exaggerate the significance of binding at extremely low concentrations. Nevertheless, the presence of either lower-affinity or nonspecific binding sites can complicate the interpretation of Scatchard plots. We have recently discussed common errors in the use of Scatchard plots and presented solutions for simple cases[41]; a more complete and detailed mathematical approach has been offered by Rodbard.[42] Finally, an alternative graphical means of interpreting binding data has been proposed by Baulieu and Raynaud.[43] Called the proportion graph, this method uses logarithmic scales to bring a wide range of steroid concentrations into the useful working area of the graph; it does not, however, give the straight lines in simple cases which make the Scatchard plot so visually useful, and it requires computer assistance for interpretation.

Because affinity analyses of the sort just described are laborious and require large amounts of tissue, many assay methods rely on a single steroid concentration chosen to saturate or nearly saturate receptor binding sites while still minimizing nonspecific binding. Needless to say, such a choice can never be completely satisfactory. There are, however, approaches available for increasing the specificity of such methods. These make use of the saturation of receptor sites at relatively low steroid concentrations: If, for example, a 100-fold excess of nonradioactive estradiol is present along with a near-saturating concentration of the radioactive hormone, then 99% of the receptor sites will be filled with the unlabeled compound. Since proteins of much lower affinity will be nowhere near saturation, the presence of the unlabeled estradiol will have little effect on binding of the label to these proteins, so that this binding in the presence of excess unlabeled estradiol is a measure of nonspecific binding and can be subtracted from the total binding. Thus, the *competible* binding of the labeled hormone provides a measure of the specific receptor sites present. This method can, of course, be used to correct for nonspecific binding in multiple-concentration methods as well as in single-dose assays. A note of caution: the higher the excess of unlabeled hormone, the greater the competition for binding to *low-affinity* sites; no more than 50 to 100-fold excess should be used. Also, the unlabeled hormone should be added either before or with the labeled, never after, since it will replace the label only very slowly if added afterward. Some theoretical objections based on the possibility that the large excess of unlabeled hormone will perturb the assay system have been presented and demonstrated,[44] but this approach remains the most accepted reasonably quantitative way of determining specific binding.

Specificity of the assay can be further enhanced by the appropriate choice of radioactive ligand and competitors. Labeled estradiol, for example, binds estrogen receptor with very high affinity but also has considerable affinity for SHBG. The possibility of SHBG interference in a receptor assay can be reduced by using not unlabeled estradiol but rather diethylstilbestrol as competitor, since diethylstilbestrol has equal affinity for receptor but far lower affinity for SHBG. Many have successfully used antiestrogens, usually nafoxidine (Upjohn U11,100A) or CI 628 (Parke-Davis) for the same purpose and the same reasons, but the possibility that these compounds act allosterically at a secondary site on the receptor[45] could complicate interpretations. Another approach is to use a synthetic steroid with more desirable specificity properties. For instance, [^{3}H]estradiol can be replaced with the synthetic estrogen [^{3}H]-R2858, which approaches estradiol in its affinity for the estrogen receptor but has very low affinity for SHBG and other interfering binding proteins.[46,47] (Use of [^{3}H]diethylstilbestrol would have a similar result, except that the labeled form of this compound is not very stable.) As will be seen below, useful synthetic compounds are now available for the assay of progesterone, androgen, and glucocorticoid receptors as well; the use of [^{3}H]-R5020 for progesterone receptor has been particularly valuable. A third approach, where the nature of the potential interfering binder is known, as in the case of SHBG, is to include in all parts of the assay an unlabeled ligand that binds SHBG but not the receptor in question; testosterone or dihydrotestosterone (DHT) have been suggested for this purpose in the assay of estrogen receptor,[37] though their weak but definite affinity for the estrogen receptor should not be ignored.[48-50] Another example of this approach is seen in the assay of progesterone receptor, where unlabeled cortisol can be added to prevent CBG from interfering.[51]

In cases where the receptor is not very stable, the presence of the ligand frequently stabilizes it. This means that the earliest possible addition of ligand can be very helpful; for instance, in one androgen receptor procedure, [³H]-DHT is added right after homogenization and before high-speed centrifugation.[52]

Finally, some assay methods physically separate the receptor with its bound labeled hormone from some of the other proteins that also bind the labeled hormone. The precipitation of the receptor by protamine sulfate or its adsorption on hydroxylapatite or DEAE filters are examples of such methods, as are methods involving electrophoresis or density gradient sedimentation. All of these, along with others, will be discussed in detail later.

An example of the importance of attention to these general considerations is given by the recent discovery by Clark et al.[53] of relatively large amounts of an anomalous estrogen binder which they call Type II in both cytoplasm and nuclei of uterine cells. This binder has considerable affinity for estradiol and diethylstilbestrol, though less than the receptor, and is clearly revealed when Scatchard plots are extended to higher ligand concentrations than usual. It may well cause high estimates of receptor levels if single-concentration assays are used, especially with excessive competitor. Type II binding has not yet been described in breast cancer tissue but it may well be present, emphasizing the necessity of care in defining each assay variation.

Another problem that must be considered is that most methods depend on the binding of a labeled ligand to *unoccupied* receptor sites; if many of these sites are already occupied by endogenous ligand, receptor could be underestimated or even missed completely. This may not be a serious problem in the case of cytoplasmic estrogen receptor, since Sakai and Saez found at most 30% of the receptor to be occupied, even with high plasma estrogen levels, in a series of breast cancer specimens.[54] Also, Fishman et al. have reported no correlation between high plasma estrogen levels and reduced estrogen receptor measurements.[55] In the case of progesterone receptor, however, the problem is apparently much more serious. The apparent incidence of tumors with this receptor is very much reduced in the second half of the menstrual cycle, when progesterone levels are high, and when plasma progesterone levels exceed 1.0 ng/ml no receptor at all is detected.[56] In addition, receptors for all steroids would be expected to be occupied when found in nuclei after translocation. To measure such occupied receptors, conditions must be found under which the radiolabeled ligand will not only fill unoccupied sites but also exchange for endogenous ligand in occupied sites. Such exchange conditions usually involve increased temperatures and/or longer exposure times, with attendant danger of inactivating the receptor being sought. Nonetheless, exchange assays have been developed for cytoplasmic and nuclear estrogen receptors and are under development for other receptors, as will be discussed in the appropriate sections below.

2.2. Tissue Storage and Preparation

There is general agreement that breast tumor tissue for receptor assay must be chilled immediately upon removal and either processed within hours or quick-frozen in liquid nitrogen.[16,26,57,58] (Brown et al.[58] have found the fluorinated hydrocarbon spray Cryokwik to be as effective as liquid nitrogen.) The importance of this matter has been emphasized by LeClerq et al.,[59] who attribute a higher percentage of receptor-positive tumors in more recent assays to better coordination of tissue handling from the operating room to the laboratory freezer. The tumors should be stored at $-70°C$ or below and shipped, if necessary, in dry ice. There are some reports of partial estrogen[60-62] or progesterone[63] receptor loss even under these conditions, while others find no detectable loss on freezing.[64-67] Those losses which occur might be prevented by freezing in the presence of a thiol reagent.[59,68] Also, even though receptor itself is preserved, there may be some dissociation of endogenous ligand from the receptor due to freezing.[54] It is probably *not* possible to prepare cytosol and then freeze it for storage or shipment without major receptor losses,[60,63,66,69] though Barnes et al.[67] report successful preservation of estrogen and progesterone receptor activity in cytosols in liquid nitrogen, and Saez (personal communication) has found storage at 4° after lyophilization satisfactory for estrogen but not progesterone receptor.

There is remarkable uniformity in the selection of buffers for estrogen receptor assay. Though the receptor has been reported to be stable in the range pH 7–9,[66] pH 7.4 has usually been chosen. Tris [tris (hydroxymethyl)aminomethane] at 10–50 mM is the common buffering agent, often supplemented with 1–2 mM EDTA (or EGTA) to prevent receptor aggregation. Tris, however, is notorious for the variation of its pH with temperature (a solution of pH 7.4 at 0°C, for example, would be pH 6.5 at the 30°C often used for exchange assays)[70]; it is in any case a rather weak buffer at pH 7.4. Some, therefore, have preferred to use 5 mM sodium phosphate, still at pH 7.4, with no adverse effect on activity.[71,72] A few have added 0.25 M sucrose to their buffers, primarily to stabilize nuclei and lysosomes. Sodium azide, usually 1 mM, is sometimes added as a preservative. Glycerol at 10% or more is not known to have any effect on estrogen receptor assays but it is very important for progesterone and probably androgen receptor (see individual sections below) and is therefore often included. Finally, a number of reports emphasize the receptor's dependence on sulfhydryl groups[73,74] and therefore the importance of thiol reagents[59,61,69,75-77]; 0.5–5 mM dithiothreitol or 1–12 mM thioglycerol are common choices.

Ideally the entire tumor specimen is pulverized while still frozen in preparation for homogenization in buffer. This not only breaks up the fibrous tissue so common in human breast tumors but also permits thorough mixing, so that a sample representative of the entire tumor can be obtained if only a portion is to be used. The importance of this treatment is emphasized by the large variations reported in estrogen receptor assays of different portions of the same tumor[59,78]; the great heterogeneity of receptor distribution has been confirmed by the immunofluorescence technique of Pertschuk et al.,[79] to be discussed later. Suitable devices for pulverizing the specimen are the Thermovac device or the Braun "microdismembrator." After this treatment, the sample is then further homogenized in a few volumes of buffer, or in some cases is merely allowed to thaw in the buffer. Any of several types of homogenizers can be used; our own laboratory employs a Polytron PT-10-ST (Brinkman), although one report indicates that a pressure homogenizer (or "bomb") may give a better receptor yield than the rotating-blade type.[77] A critical point is to keep the sample cold at all times[57,80]; this requires keeping the sample on ice and allowing rest periods during homogenization to dissipate any heat built up by friction.

The cytosol is then separated from particulate fractions and debris by centrifugation. Following Toft and Gorski,[13] many use the ultracentrifuge at 100,000g or more for up to an hour to make this separation. In the interests of simplicity and considerations of expense, however, others have used ordinary low-speed centrifugation at 800–2000g for 10–20 minutes without adverse results. There are claims of a substantially greater yield of receptor by the latter method[81,82]; whether this is due to the presence of a form of receptor in the microsomal fraction as recently reported[83] or to some other reason is not yet known.

2.3. Protein and DNA Determinations

Receptor values have been reported per milligram wet weight of tissue, per milligram cytosol protein, or per milligram DNA. Hähnel and Twaddle recently have compared results calculated by all three methods,[84] noting substantial differences in some cases. The use of the cytosol-protein concentration to normalize results does correct for variable amounts of fibrous tissue and variable yields from homogenization, but Hawkins et al. have noted that this does little to improve the reproducibility of results.[78] Masters et al.[85] report that apparent estrogen receptor levels are strongly correlated with the cellularity of the tumor specimen, which presumably would be most closely correlated in turn with the DNA content. The DNA content, in fact, varies widely from 1 to 15 mg per mg wet weight in a series of breast cancers examined by Mobbs and Johnson.[86] DNA may therefore be the best basis for reporting receptor measurements, in spite of the fact that DNA must be determined from the residual pellet after centrifugation rather than from the cytosol itself.

DNA determinations can be made by the Burton modification of the diphenylamine method[87]; a modification of the indole color reaction has also been used.[88]

For protein the method of Waddell[89] is occasionally used, but protein is usually determined by the method of Lowry et al.,[90] though the presence of thiol reagent can interfere with this method[91] and a modification has been recommended.[92] In most cases the method of Lowry et al. is probably adequate, as long as standards are prepared in the same buffer as the cytosol. Such standards are also important when the buffer contains a high concentration of glycerol, which also interferes to some extent.[67] The total cytosol protein frequently includes a considerable amount of plasma protein, as already noted; in one series, plasma protein averaged 40% of the total "cytosol"[84] protein. About 60% of human plasma protein is albumin, which can be measured by an immunodiffusion assay[93] and used to correct for plasma contamination of tissue protein.[57]

3. Estrogen Receptor

3.1. Cytoplasmic Receptor: Established Methods

3.1.1. Tissue-Slice Uptake

This method, the first in vitro test devised, measures the binding of [³H]estradiol to thin slices of tumor tissue rather than to soluble cytoplasmic receptor as do all the remaining techniques. It was first applied to human breast tumors by Jensen's group,[14] who took a number of 0.5-mm slices of 10–20 mg each for incubation at 37°C in Krebs–Ringer–Henseleit buffer with glucose and 10^{-10} M [³H]estradiol. Nafoxidine at 10^{-5} M was the competitor. This estradiol concentration is nowhere near that needed to saturate receptor and therefore prevents a truly quantitative assessment of receptor in the tissue; incomplete access of estradiol to all parts of the tissue and receptor degradation during incubation also contribute to this problem. Most other investigators who have employed this technique used similar low concentrations in order to minimize nonspecific binding,[12,60,94,95] though Johansson et al.[96] and Hoge et al.[97] were able to use 2×10^{-9} M successfully.

This in vitro slice method has been compared with cytosol techniques.[77,98,99] The results agree as to the presence or absence of receptor in most of the tumors studied, but the overall percentage of positive results in larger series is somewhat less with the slice technique. Correlations with tumor response to endocrine therapy are also basically parallel.[100] Most investigators note the importance and also the difficulty of obtaining truly representative slices from the extremely heterogeneous tissues comprising most human breast tumors. The requirement for fresh tissue is also a negative feature of this method; apparently much of the cytoplasmic receptor leaks out of frozen cells upon thawing.[98] The method requires up to 0.5 g of tissue for sufficient slice samples, as compared to 0.1–0.2 g for most of the cytosol procedures. The 37°C incubation allows [^{3}H]estradiol to replace any endogenous hormone which may have occupied receptor sites in cytoplasm or nuclei, as opposed to the usual cytosol procedures which measure only unfilled cytoplasmic receptors. Nevertheless, there are now newer techniques for evaluating these other receptor compartments, and most laboratories have replaced the tissue-slice method with more quantitative assays.

3.1.2. Sucrose Density Gradient Centrifugation

This technique, which was employed in the first direct demonstration of cytoplasmic estrogen receptor,[13] was also among the first used for quantitative assay of receptor in human breast cancer tissues.[15] Two examples of results appear in Fig. 1. The cytosol is first incubated with [^{3}H]estradiol, then layered as a narrow band on a prepared gradient of sucrose (5–20% sucrose is often used, though 10–30% may offer some improvement in results[15]; the same buffer chosen for homogenization is usually employed). A parallel gradient is layered with cytosol incubated with an excess of unlabeled competitor along with the [^{3}H]estradiol to determine nonspecific binding. The gradients are centrifuged at least 15 hours, the exact time depending on the g force available and the tube length, and then collected by any of several techniques and the fractions counted to reveal the peaks of bound [^{3}H]estradiol. Unbound ligand remains at the top of the gradient; much of it is often removed by brief exposure to a pellet of dextran-coated charcoal (see below) after incubation and before layering on the gradient.[101,102] The sedimentation velocities are calculated by the method of Martin and Ames.[103] This method requires a standard, which can be bovine serum albumin (4.6 S) or some other known pure protein run in a parallel gradient, but the inclusion of ^{14}C-labeled bovine serum albumin in the same gradient tube as the cytosol sample eliminates any possible variation.[104]

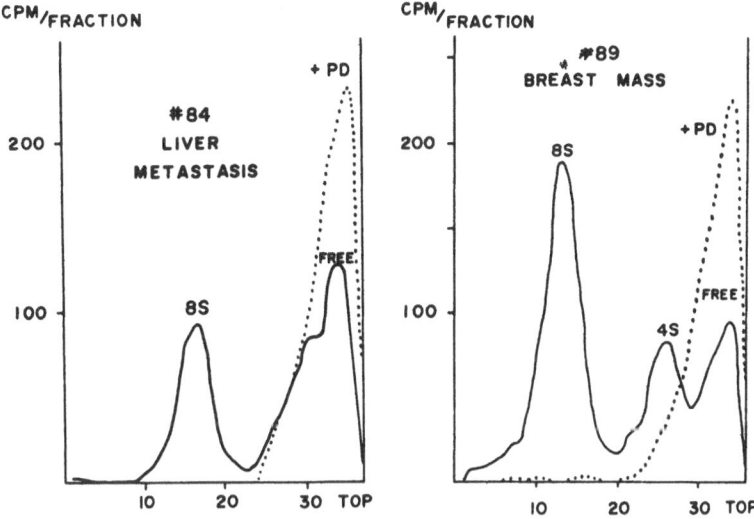

Fig. 1. Sucrose density gradient sedimentation patterns of typical human breast cancer cytosols containing estrogen receptor. Cytosols contain 0.5 nM [³H]estradiol in the absence (solid curve) or presence (dotted curve) of 0.2 μM Parke-Davis Cl 628. (From Jensen *et al.*[15])

This assay makes use of the fact that all cytoplasmic steroid receptors sediment primarily at 8 S in low salt concentrations, whereas albumin, SHBG, and other nonreceptor binding proteins sediment at 4 S. This fact is probably fortuitous, since there is evidence that the receptor sediments at 6 S at physiological ionic strength and at 4 S in higher salt concentrations,[104,105] but it does allow the convincing distinction of receptors from other steroid binders. Nonetheless, a considerable amount of competible 4 S binding is often found when 8 S binding is present, suggesting that the receptor may sometimes be partially dissociated even in low-salt conditions.

This technique has been adopted by a number of laboratories studying human breast cancer,[101,106,107] and estrogen receptors determined by this method in extensive series of cases have been correlated with clinical response to endocrine therapy.[61,64,108–110] The series reported by Wittliff's group contained a number of examples with competible 4 S binding but no 8 S[62]; 10 out of 10 of these cases failed to respond to endocrine therapies.[111] It was suggested that the 4 S peak represents an inactive form of the receptor, perhaps produced by proteolysis,[112] for which the stable 4 S receptor sometimes seen in rat uteri[113,114] could be a model. This rat 4 S form is unable to bind to nuclear fractions,[115,116] and if the human 4 S were also ineffective, as suggested by Wittliff, then it would be important to have a technique such as sucrose gradient centrifugation capable of distinguishing it from the 8 S form. It has not been proved, however, that this 4 S competible binding has the properties of receptor or that it would actually be measured by the techniques to be discussed below. Tissue such as stomach and kidney which have not been shown to have any true estrogen receptor sometimes do have 4 S competible binding,[117,118] while the extensive series of breast tumors analyzed by Jensen's group[109] included no examples of 4 S competible binding in the absence of the 8 S receptor. The difference could be one of methodology; the latter series used 5×10^{-10} M [³H]estradiol with the antiestrogens nafoxidine or CI 628 as competitors, so that binding to nonreceptor proteins would be low and could not be competed with, whereas the former group apparently employed $4-5 \times 10^{-9}$ M [³H]estradiol with $2-20 \times 10^{-6}$ M unlabeled estradiol (or sometimes CI 628) as competitor, leading to both greater nonreceptor binding and greater competition for this binding. Others [101] have used the higher concentration of [³H]estradiol—indeed, Jensen et al. have noted that their own low concentration does not fully saturate the receptor and therefore is not fully quantitative—but with much less unlabeled estradiol as competitor (4×10^{-7} M). Probably diethylstilbestrol, with its low affinity for nonreceptor estradiol binders, would be an even better choice as competitor. In any case, this question may provide an example of the importance of appropriate selection of ligands, competitors, and concentrations for each assay situation.

The sucrose gradient method assures that 8 S competible binding represents true receptor, but it is rather cumbersome and almost impossible for other than a one-point assay. The long centrifugation time required in the usual swinging-bucket rotor allows the possibility of considerable dissociation of the receptor–steroid complex, especially when the ligand is of lower affinity than estradiol. This problem may be much reduced by the availability of vertical-tube or other rotor systems designed to reorient the gradient within the tube during the centrifuge run, thus providing a far shorter path and reducing running time from 16 hours to perhaps 2 hours.[119] In fact, the binding of [³H]tamoxifen to 8 S estrogen receptor can be demonstrated clearly with a vertical-tube rotor but not at all with a swinging-bucket rotor.[120] We will see later that this new technique is also important for the quantitative measurement of 8 S progesterone receptor.[121]

3.1.3. Dextran-Coated Charcoal (DCC)

Korenman in 1968[122] first used charcoal to adsorb free steroids in an estrogen receptor assay, and applied this assay two years later[123] to several human breast cancer specimens. Because of its relative simplicity, a number of laboratories quickly established their own versions,[81,101,124–130] and the assay has been responsible for a considerable portion of our present data on estrogen receptors in human breast cancer.

The procedure is straightforward. In our own version, after incubation of 250 μl of cytosol with [³H]estradiol, 1 ml of a suspension of 2.5 g/liter charcoal (Norit A) and 0.025 g/liter dextran in buffer is added and shaken vigorously for 30 minutes in the cold. (The dextran reduces adsorption of proteins without interfering with adsorption of free steroids, though at low protein concentrations some protein loss may still occur; 0.1% gelatin is also added by some.[67,131]) Brief centrifugation pellets the charcoal with adsorbed free [³H]estradiol; an aliquot of the supernatant is counted to determine the receptor-bound [³H]estradiol. As a control, identical amounts of [³H]estradiol are incubated with buffer rather than cytosol and then treated with DCC to measure the small amount of free ligand left behind by the charcoal step. We find it desirable to make new DCC every two weeks and to test each preparation with both control [³H]estradiol alone and with a standard cytosol (rat uterus) before use for tumor assays, since very occasional DCC preparations may show higher blanks or other irregularities. Indeed, the method may be more sensitive than some to uncontrolled variables; for example, serious problems have been known to arise due to a bad water filter, to a compound present in certain anesthetic preparations, and to dextran infused during surgery (S. Saez, personal communication).

The exposure to DCC actually removes [³H]estradiol from many nonreceptor proteins such as albumin[69] and probably SHBG.[127] Of course, it may also dissociate a certain number of receptor–estrogen complexes depending on the time and temperature of exposure. (This dissociation has been reported to be especially serious in buffers of high ionic strength,[132] though others have not always observed this phenomenon.) Theoretically, the dissociation can be corrected for by incubating with DCC long enough to dissociate all of the nonreceptor binding, then continuing the incubation for a time, observing the slow dissociation of [³H]steroid from the receptor, and extrapolating back to zero time.[133] In practice this is seldom done. With the estrogen receptor, at least, it is possible to choose conditions which effectively reduce nonspecific binding without much loss of receptor-bound estradiol. With other steroid receptors having somewhat lower affinities for their ligands, the problem is more serious, and the exposure to DCC must be much reduced or even abandoned in favor of other methods.[134]

In general, all of the procedures noted are carried out at 0–4°C. At least 3–4 hours are required to approach equilibrium binding of [³H]estradiol to receptor at this temperature, and many continue this incubation overnight. At somewhat higher temperatures, however, a much more rapid equilibration can be achieved. LeClerq et al.[127] use 30 minutes at 18°C, for example, with no apparent loss of receptor as compared with 2°C; the data of Feherty et al. [124] agree with both equilibration and stability under these conditions. Unfortunately, the latter group elected to use 30°C for 30 minutes as their standard incubation condition, and their own data as well as that of others [76,81] show clearly that maximum binding of [³H]estradiol to receptor cannot be reached or maintained at this temperature before degradation of receptor becomes significant. The 30°C temperature is continued by Feherty et al. through 10 minutes of shaking with DCC to enhance dissociation of nonspecific binding, but this step may also contribute to further receptor loss. Nonetheless, Braunsberg finds one of the highest reported percentages of receptor-positive tumors in her case series using this technique, [69] suggesting that these receptor losses rarely convert a positive result to a negative. The same is probably true of shaking with DCC in the cold, though Korsten and Persijn [131] recommend shaking 10 seconds every 3 minutes, claiming that the EORTC standard 90 minutes of continuous shaking causes some receptor losses.

Most of the proponents of the DCC method have used a range of [³H]estradiol concentrations and have constructed Scatchard plots to interpret the results; some further guarantee specificity by employing unlabeled competitors at one or all concentrations of the labeled hormone. The desire to simplify this procedure and to reduce the amount of tissue required led Leung et al. to propose a one-point assay [128]—more properly, a one-concentration assay—measuring DCC-resistant binding of [³H]estradiol with and without competitor using a single [³H]estradiol concentration. Because their ligand concentration was not sufficient to saturate the receptor, the true concentration of receptor sites could not be calculated, but the "binding index" which these authors devised was shown to correlate with results of more conventional and cumbersome procedures. Another simplified method used only two nonsaturating ligand concentrations, constructing a Scatchard plot to extrapolate from these two points to the receptor number and K_d [65]; the potential error in such a procedure is quite large, and a one-point method using a low but essentially saturating ligand concentration without the necessity of extrapolation seems preferable even though K_d cannot be estimated. LeClerq et al. [127] and Mobbs and Johnson [86] employed such a one-point procedure with a few tumors and showed agreement with their Scatchard results. A much more extensive series from McGuire et al. [72] demonstrates excellent quantitative correlation of receptor number between the one-point DCC assay, Scatchard DCC assay, and sucrose density gradients; one of these correlations is shown in Fig. 2. Nevertheless, the finding of an appropriate K_d by Scatchard plot or an 8 S peak by sucrose gradient gives added confidence that one is truly measuring receptor.

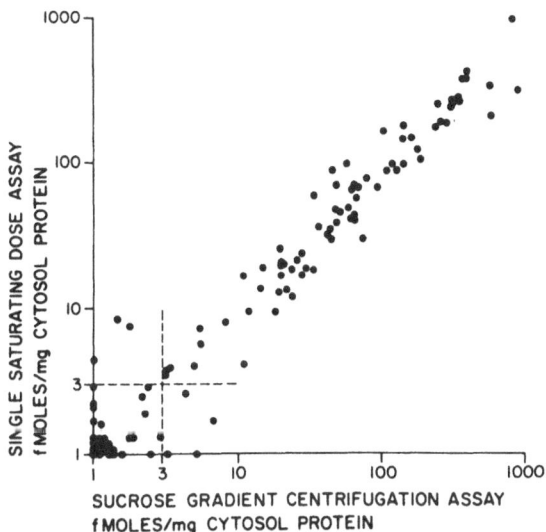

Fig. 2. Comparison of sucrose density gradient and single-dose charcoal assay results on 115 human breast tumor cytosols. (From McGuire *et al.*[72])

Probably no laboratory should rely exclusively on a one-point DCC assay for estrogen receptor, at least until considerable experience is obtained with the other methods.

All of the foregoing procedures measure only unoccupied cytoplasmic receptors. In the rat uterus, occupied cytoplasmic receptors are usually neglected, since virtually all estrogen-filled receptors are found in the nucleus[135]; techniques for measuring these will be considered later. As discussed earlier, however, one could consider the possibility that a substantial fraction of filled receptor sites in tumors may remain in the cytoplasm. Katzenellenbogen *et al.*[136] have described a method for determining such sites. (Another exchange assay for cytoplasmic receptor is considered later in Section 3.2.1.) According to Katzenellenbogen *et al.*, the [³H]estradiol concentration is first raised to 3×10^{-8} M. Then, after unoccupied sites have been filled (and thereby stabilized), the temperature is brought to 30°C for 8 hours or more, permitting replacement of unlabeled endogenous ligand by the radioactive hormone. Excess free hormone is then removed by DCC. Application of this procedure to tumor cytosols might require some modifications; nonspecific binding would often be unacceptably high with such a high [³H]estradiol concentration, though at least 1×10^{-8} M is probably necessary to maintain saturation (unfilled sites are markedly labile at 30°C). Also, some tumor cytosols contain proteases which could destroy much of the receptor at 30°C. Sakai and Saez[54] used 5 hours at 26°C, reporting that 2 hours was sufficient for full exchange; as noted before, their tumor specimens contained at most 30% apparently occupied cytoplasmic estrogen receptor, and usually much less. No other series has yet been examined by a cytoplasmic exchange assay.

3.1.4. Gel Filtration

Gel filtration, or gel exclusion chromatography, was exployed by many in the characterization of estrogen receptor, but it was not adopted at first as a receptor assay procedure. Hähnel,[71] for instance, compared it with the DCC method and concluded that though equally valid, it offered more difficulties and no advantages, and it was therefore rejected.[77] Godefroi and Brooks, however, adapted the technique for use on human breast cancer specimens[137] and with their colleagues have reported a large series correlating the assay with treatment response.[61,138]

In the procedure according to Godefroi and Brooks, cytosol is incubated in the cold with [³H]estradiol, then applied to a column of 3.0 g Sephadex G25. The void volume (indicated by blue dextran) contains the receptor-bound radioactivity; it is extracted three times with ethyl acetate, and the extract is evaporated and redissolved in ethanol for counting. Sephadex itself has considerable affinity for estradiol; the amount of Sephadex was chosen to maximize the relatively rapid dissociation of nonspecifically bound ligand while not excessively removing the receptor-bound ligand. In fact, about 15% of the receptor-estradiol complex is dissociated by this procedure. This can be determined and corrected for by running parallel columns with up to 7.0 g Sephadex and extrapolating back to zero, though this cumbersome procedure is not routinely performed. Sephadex G100, which theoretically could separate 8 S and 4 S receptor forms, can also be used but causes more dissociation.

Values obtained by this assay have been reported to be several times those of sucrose density gradient determinations on the same cytosol,[61,139] though in these cases the cytosol was treated with DCC and then subjected to the long sucrose gradient run in the absence of any thiol reagent, so that the best results possible with the gradient procedure were probably not achieved.

The gel filtration technique just described is somewhat involved, and several variations have been suggested for simpler, more rapid assays. Gore-Langton et al.[140] have demonstrated the use of the thin-layer gel filtration procedure for receptor assays. Sephadex G150 was used, which allows distinction of 8 S and 4 S receptors in case this should turn out to be important as suggested by Wittliff.[111] Results could be obtained using the low-speed supernatant from only 50 mg of tissue. Radioactivity had to be recovered from the gel by replica absorbtion on a strip of filter paper, which may explain why values resulting from this technique were considerably less than those from parallel runs by sucrose gradient. Nor was there an attempt to quantitate losses due to the affinity of the Sephadex for estradiol, though it was reported that nonspecific binding present in the cytosol was dissociated during the procedure.

Another thin-layer gel filtration procedure by Töpert et al.[141] used a cellulose film between the glass supporting plate and the gel, permitting cutting of the gel into strips for quantitative recovery of radioactivity in scintillation vials. These workers employed Sephadex G75 or G100 and reported good separation of receptors from plasma binders, though no competitor was present to show whether specific binding of the 4 S type might be present. This variation has been used for androgen[141] and glucocorticoid[142] receptors, but not yet for breast cancer tissue or for estrogen receptor.

Another variation has been proposed recently by Cochet et al.[143] Very small G200 columns permit small samples and avoid the necessity of extracting radioactivity from large volumes for counting. The column separation requires only 2 hours, which may be a definite advantage in view of the receptor's tendency to dissociate and to lose its binding capacity. No study of dissociation due to the Sephadex itself was made. Initial results of this procedure with both rat uterus and human breast cancer cytosols suggest a possible unexpected solution to the 4 S receptor question; both low-salt (8 S) and high-salt (4 S) conditions produce apparently identical receptor peaks which are well separated from human SHBG. The physicochemical meaning of this result in terms of the multiple forms and combinations of receptor subunits has been discussed elsewhere.[144] In any case, it is not clear whether the 4 S form produced by salt dissociation of 8 S receptor is the same as that sometimes seen in low-salt sucrose gradients and discussed earlier,[111] but the observation deserves further attention.

Finally, Ginsburg et al.[145] have demonstrated certain advantages of the hydroxypropylated Sephadex LH20 over G25. Very small columns are possible, and the enhanced affinity of the gel for estradiol encourages dissociation of low-affinity binding without appearing to affect receptor-bound radioactivity. This dissociation is enhanced by allowing the cytosol to remain in contact with the gel for 30–120 minutes before elution is completed; Godefroi and Brooks[137] had achieved the same result by increasing the amount of gel. The LH20 gel filtration assay has been applied primarily to the difficult problem of measuring very low levels of estrogen and androgen receptors in regions of the brain; it has been used also for estrogen receptors in dimethylbenz(α)anthracene (DMBA)-induced rat mammary tumors.[146,147] Barnes et al.[67] examined both estrogen and progesterone receptors in a series of human breast cancer specimens by this method, and report good quantitative correlations with dextran-coated charcoal results for both receptors.

3.1.5. Agar Gel Electrophoresis

The foregoing procedures have made use of molecular size and/or high binding affinity of receptors to distinguish them from free and nonreceptor-bound estradiol. In 1972, Wagner[148] presented a new method in which receptor is separated by its distinctive electrophoretic mobility. A 1% agar gel is prepared in barbiturate–acetate buffer at pH 8.2, and small wells are punched along the centerline to contain about 50 μl of cytosol (prepared in tris buffer, usually at pH 7.5 and often with the addition of 1 mM NaN_3, and preincubated with [^{3}H]estradiol). The gel is placed on a Teflon-coated brass plate over a coolant such as chilled methanol at about $-1°C$; it is important to prevent heating during the run, and this technique has been shown to maintain the temperature of the gel at or below 3–4°C. Electrophoresis usually proceeds for 90 minutes. The gel is then sliced and extracted or dissolved for counting. Receptor-bound radioactivity is found on the anodal side of the starting well, while SHBG forms a distinctive peak on the cathodal side and free steroid is swept by electroendosmotic flow even farther toward the cathode. Albumin moves beyond the receptor toward the anode, but complete dissociation of steroid from albumin takes place during electrophoresis. Unfortunately, this dissociation can leave a certain amount of radioactive steroid in the receptor region of the gel, and to measure this Wagner used a control cytosol heated to 48°C for 60 minutes (which destroys receptor but not plasma binding components). One example of the results of this method appears in Fig. 3.

Results of this procedure were compared with a number of other techniques by Jungblut et al.,[139] using both calf uterus and human breast tumor preparations. Agar gel electrophoresis and Sephadex G25 gel filtration gave the highest receptor values, whereas the DCC value was 49% of these and sucrose gradients 30%. It is worth noting that no thiol reagent was present, providing a significant disadvantage for the sucrose gradient method with its relatively long separation run; the authors also believed that modification of their DCC procedure would produce 100% results. Nevertheless, the agar gel electrophoresis assay was clearly at least the equal of the others. Other less quantitative comparisons from Maass et al. showed qualitative agreement with the slice technique in 9 out of 11 cases[95] and with a hydroxylapatite method in 28

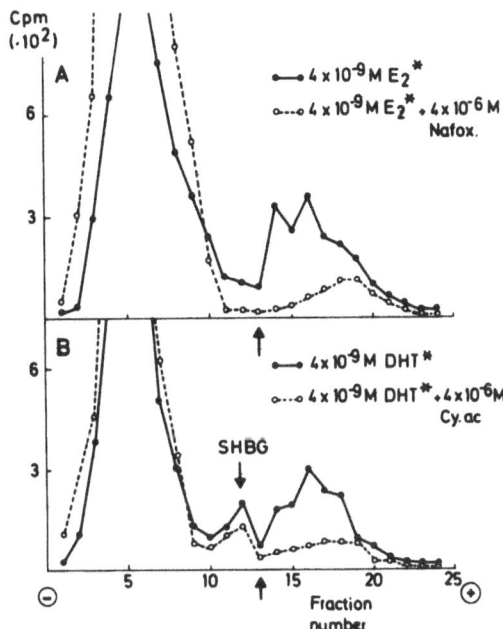

Fig. 3. Agar gel electrophoresis determination of estradiol and DHT binding in human breast cancer tissue (axillary lymph node). Both receptors move to the right of the origin. The amount of DHT binding to SHBG is often much greater than in this 83-year-old patient. (From Trams and Maass.[152])

out of 31 cases[36,99]; the latter also reported a somewhat higher percentage of receptor-positive tumors with this method or DCC as compared to slice or hydroxylapatite techniques. Another report by Korsten *et al.* included 4 out of 32 "false negatives" (objective remissions with endocrine therapy in spite of zero estrogen receptor values) with DCC and only 1 out of 24 with agar gel electrophoresis,[149] but this observation was, of course, only suggestive. A later direct but semiquantitative comparison of the two methods by this group also showed good agreement.[131] A similar series from Van Netten *et al.*[82] also showed general agreement; the somewhat lower electrophoresis values probably followed from too short an incubation with nonsaturating [³H]estradiol. This group did note that cytosol-protein concentrations below 2.5 mg/ml prevented interference from serum binders in the agar gel electrophoresis procedure.

Recently some improvements in this method were proposed by Wagner and Jungblut.[150] A brief treatment of the cytosol with DCC before electrophoresis probably removed much of the albumin-bound steroid as well as free steroid, and the resolution with a large number of human breast tumors was somewhat improved. A passage through 0.45-μm Millipore filters after heating of the control cytosol removed microaggregates which might clog the agar gel pores, but the heated control was then eliminated entirely in favor of competition with excess unlabeled estradiol or nafoxidine. Similar modifications have been adopted by Teulings *et al.* for their breast cancer series,[151] while Trams and Maass continue to experience satisfactory results with the original procedure.[152] Perhaps the most novel recent use of this assay showed that estrogen and androgen receptor levels are not changed from the original breast cancer biopsy when the human cancer tissue is caused to grow in athymic *nu/nu* mice; about 85% success in transplantation is reported.[153]

Surprisingly, polyacrylamide gel electrophoresis has had little success in steroid receptor assays in spite of the higher resolution usually attainable. Under most conditions, the cytosol receptor seems to aggregate upon entering the small-pore gel. The method did find application in final purification of calf uterine nuclear estrogen receptor,[154] and it has been used in studies of human plasma SHBG[155] and of progesterone receptor.[156] Very recently, measurement of human breast cancer cytosol estrogen receptor and its clear separation from SHBG by a polyacrylamide gel electrophoresis procedure have been reported[157]; it remains to be seen whether this promising technique will prove valuable.

3.2. Cytoplasmic Receptor: Newer Methods

We will now proceed to a brief discussion of several receptor assays which have not yet gained wide acceptance and which in many cases have not been applied directly to the measurement of estrogen receptor in breast cancer tissue. Nevertheless, each of them offers certain advantages which may recommend them for more thorough examination.

3.2.1. Protamine Sulfate

The precipitation of estrogen receptor by protamine sulfate was first reported by Steggles and King.[113] They proposed an assay in which cytosol was first incubated with [3H]estradiol, then precipitated with protamine to leave unbound hormone in solution; it appeared that nonreceptor binding proteins might also fail to precipitate. Using this method, Jungblut *et al.*[139] found a receptor value in a human breast tumor only 23% of that from agar gel electrophoresis on the same tumor. The procedure was modified and employed by Korach and Muldoon in studies of hypothalamic receptors of the rat,[158] but it did not receive wide acceptance as an assay. Nevertheless, protamine precipitability became one of the accepted distinctive properties of steroid receptors.

We developed a variation of this assay by showing that after protamine precipitation the receptor retained the ability to bind and, at elevated temperatures, to exchange [³H]estradiol.[159] In addition to its convenience, this procedure separated the receptor very quickly from both interfering plasma proteins and potentially destructive enzymes. Incubation at 4°C permitted only unfilled receptor sites to bind radioactive estradiol, while 3 hours at 30°C also allowed the labeled ligand to replace endogenous unlabeled estradiol already present on the receptor, thus providing a measure of both bound and free cytoplasmic receptors. Another exchange assay was mentioned previously,[136] but the protamine assay has the advantage of stabilizing and protecting the receptor while apparently permitting a somewhat faster exchange. Lippman and Huff[160] have used the assay with human breast cancer tissue, showing as we did identical values for protamine and DCC assays of cytoplasmic estrogen receptor, and also demonstrating equally good results for androgen receptor. Our laboratory demonstrated both androgen and progestin receptors in a human breast cancer cell line with this assay,[161] and its application to the assay of nuclear estrogen receptor will be discussed later, but no extensive series of estrogen receptor measurements in breast cancer has been reported.

3.2.2. Hydroxylapatite

In 1970, Erdos et al.[162] showed that hydroxylapatite in very small columns adsorbs [³H]estradiol-charged estrogen receptors. Most of the free ligand can be removed by washes, so that remaining adsorbed radioactivity is a measure of receptor. As noted previously, 31 tumors assayed by this method and simultaneously by agar gel electrophoresis by Maass et al.[36] produced 3 qualitative disagreements (2 positive only by agar gel and 1 only by hydroxylapatite) and considerable quantitative inconsistency, while the percentage of receptor-positive tumors in a larger series assayed by hydroxylapatite was somewhat lower than that assayed by either agar gel or DCC.

A more convenient and reproducible batch-adsorption procedure replaced the hydroxylapatite column in the modification developed by Williams and Gorski[163]; the method has been further studied and slightly modified by Pavlik and Coulson,[164] by Clark et al.,[39] and by ourselves.[165] The method offers some selectivity in that plasma contaminants adsorb weakly. Residual contaminants can perhaps be removed by washing with low concentrations of phosphate. Garola and McGuire[166] adapted this to produce a single-saturating-dose micromethod for breast cancer cytosols which agrees well with multiple-dose Scatchard plot determinations and DCC measurements at the usual cytosol-protein concentrations and is far more reliable at low concentrations. Less than 50 mg of tissue are required.

Adsorption of receptor to hydroxylapatite is not affected much by monovalent ions, so that unlike protamine sulfate or ion exchange methods, no dilution is required for salt extracts from nuclei. In fact, though the modified hydroxylapatite assay has not been used for cytoplasmic estrogen receptor determination in breast cancer, it provides the basis for a promising breast cancer nuclear receptor assay to be described later.

3.2.3. Isoelectric Focusing

Isoelectric focusing has been proposed as an alternative to electrophoresis for separating receptors from other steroid binders on the basis of their charge properties. The technique involves the use of ampholines, families of small molecules with a range of isoelectric points which arrange themselves in an electric field so as to establish a gradient of pH. Proteins also migrate to the region of pH corresponding to their own isoelectric points, thus providing separation on the basis of pI. A stabilizing matrix is required; sucrose or glycerol gradient columns, polyacrylamide gels, or flat beds of Sephadex have been used. Coffer and King[167,168] chose the last for its relative simplicity, ease of cooling, and speed. They found that free [³H]estradiol tended to remain at the point of application due to its affinity for Sephadex, which was an advantage as long as a prefocusing period was used to establish the pH gradient prior to applying the sample well away from the final pI. Regions of pH at which receptor is unstable also had to be avoided. The 8 S form of the rat uterine receptor focused at pH 5.8, while the 4 S form seemed to be heterogeneous around pH 6.6. The pI found for SHBG was 5.4, which may be too close to the 8 S receptor for convenient resolution, but no attempts were made to demonstrate this resolution or to compare results for human material.

A somewhat different focusing procedure was employed by Wrange et al.[169] in a comparison with sucrose gradient results in 26 human breast cancer specimens. The pH gradient was established in a 10–60% glycerol gradient without prefocusing. A competible binding peak appeared at pH 6.6 and was considered to be receptor, but aggregation and precipitation obscured the pH 4–5.5 region which probably includes the 8 S receptor form. Perhaps for this reason, nearly all values were considerably lower than corresponding values by sucrose gradient, and results did not correlate well with the presence of 8 S specific receptor on gradients. To correct this problem they modified the procedure to include a limited digestion with trypsin (7mg/mg cytosol protein, 10°C for 30 minutes) in order to convert 8 S receptor to the sharply focused, fully competible 4 S form[170] (see Fig. 4). The modification uses prefocused polyacrylamide gel slabs which can accommo-

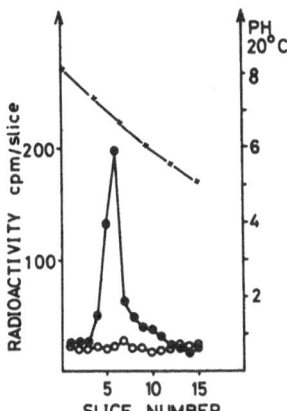

Fig. 4. Isoelectric focusing analysis of a human breast cancer cytosol after limited trypsin digestion. The cytosol was first incubated with 2 nM [³H]estradiol in the absence (●———●) or presence (O———O) of 1 μM unlabeled estradiol. The pH gradient is also shown (×———×). (From Wrange et al. [170])

date 8 samples of up to 3 mg cytosol protein each and require only 2 hours for final focusing. In comparison with sucrose density gradient determinations on the same samples, this procedure is claimed to achieve higher receptor values, though with a general positive correlation. Though the usefulness of isoelectric focusing as an analytical tool is unquestionable, it is too early to say whether the new modification will permit broad routine application.

3.2.4. DEAE Filters

An assay by Santi et al. [171] makes use of DEAE-cellulose filters to adsorb receptor–[³H]steroid complexes while allowing unbound steroid to be washed through with buffers of low ionic strength. The method was designed for [³H]dexamethasone binding to glucocorticoid receptors, and was carefully validated. Its suitability for estrogen or androgen receptors has been questioned, however, because of higher affinity of the respective free ligands for the DEAE-cellulose. [39] A variation has nevertheless been developed for estrogen receptor by Barbanel et al., [172] who spot their samples on DE-81 paper strips and then wash for precisely 1 hour in a 4°C bath of Tris–EDTA buffer. The method tolerates pH 6.9–9.0 and up to 10% glycerol, 2.5% ethanol, or 0.25 M sucrose, but not, of course, high ionic strength. It was well characterized for lamb uterine receptor but like other DEAE methods has not been applied to human breast cancer specimens.

3.2.5. Immobilized Antisteroid Antibodies

Three laboratories have reported the use of specific antisteroid antibodies to remove remaining free steroid from solution after incubation with receptor-containing cytosol. Success depends on the fact that such antibodies generally have much lower affinity for the steroid than the receptor, but higher affinity than nonreceptor proteins. A somewhat variable method blank necessitates the use of controls with excess non-radioactive competitor, just as with other methods.

Castaneda and Liao[173] performed many of their experiments with soluble antibody and examined the results on sucrose gradients with 0.4 M KCl present so that labeled receptor sedimented at 4 S and the steroid–antibody complex at about 8 S. They showed clearly by this method that all 4 S protein-bound 5α-dihydrotestosterone, cortisol, or progesterone in human serum was dissociated by antibody treatment, thus eliminating the problem of the serum binding proteins. For assays they used commercially available antibody and immobilized it on Sepharose beads for easy separation.

Floridi et al.[174] chose polyacrylamide beads for their insoluble matrix and concentrated their efforts on estrogen binding, unlike the preceding group, but their results, though less extensive, were similar.

Fishman and colleagues[175,176] were the only group to examine a considerable series of human breast cancers with their antibody assay. The technique was a bit different in that the antibody was adsorbed onto polyvinylidene fluoride strips and dried, in which condition it could be stored at room temperature with no loss of activity for at least 6 months. In 27 comparisons with the DCC assay and 15 with sucrose gradients, they reported few major discrepancies. Nonetheless, the method as reported is not truly quantitative, in part, perhaps, because of the relatively low nonsaturating concentrations of both [^{3}H]estradiol (10^{-10} M) and competing nafoxidine ($\sim 2.5 \times 10^{-8}$ M). Both the rapidity and low tissue requirement of the procedure is attractive; one result was obtained in 4 hours using only 25 mg of tissue. The future of this specific antibody method is not yet clear.

3.2.6. Immunofluorescence

In an elegant study, Nenci and associates[177–179] were able to use antiestradiol antibody to localize estrogen receptor in cells from human breast tumors or other tissues. Cell suspensions were prepared, usually without the use of trypsin or collagenase, incubated with estradiol, dried in the cold on slides, and then treated first with rabbit antiestradiol antiserum and second with fluorescein-conjugated goat anti-rabbit-immunoglobulin antiserum. After washing, the cells could be stained to enhance cellular details and viewed under a fluorescence microscope. Many human breast cancer cells showed strong fluorescence, while non-target cells or breast cancer cells treated with an excess of nafoxidine, tamoxifen, or diethylstilbestrol together with the usual estradiol all failed to fluoresce. Some cells showed slight fluorescence even without estradiol addition, perhaps indicative of endogenous estradiol present in the tumor. Many tumors were extremely heterogeneous in the ability of cells to bind added estradiol. Even more striking, when incubated with estradiol in the cold, cells showed fluorescence only in the cytoplasm, whereas warming during or after the exposure to estradiol allowed translocation to the nuclei. In newborn rats, however, fluorescence accumulated at the periphery of the nuclei in distinctive rings rather than entering, as in older animals; the finding of a similar defective translocation in some breast cancer cells suggested a possible correlation with the reappearance of fetal or embryonic antigens and other dedifferentiated characteristics often observed in malignant cells.

One question arises from the comparison of this technique with the immobilized antibody procedure[173–176]: In the latter, estradiol bound to receptor is apparently not available to antibody, whereas the present method depends totally on this availability. A discussion between Nenci et al. and Jungblut at the presentation of one of their papers[178] suggested the explanation that estradiol may be released from the receptor during drying of the cells on the slide, thereby making the hormone accessible to the antibody. Diffusion apparently is not a problem under these conditions, but it must be considered in any proposed modification.

An independent proposal of a similar procedure has been made by Pertschuk.[180] His technique employs 4-μm sections rather than cell suspensions, and includes the novel use of polymerized estradiol phosphate rather than estradiol itself in order to enhance sensitivity. In a series of just over 100 breast cancer biopsies examined by this technique,[79] less than 5% were completely negative or completely positive. Comparison with a DCC assay showed that specimens with fewer than 10% positive cells by immunofluorescence were usually negative by DCC, while those with 10–20% positive cells tended to yield borderline DCC values. Eight of the specimens submitted for receptor assay showed no apparent tumor cells, a point which might not have been noticed using other techniques, and four (all from premenopausal patients) showed substantial fluorescence due to endogenous bound estrogens without addition of polyestradiol phosphate. No fluorescence was found in any tumor section if the competitor CI 628 was also present. Mercer et al.[181,182] used a similar method but with estradiol instead of polyestradiol phosphate. In a series of human breast cancers, 42% appeared wholly negative but only 10% showed essentially all positive cells; the remainder were mixed. Interestingly enough, in a group of DMBA-induced rat mammary tumors, the wholly positive tumors regressed and vanished after ovariectomy while the mixed tumors showed an incomplete response. It may be that the extremely variable quality of response and duration of remission found in human patients is at least partly due to this heterogeneity, as has been proposed on theoretical grounds. This group also found at least one case from a premenopausal woman in which all of the normal cells contained receptor while the malignant cells did not[183]; this case, which would have been considered positive by the usual techniques, illustrates the discriminatory power of this approach.

An immunoperoxidase method rather than fluorescent second antibody was used by Ghosh et al.[184] to reveal the binding of the antiestradiol antibody to human breast cancer sections. A greater variation is that of Lee,[185] who prepared an estradiol–albumin–fluorescein conjugate (the preparation is reported in detail) and incubated this conjugate with unfixed frozen sections to detect receptor binding. This study, like those discussed above, revealed highly heterogeneous populations of receptor-positive and receptor-negative cells in human breast tumors.

It is clear that these techniques hold promise of providing much more information than simply the presence or absence of receptor in a tumor specimen; the distribution of receptor among tumor cells and even its normal or abnormal translocation and intranuclear localization can also be examined. As a further advantage, extremely small amounts of tissue should be sufficient to obtain these results. It is not necessary to prepare a cell suspension, since results have also been demonstrated using thin sections of tissue. The principal disadvantage of these methods is the difficulty of quantitating the results in terms of receptor concentration. Nevertheless, the potential sensitivity and range of information available from these methods suggest great possibilities for further application.

3.2.7. Direct Radioimmunoassay

Radioimmunoassay using a specific antireceptor antibody would clearly provide a sensitive measure of receptor without the problems of plasma binding components, etc. Until now, such an assay has been impossible because of the lack of purified estrogen receptor which could serve as an antigen in preparing the antibody. Jensen's laboratory, however, has now developed a rabbit antibody to a highly purified calf uterine nuclear estrogen receptor.[186] The antibody cross-reacts with estrogen receptor from other sources including human breast cancer, but not with receptors for other steroids. Such an antibody could be used to confirm and extend the results obtained with antiestradiol antibody by immunofluorescence (discussed above) in addition to measuring receptor levels.

3.3. Nuclear Receptor

Up to the present, virtually all of the studies of estrogen receptor in human breast cancer tissue have focused on cytoplasmic receptor unoccupied by estradiol. Although exchange methods suitable for measuring filled cytoplasmic receptors have been noted,[136,159] most filled receptors are rapidly translocated to the nucleus, at least in normal cells.[135] It seems, then, that the finding of filled *nuclear* estrogen receptor in a tumor biopsy would provide considerable additional information: first, that the receptor system is intact at least to the point of translocation; second, that sufficient estrogen is present in the patient to be affecting tumor growth; and third, that the patient's tumor cannot be wrongly ruled receptor negative because all of its receptors are bound in the nuclei rather than being available for assay in the cytoplasm.[23,24] Nevertheless, there is evidence that most of the estrogen receptor which enters the nucleus is depleted relatively rapidly; this "processing" does not return receptor to the cytoplasm and therefore results in a net loss of total estrogen receptor from the cell,[187] although new receptor synthesis eventually replenishes the cytoplasmic levels. This means that nuclear receptor levels might never be very high, and may incidentally provide an explanation for the universal finding of lower average estrogen receptor levels in tumors from premenopausal women.

The first approach to determination of nuclear estrogen receptors was made by Anderson *et al.*[188] They incubated whole nuclei with 13 nM [³H]estradiol at 30°C for 1 hour to permit exchange, then washed the nuclei several times to remove unbound ligand and extracted the remainder with ethanol for counting. Though this technique made possible some very important studies in the rat uterus and other normal tissues, it has not had wide application to human tumors, partly perhaps because of a recently discovered proteolytic activity found in a large number of tumor nuclei.[189] However, a study by Laing *et al.*[190] did use incubation of crude breast tumor nuclei with [³H]estradiol at 4°C for 18 hours, claiming that these conditions allowed exchange and measured occupied nuclear estrogen receptor; they reported a rough correlation between cytoplasmic and nuclear receptor levels, with only 7% containing nuclear without detectable cytoplasmic receptor out of a total of 40% with nuclear receptor. Others have pointed out that their procedure almost certainly measured only unoccupied nuclear receptor, [191,192] whose presence agrees with the results of other studies to be discussed below.

The remaining approaches to measuring nuclear receptor require extraction of receptor from isolated nuclei with buffers containing at least 0.4 M KCl. (It should be noted that there are recent suggestions that the very small amount of nuclear receptor which appears to resist salt extraction may actually be the most significant in terms of function,[193,194] though others disagree.[195] This salt-resistant nuclear receptor has been reported to be associated with the nuclear matrix, a protein structure remaining behind after DNA, RNA, and nucleoplasmic and chromosonal proteins are removed from purified nuclei.[196]) Capony and Rochefort have exchanged such KCl nuclear extracts with [³H]estradiol at elevated temperature and then used dextran-coated charcoal to separate unbound ligand[197]; the possible dangers of using charcoal at high ionic strength have been mentioned previously,[132] and in any case this procedure has not been applied to human tumors. Panko and MacLeod,[192] however, did incubate KCl nuclear extracts with [³H]estradiol at 4°C for 4 hours, labeling unoccupied nuclear estrogen receptor sites without exchanging occupied sites. Free ligand was removed with dextran-coated charcoal before sucrose gradient centrifugation. Of 139 human breast cancer specimens, 29% contained significant unoccupied nuclear receptor; controls showed that neither cytoplasmic receptor nor occupied nuclear receptor seemed to contribute artifactually to this apparent unoccupied receptor.

In another approach, the protamine precipitation technique was modified by Zava et al.[198] for salt-extracted nuclear receptors of the rat uterus; the extract was first diluted, because salt concentrations of greater than 0.1 M interfere with receptor precipitation by protamine. Exchange was complete in 2.5 hours at 37°C with 2 nM [³H]estradiol, whereas virtually no exchange occurred at 4°C. Results were superior to those of the direct nuclear exchange in mature rat uterus, but unfortunately the protamine precipitation did not eliminate the proteolytic activity found in human tumor nuclear extracts.[189] Garola and McGuire[189,199] therefore used a similar tactic with hydroxylapatite, adsorbing receptor from the nuclear extract and washing before incubation with 5 nM [³H]estradiol (with or without 500 nM diethylstilbestrol) at 30°C for 5 hours. The protease effect was eliminated, and they showed that this one-point assay gave essentially identical results to multipoint assays with Scatchard plots using the same technique. They presented a preliminary series of 28 cases with values for free and occupied nuclear estrogen receptor and for cytoplasmic receptor; nuclear receptor was present in the majority of these, including a large amount of unoccupied nuclear receptor in some and a substantial excess of nuclear over cytoplasmic sites in several. Kiang found similar results using a variation of the protamine procedure, though details were not given.[191]

Finally, a novel technique has been presented by Hospelhorn et al.[200] for the total exchange of nuclear estrogen receptor at 2°C. The receptor is extracted with KNO₃ and bound estradiol is released by the action of $AgNO_3$ on the groups required for binding. These sulfhydryl groups are then rereduced by the addition of dithiothreitol, so that [³H]estradiol can be bound to the newly freed binding sites without ever raising the temperature to force exchange in the usual way. This interesting procedure has not yet been applied to human breast tumor nuclei.

4. Progesterone Receptor

The role of progesterone in the control of breast cancer still remains somewhat obscure; the subject has been reviewed recently.[201] Ellis et al. injected [³H]progesterone before breast biopsy and found no retention by the tumors, though similar experiments showed significant binding of [³H]estradiol.[11] Terenius[202] found charcoal-resistant [⁰H]progesterone binding in tumor cytosols, usually in cytosols that contained estrogen receptor, though the converse was not always true. Without a clearcut connection between progesterone receptor (PgR) and the regulation of tumor growth, there was little impetus to pursue the problems of this receptor vigorously.

The situation changed sharply when, with the finding that PgR levels in animal and human uteri are controlled by estrogen,[203-205] it was proposed that PgR might be used as a marker of estrogen responsiveness in human breast cancer.[25] Tumors that were being stimulated by estradiol should possess PgR, whereas those that were not should lack it, whether the failure was due to absence of estrogen receptor, absence of estrogen, or a breakdown of the response system. It was known that many tumors with estrogen receptor nevertheless failed to respond to endocrine treatment,[16] and the hope that PgR could distinguish with more certainty those tumors likely to respond to hormone therapy led quickly to a refinement of assay methods and the appearance of preliminary clinical correlations. Many of these were discussed at a recent published symposium.[206]

The assay of cytoplasmic PgR is beset with a number of problems. Progesterone has a high affinity for glucocorticoid receptor and for corticosteroid-binding globulin (CBG) as well as for PgR,[33] while its affinity for PgR itself, though high, is not high enough to prevent considerable dissociation during many of the procedures useful for estrogen receptor. Furthermore, the receptor itself is rather unstable, especially in the absence of ligand.

Terenius[202] attacked the specificity problem by including 6×10^{-8} M unlabeled cortisol in his incubations to block glucocorticoid receptor and CBG, and many have since followed this approach.[51,63,207-209] The affinity problem required a new ligand, a synthetic progestin which would bind PgR with higher affinity than progesterone itself while possessing little attraction to other binding proteins. Such a ligand was produced by Raynaud's group at Roussel-Uclaf.[210-212] Designated R5020, this compound revealed 7–8 S PgR on sucrose density gradients of human tumor cytosols,[213] which had not been consistently possible with [³H]progesterone. A number of laboratories have therefore employed [³H]-R5020, generously provided by Roussel-Uclaf and now also commercially available from New England Nuclear, in PgR assays. One disadvantage has been noted, however; although R5020 does not bind CBG, it has a higher affinity than progesterone for other serum binders including albumin.[209]

The actual assay techniques are variations on those generally used for estrogen receptor, primarily dextran-coated charcoal and sucrose density gradients. Buffers are pH 7.4–8.0 Tris or phosphate, always with a thiol reagent (thioglycerol, dithiothreitol, or mercaptoethanol), often with EDTA, and often with at least 10% glycerol. The importance of glycerol is just now being fully recognized, though earlier work with mouse, rat, and human uteri had shown that glycerol stabilizes [³H]progesterone binding.[214,215] Pichon and Milgrom[51] have now shown that glycerol greatly slows the dissociation of ligands, especially progesterone, from PgR of human breast cancer, so that even [³H]progesterone can reveal 8 S PgR peaks on glycerol gradients and 64% of tumors show specific PgR with DCC in 30% glycerol. Cortisol at 1 μM prevents binding to CBG or glucocorticoid receptor, while 30 minutes of agitation with DCC removes progesterone bound weakly to other proteins. Similar DCC procedures used by other laboratories take advantage of the properties of R5020 and omit these large concentrations of glycerol; LeClerq et al.[216] and Levy and Glick[217] take a number of [³H]-R5020 concentrations and construct Scatchard plots, while Raynaud et al.[63] have found 5 × 10⁻⁹ M [³H]-R5020 with 500-fold excess unlabeled R5020 as competitor to be satisfactory. (The last group also examined the effects of freezing: No more than 20% loss of PgR occurred if tumors were frozen in liquid nitrogen for 2 months, but 60% loss was experienced if tumors were stored at −40°C, and cytosol could not be successfully stored even in liquid nitrogen.) May-Levin et al.[218] have reported results with 379 human tumors using the last procedure. A different single-concentration method employed by Liskowski et al.[219] used [³H]progesterone as ligand and considered only the binding not competed with by norethindrone or medroxyprogesterone acetate (which do not bind CBG or glucocorticoid receptor) as PgR; unfortunately, less than 2 × 10⁻¹⁰ M [³H]progesterone was used, which is far less than saturating and probably explains the very low quantitative values reported.

Sucrose gradient procedures with [³H]-R5020 as ligand are used by several laboratories including our own.[207,213,220,221] A minor technical problem arises from the tendency of R5020 to stick to the cellulose nitrate tubes often used for sucrose gradients, necessitating a change to other tubes such as polyallomer. The presence of 7–8 S competible R5020 binding is specific for PgR.[213] This binding peak is often accompanied by competible 4 S binding, which may also represent PgR; the occasional appearance of 4 S competible R5020 binding in the absence of 8 S could possibly be due to PgR as well, but this point is in question.[221] The possibility that a considerable portion of the 8 S PgR-bound [³H]-R5020 dissociates during the usual 16-hour centrifugation, perhaps rebinding to plasma proteins in the 4 S region, has been investigated by Powell *et al.*[121] The use of a vertical-tube rotor[119] permitted centrifugation times of less than 2 hours, and, indeed, substantially more 8 S binding appeared with a comparable reduction in competible 4 S binding. Furthermore, nearly all of this 8 S but very little 4 S was adsorbed by hydroxylapatite, arguing that the latter may not represent true PgR.

The quantitative adsorption of PgR by hydroxylapatite was further used by Powell *et al.*[121] as the basis for another assay technique similar to that discussed earlier for estrogen receptor. A comparison of [³H]-R5020 binding in 27 human tumor cytosols using 8 S sucrose gradient, hydroxylapatite, and DCC techniques produced good correlations, though the authors felt that the 8 S sucrose gradient peak (vertical-tube-rotor technique) is still the most reliable measure of PgR.

Another technique used in estrogen receptor assays, the LH20 gel filtration method,[145] was applied to [³H]-R5020 binding to PgR in human breast cancer specimens in a careful study by Barnes *et al.*[67] The results were very well correlated with parallel analyses by DCC.

Other techniques, including isoelectric focusing, gel filtration, polyacrylamide gel electrophoresis, and ion exchange chromatography, have been applied to the measurement of cytoplasmic PgR in human uterus and endometrial carcinoma, though not in breast cancer.[222,223] The agar gel electrophoresis method as used for estrogen and androgen receptors does not normally separate PgR from CBG, but Wagner and Jungblut were able to effect this separation by first treating the cytosol with neuraminidase, which altered the mobility of CBG without injury to its binding properties or to PgR.[224] The modified procedure detected PgR in human uterus but not in breast cancer. Though interesting, none of these techniques appear to offer exceptional advantages.

Nuclear PgR has not been determined in human breast cancers, though progesterone-bound cytoplasmic PgR from human breast cancer or mouse uterus is fully exchanged by 5 nM [³H]-R5020 in 4 hours at 0°C.[63,225] In the rat uterus, however, exchange assays for PgR in nuclei have been developed. Clark's laboratory has replaced an earlier 5-hour

15°C exchange method[226] with one using 4°C; washed nuclei are incubated at 4°C for 18–24 hours with 20 nM [³H]-R5020 or [³H]progesterone in Tris buffer with 30% glycerol.[227,228] They note significant exchange even in 1 hour at 4°C, so that washing must be rapid. Milgrom et al.[229] use a very similar procedure with 10 nM [³H]-R5020 and 6 hours at 0°C. It is tempting to speculate that the apparently faster exchange in the latter study results from the use of 10% rather than 30% glycerol. Investigations of nuclear PgR in human mammary tumors will very likely appear soon.

5. Androgen Receptor

Androgen receptor has usually been assayed using [³H]-5α-dihydrotestosterone (DHT) as the ligand. The usual problems of binding to SHBG and to albumin occur, together with the relatively unexpected problem of DHT conversion to androstanediol even at 0°C by enzymes present in many cytosols.[230] Wagner's agar gel electrophoresis assay separates receptor-bound DHT from SHBG[148] and from the specific androgen-binding protein of epididymis,[231] though DHT may dissociate from albumin and remain in the receptor region of the gel.[232] A control for nonspecific binding is therefore necessary, and was at first provided by running a parallel aliquot of the cytosol in which receptor was denatured by heating at 45°C for 60 minutes. Later this heated extract was passed through 0.45-μm Millipore filters to remove microaggregates which could clog the agar gel pores, and still later the heated cytosol aliquot was replaced by one incubated with excess unlabeled competing steroid.[150] A short treatment with DCC prior to electrophoresis served to remove unbound [³H]-DHT and also most of that bound to albumin.[150,232]

Slightly varying versions of this agar gel electrophoresis technique have been used to measure androgen receptors in several series of human breast cancers[150,152,233–235]; it is the principal technique thus far used for this purpose. A surprising variation in results has appeared: Trams and Maass[152] and Wirtz et al.[234] found only about 20% of all mammary tumors to contain androgen receptor, whereas Persijn et al.[235] found about 40% to be positive, and Wagner et al.[150,233] report 50% or more. No explanation for the differences has appeared. Very preliminary results suggest that tumors with both estrogen and androgen receptor are more likely than those with estrogen receptor alone to respond to endocrine therapy,[152,235] but no obvious explanation has been offered and the results are as yet highly tentative.

The protamine sulfate precipitation assay separates androgen receptor from SHBG and also from the 3-ketoreductase responsible for metabolism of DHT. It has been used for androgen receptor in rat and human prostate tissues[236-238] and in cell lines derived from human breast cancers,[160,161] though not for the breast cancers themselves. An exchange assay for nuclear androgen receptor has been presented using protamine sulfate and [³H]-DHT at 15°C for 6 hours[238]; it has not been tested on breast cancer tissue.

A synthetic androgen has now been prepared by Roussel-Uclaf which may alleviate both nonreceptor binding and ligand metabolism problems. Designated R1881, or methyltrienolone, this compound is comparable to DHT in its affinity for androgen receptor while possessing very low attraction to serum binding proteins[239] and little metabolism. [³H]-R1881 is now available from New England Nuclear. In spite of its desirable properties, however, R1881 cannot be used for most androgen receptor measurements without blocking PgR, which also has a high affinity for R1881. Low concentrations of unlabeled R5020 have been used for this purpose,[240] but R5020 also binds weakly to the androgen receptor itself. The synthetic glucocorticoid triamcinolone acetonide is a better choice, since a 500-fold excess will efficiently block PgR without affecting [³H]-R1881 binding to androgen receptor.[241]

Though DCC does not remove [³H]-DHT from SHBG and is therefore not a good method for androgen receptor assays with DHT, R1881 is not subject to this problem. A series of specimens from Japanese breast cancer patients was therefore assayed with [³H]-R1881 by Ochi et al.,[240] employing a DCC method and constructing Scatchard plots. They report 36% of their samples to contain androgen receptor, and agree with Trams and Maass[152] but not with Persijn et al.[235] in finding a higher incidence of androgen receptor in those tumors with estrogen receptor. Correlations with response to therapy are not yet available in this series.

6. Glucocorticoid Receptor

Glucocorticoid receptor has been determined in one series of 122 human breast cancers by Fazekas and MacFarlane.[242] The ligand was 10^{-8} M [³H]dexamethasone, which has a considerably higher affinity for the receptor than does the native ligand cortisol but possesses little affinity for CBG.[243] A 100-fold excess of unlabeled dexamethasone was the competitor. Dextran-coated charcoal was used to separate bound and free steroid; the incubated cytosol was exposed to DCC for 20 minutes at 4°C with vigorous shaking. Only about 20% of the tumors contained glucocorticoid receptor by this assay, though most also contained a CBG-like cortisol binder which could not be accounted for by plasma contamination as determined by albumin assay. No information on endocrine therapy was available, though most of the glucocorticoid-receptor-positive tumors also contained estrogen receptor.

Another series of 142 has been examined by Allegra *et al.* Their preliminary report[244] does not present methods, but notes a 34% incidence of tumors with glucocorticoid receptor as compared with 44% for estrogen receptor. The presence of glucocorticoid receptor, like that of progesterone receptor, was correlated with the presence of estrogen receptor. Of 53 treatment trials in this group, the response rate for all cancers possessing estrogen receptor was 66%; the subgroups containing either progesterone or androgen receptor as well showed about the same rate, while the subgroup with both glucocorticoid and estrogen receptors experienced a 90% response rate. Although the series is far too small for any conclusions, accurate determination of glucocorticoid receptor in more breast cancer specimens will clearly be important.

Glucocorticoid receptor has also been assayed by a procedure very similar to that of Fazekas and MacFarlane[242] in cell lines derived from human breast cancer.[161,245] A gentler exposure to DCC than for estrogen receptor was recommended.[161] Growth of those cell lines which possessed glucocorticoid receptor seemed to be inhibited by glucocorticoid in the medium[245]; whether this finding can be extrapolated to human breast cancer patients has not been determined.

Finally, glucocorticoid receptor has also been demonstrated in two breast cancers by an agar gel electrophoresis procedure.[246] The problem of CBG noted earlier was again circumvented by use of [^{3}H]dexamethasone as the ligand.

7. Comments on Choice and Interpretation of Receptor Assays

With regard to cytoplasmic estrogen receptor assays, most workers have taken the lower detection limit of their assay as their cutoff point between receptor-positive and receptor-negative tumors. This often falls between 1 and 10 fmol/mg cytosol protein; in our own laboratory this limit of reliable detection is about 3 fmol/mg.[72] The percentage of tumors found to be positive by this criterion seems to be steadily increasing, leading LeClerq *et al.*[59] to hypothesize that all tumors in fact contain receptor, with only the quantity being variable. Indeed, none of the extensive series now available show evidence of two distinct tumor populations; instead, receptor levels seem to fall into a single log normal distribution whose lower ranges are just becoming defined with improving methodology.

Jensen *et al.*[109,110] approached this problem by redefining positive and negative in terms of a new, higher cutoff level. Because of the higher receptor levels generally found in postmenopausal women, the new cutoff for these cases was set much higher than for premenopausal women. By this criterion, patients with "receptor-rich" tumors experienced a 74% remission rate in Jensen's series of 98, whereas the enlarged "receptor-poor" and borderline groups together experienced only a 3% remission.

Rather than attempting to establish a single cutoff value, McGuire *et al.*[23] have grouped their patients according to receptor level and have shown that the probability of remission increases with increased receptor values. Heuson *et al.*[247] have reported similar observations and have even proposed a formula for computing the remission probability primarily from the receptor value, though other factors are included; based as it is on a relatively small number of cases, this formula will undoubtedly need refinement.

While discussing the value of quantitating receptor levels rather than merely classifying positive and negative tumors, one should also consider the nature of the *response* to endocrine therapy. Stoll, for instance, has argued that at least an additional 30% of patients receive considerable benefit from endocrine treatment without meeting all of the rigid criteria for an objective response,[248] and LeClerq and Heuson have suggested that since nearly all breast cancers appear to have some estrogen receptor and most patients may therefore receive some benefit, perhaps all should receive both endocrine and cytotoxic therapy, appropriately sequenced.[34]

Given the clear necessity for a quantitative rather than a merely qualitative evaluation of cytoplasmic estrogen receptor in human breast cancer specimens, has a "best" assay emerged? The answer must be negative. Some procedures, such as the tissue-slice technique, do not give truly quantitative results and may therefore be rejected for the future without negating the contribution they have already made. Of the established cytosol assays, all are quantitative given careful attention to conditions and to ligand and competitor selection and concentration, and all seem to give generally similar results when compared in the hands of those most experienced in the methods in question. Nevertheless, several more such comparisons of various methods on the same tumor cytosols are needed before even some of the established assays can be fully accepted as quantitatively equivalent, and of course those of the newer methods which seem to hold promise must be subjected to the same scrutiny. The remaining qualification must be simplicity and reliability, since ideally the procedure should be adaptable to inexpensive but accurate repetition in the clinical laboratory; probably the dextran-coated charcoal assay has been chosen more often than any other for these reasons. If possible, the amount of tissue required should also be reduced so that very small tumors and perhaps even needle biopsies can be assayed, and so that other receptor determinations can be performed on the remaining sample. Our recent demonstration that a one-point dextran-coated charcoal assay can be made quantitatively equivalent to more complex sucrose gradient procedures or multipoint charcoal methods[72] is a step in this direction, as is the hydroxylapatite microassay.[166]

In spite of this emphasis on quantitative estrogen receptor values, one should not ignore the rapidly emerging immunocytochemical techniques. Although these techniques do not provide an accurate value for average receptor concentration throughout the tumor specimen, they do provide important information on the percentage of receptor-containing cells and their distribution, on nuclear localization of receptor, and even on whether the receptor is concentrated in tumor cells or in normal epithelial cells also present in the sample. Also, very little tissue is required, so that perhaps one of these techniques can be combined with one of the quantitative assays to provide a complete qualitative and quantitative picture of the estrogen receptor status of the tumor.

With regard to "best" assays for nuclear estrogen receptor and for other steroid receptors, even less can be said. In some cases a number of assays appear to give similar results and may therefore be considered reliable, but the number of such quantitative comparisons is small, and in any case newer and perhaps more informative assays requiring less tissue may well replace those now in use. Careful selection of ligand, competitors, concentrations, and separation methods will always be required. Given reliable assays, the same qualitative and quantitative considerations discussed above for cytoplasmic estrogen receptor will probably become relevant. Only with such rigorous and quantitative approach will further understanding of steroid receptors and their relationship to hormone dependence in breast cancer be attainable.

ACKNOWLEDGMENTS: This work was supported by grants from the National Institutes of Health (CA-22343, CA-11378, CB-23862, and P30-HD-10202) and the American Cancer Society (BC-23).

8. References

1. G. T. Beatson, On the treatment of inoperable cases of carcinoma of the mamma: Suggestions for a new method of treatment with illustrative cases, *Lancet* **2**, 104–107; 162–165 (1896).

2. C. Huggins and D. M. Bergenstal, Inhibition of human mammary and prostatic cancers by adrenalectomy, *Cancer Res.* **12**, 134–141 (1951).

3. R. F. Glascock and W. G. Hoekstra, Selective accumulation of tritium-labeled hexoestrol by the reproductive organs of immature female goats and sheep, *Biochem. J.* **72**, 673–682 (1959).

4. E. V. Jensen and H. I. Jacobson, Fate of steroid estrogens in target tissues, in: *Biological Activities of Steroids in Relation to Cancer* (G. Pincus and E. P. Vollmer, eds.). pp. 161–178, Academic Press, New York (1960).

5. E. V. Jensen and H. I. Jacobson, Basic guides to the mechanism of estrogen action, *Recent Prog. Horm. Res.* **18**, 387–414 (1962).

6. P. J. Folca, R. F. Glascock, and W. T. Irvine, Studies with tritium-labeled hexoestrol in advanced breast cancer, *Lancet* **2**, 796–802 (1961).

7. J. A. Demetriou, L. G. Crowley, S. Kushinsky, A. J. Donovan, P. Kotin, and I. MacDonald, Radioactive estrogens in tissues of postmenopausal women with breast neoplasms, *Cancer Res.* **24**, 926–934 (1964).

8. N. Deshpande, V. Jensen, and R. D. Bulbrook, Accumulation of tritiated oestradiol by human breast tissue, *Steroids* **10**, 219–232 (1967).

9. H. Braunsberg, W. T. Irvine, and V. H. T. James, A comparison of steroid hormone concentrations in human tissues including breast cancer, *Br. J. Cancer* **21**, 714–729 (1967).

10. W. H. Pearlman, R. DeHertogh, K. R. Laumas, and M. R. J. Pearlman, Metabolism and tissue uptake of estrogen in women with advanced carcinoma of the breast, *J. Clin. Endocrinol.* **29**, 707–720 (1969).

11. F. G. Ellis, T. V. Berne, N. Deshpande, F. O. Belzer, and R. D. Bulbrook, The uptake of tritiated steroids by human breast carcinoma, *Surg. Gynecol. Obstet.* **28**, 975–984 (1969).

12. F. James, V. H. T. James, A. E. Carter, and W. T. Irvine, A comparison of *in vivo* and *in vitro* uptake of estradiol by human breast tumors and the relationship to steroid excretion, *Cancer Res.* **31**, 1268–1272 (1971).

13. D. O. Toft and J. Gorski, A receptor molecule for estrogens: Isolation from the rat uterus and preliminary characterization, *Proc. Natl. Acad. Sci. U.S.A.* **55**, 1574–1581 (1966).

14. E. V. Jensen, E. R. DeSombre, and P. W. Jungblut, Estrogen receptors in hormone-responsive tissues and tumors, in: *Endogenous Factors Influencing Host–Tumor Balance* (R. W. Wissler, T. L. Dao, and S. Wood Jr., eds.). pp 15–30, University of Chicago Press, Chicago (1967).

15. E. V. Jensen, G. E. Block, S. Smith, K. Kyser, and E. R. DeSombre, Estrogen receptors and breast cancer response to adrenalectomy, *Natl. Cancer Inst. Monogr.* **34**, 55–70 (1971).

16. W. L. McGuire, E. P. Vollmer, and P. P. Carbone (eds.), *Estrogen Receptors in Human Breast Cancer*, Raven Press, New York (1975).

17. E. V. Jensen and E. R. DeSombre, Estrogen-receptor interaction, *Science* **182**, 126–134 (1973).

18. B. W. O'Malley and A. R. Means, Female steroid hormones and target cell nuclei, *Science* **183**, 610–620 (1974).

19. J. Gorski and F. Gannon, Current models of steroid hormone action: A critique, *Annu. Rev. Physiol.* **38**, 425–450 (1976).

20. K. R. Yamamoto and B. M. Alberts, Steroid receptors: Elements for modulation of eukaryotic transcription, *Annu. Rev. Biochem.* **45**, 721–746 (1976).

21. E. V. Jensen, T. Suzuki, T. Kawashima, W. E. Stumpf, P. W. Jungblut, and E. R. DeSombre, A two-step mechanism for the interaction of estradiol with rat uterus, *Proc. Natl. Acad. Sci. U.S.A.* **59**, 632–638 (1968).

22. J. Gorski, D. O. Toft, G. Shyamala, D. Smith, and A. Notides, Studies on the interaction of estrogen with the uterus, *Rec. Prog. Horm. Res.* **24**, 45–80 (1968).

23. W. L. McGuire, K. B. Horwitz, D. T. Zava, R. E. Garola, and G. C. Chamness, Hormones in breast cancer—update 1978, *Metabolism* **27**, 487–501 (1978).

24. P. W. Jungblut, A. Hughes, W. Sierralta, and R. K. Wagner, A proposal for assessment of hormone sensitivity and consequent endocrine therapy of breast cancer, *Eur. J. Cancer* **13**, 1201–1202 (1977).

25. K. B. Horwitz, W. L. McGuire, O. H. Pearson, and A. Segaloff, Predicting response to endocrine therapy in human breast cancer: A hypothesis, *Science* **189**, 726–727 (1975).

26. S. G. Korenman, Estrogen receptor assay in human breast cancer, *J. Natl. Cancer Inst.* **55**, 543–545 (1975).

27. R. J. B. King, Clinical relevance of steroid-receptor measurements in tumours, *Cancer Treat. Rev.* **2**, 273–293 (1975).

28. J. L. Wittliff, Steroid binding proteins in normal and neoplastic mammary cells in: *Methods in Cancer Research* (H. Busch, ed.), Vol. 11, pp. 293–354, Academic Press, New York (1975).

29. W. L. McGuire, G. C. Chamness, M. E. Costlow, and K. B. Horwitz, Hormone receptors in breast cancer, in: *Hormone–Receptor Interaction: Molecular Aspects (Modern Pharmacology–Toxicology*, Vol. 9), (G. S. Levey, ed.), pp. 265–299, Marcel Dekker, New York (1976).

30. K. M. Menon and J. R. Reel (eds.), *Steroid Hormone Action and Cancer (Current Topics in Molecular Endocrinology*, Vol. 4), Plenum Press, New York (1976).

31. J. C. Heuson, W. H. Mattheiem, and M. Rozencweig, eds., *Breast Cancer: Trends in Research and Treatment*, Raven Press, New York (1976).

32. E. E. Baulieu, M. Atger, M. Best-Belpomme, P. Corvol, J. Courvalin, J. Mester, E. Milgrom, P. Robel, H. Rochefort, and D. deCatalogne, Steroid hormone receptors, *Vitam. Horm. (N.Y.)* **33**, 649–736 (1975).

33. R. J. B. King and W. I. P. Mainwaring, *Steroid–Cell Interactions*, University Park Press, Baltimore (1974).

34. G. LeClercq and J. C. Heuson, Therapeutic significance of sex-steroid hormone receptors in the treatment of breast cancer, *Eur. J. Cancer*, **13**, 1205–1215 (1977).

35. E. B. Thompson and M. E. Lippman (eds.), *Steroid Receptors and the Management of Cancer*, CRC, Cleveland (1978).

36. H. Maass, B. Engle, H. Nowakowski, G. Stolzenbach and G. Trams, Estrogen receptors in human breast cancer and clinical correlations, in: *Estrogen Receptors in Human Breast Cancer* (W. L. McGuire, E. P. Vollmer, and P. P. Carbone, eds.), pp. 175–191, Raven Press, New York (1975).

37. T. Ratajczak and R. Hähnel, Estradiol receptors: Influence of plasma proteins on detection and quantitation, *J. Steroid Biochem.* **7**, 741–744 (1976).

38. H. Braunsberg, The determination of high affinity oestrogen receptors in human breast tumours: Critique of a method approved by the EORTC breast cancer cooperative group, *Eur. J. Cancer* **11**, 101–103 (1975).

39. J. H. Clark, E. J. Peck, Jr., W. T. Schrader, and B. W. O'Malley, Estrogen and progesterone receptors: Methods for characterization, quantification, and purification, in: *Methods in Cancer Research* (H. Busch, ed.), Vol. 12, pp. 367–417, Academic Press, New York (1976).

40. G. Scatchard, The attractions of proteins for small molecules and ions, *Ann. N.Y. Acad. Sci.* **51**, 600–672 (1949).

41. G. C. Chamness and W. L. McGuire, Scatchard plots: Common errors in correction and interpretation, *Steroids* **26**, 538–542 (1975).

42. D. Rodbard, mathematics of hormone–receptor interaction. I. Basic principles, *Adv. Exp. Med. Biol.* **36**, 289–326 (1973).

43. E. E. Baulieu and J. P. Raynaud, A "proportion graph" method for measuring binding systems, *Eur. J. Biochem.* **13**, 293–304 (1970).

44. H. Richard-Foy, G. Redeuilh, and R. Richard-Foy, A simple, rapid and precise method for calculating the steroid hormone–receptor complex concentration in the presence of saturating levels of hormone by using "differential dissociation" techniques, *Anal. Biochem.* **88**, 367–381 (1978).

45. H. Rochefort and F. Capony, Estradiol dependent decrease of binding inhibition by antiestrogens (a possible test of receptor activation), *Biochem. Biophys. Res. Commun.* **75**, 277–285 (1977).

46. G. Azadian-Boulanger and D. Bertin, Synthèse et activité utérotrophique du 11β-méthoxy estradiol, 11β-méthoxy estriol et 11β-méthoxy-17α-éthynyl estradiol, *Chim. Ther.* **8**, 451–454 (1973).

47. J. P. Raynaud, M. M. Bouton, D. Gallet-Bourquin, D. Philibert, C. Tournemine, and G. Azadian-Boulanger, Comparative study of estrogen action, *Mol. Pharmacol.* **9**, 520–533 (1973).

48. H. Rochefort and M. Garcia, Androgens on the estrogen receptor. II. Correlation between nuclear translocation and uterine protein synthesis, *Steroids* **29**, 111–125 (1977).

49. D. T. Zava and W. L. McGuire, Androgen action through estrogen receptor in a human breast cancer cell line, *Endocrinology* **103**, 624–631 (1978).

50. T. S. Ruh, S. G. Wassilak, and M. F. Ruh, Androgen-induced nuclear accumulation of the estrogen receptor, *Steroids* **25**, 257–273 (1975).

51. M. F. Pichon and E. Milgrom, Characterization and assay of progesterone receptor in human mammary carcinoma, *Cancer Res.* **37**, 464–471 (1977).

52. B. G. Mobbs, I. E. Johnson, J. B. Connolly, and A. F. Clark, Androgen receptor assay in human benign and malignant prostatic tumor cytosol using protamine sulphate precipitation, *J. Steroid Biochem.* **9**, 289–301 (1978).

53. H. Eriksson, S. Upchurch, J. W. Hardin, E. J. Peck, Jr., and J. H. Clark, Heterogeneity of estrogen receptors in the cytosol and nuclear fractions of the rat uterus, *Biochem. Biophys. Res. Commun.* **81**, 1–7 (1978).

54. F. Sakai and S. Saez, Existence of receptors bound to endogenous estradiol in breast cancers of premenopausal and postmenopausal women, *Steroids* **27**, 99–110 (1976).

55. J. Fishman, J. S. Nisselbaum, C. J. Mendendez-Botet, and M. K. Schwartz, Estrone and estradiol content in human breast tumors: Relationship to estradiol receptors, *J. Steroid Biochem.* **8**, 893–896 (1977).

56. S. Saez, P. M. Martin, and C. D. Chouvet, Estradiol and progesterone receptor levels in human breast adenocarcinoma in relation to plasma estrogen and progesterone levels, *Cancer Res.* **38**, 3468–3473 (1978).

57. E.O.R.T.C. Breast Cancer Cooperative Group, Standards for the assessment of estrogen receptors in human breast cancer, *Eur. J. Cancer* **9**, 379–381 (1973).

58. P. W. Brown, R. J. Witorsch, L. W. Banks, Jr., and W. Lawrence, Jr., Freezing and storage of breast cancer tissue for estrogen receptor protein assay: A convenient method, *Arch. Surg.* **112**, 183–185 (1977).

59. G. LeClerq, J. C. Heuson, M. C. DeBoel and W. H. Mattheiem, Oestrogen receptors in breast cancer: A changing concept, *Br. Med. J.* **1**, 185–189 (1975).

60. R. Hähnel, E. Twaddle, and A. B. Vivian, Estrogen receptors in human breast cancer. 2. *In vitro* binding of estradiol by benign and malignant tumors, *Steroids* **18**, 681–708 (1971).

61. A. Singhakowinta, R. Mohindra, S. C. Brooks, V. K. Vaitkevicius, and M. J. Brennan, Clinical correlation of endocrine therapy and estrogen receptor, in: *Estrogen Receptors*

in Human Breast Cancer (W. L. McGuire, E. P. Vollmer and P. P. Carbone, eds.), pp. 131–155, Raven Press, New York (1975).

62. J. L. Wittliff and E. D. Savlov, Estrogen-binding capacity of cytoplasmic forms of the estrogen receptors in human breast cancer, in: *Estrogen Receptors in Human Breast Cancer* (W. L. McGuire, E. P. Vollmer, and P. P. Carbone, eds.), pp. 73–91, Raven Press, New York (1975).

63. J. P. Raynaud, T. Ojasoo, J. C. Delarue, H. Magdelenat, P. Martin, and D. Philibert, Estrogen and progestin receptors in human breast cancer, in: *Progesterone Receptors in Normal and Neoplastic Tissues (Progress in Cancer Research and Therapy,* Vol. 4) (W. L. McGuire, J. P. Raynaud, and E. E. Baulieu, eds.), pp. 171–191, Raven Press, New York (1977).

64. A. Pihl, S. Sander, I. Brennhovd, and S. Olsnes, Predictive value of estrogen receptors in human breast cancers, in: *Estrogen Receptors in Human Breast Cancer* (W. L. McGuire, E. P. Vollmer, and P. P. Carbone, eds.), pp. 193–203, Raven Press, New York (1975).

65. R. B. Johnson and R. M. Nakamura, Improved estrogen receptor assay in human mammary cancer. Techniques for handling small tissue samples, *Am. J. Clin. Pathol.* **67,** 444–449 (1977).

66. Z. Chester, P. Feherty, A. E. Kellie, and D. N. L. Ralphs, Estrogen receptors in primary breast tumors in relation to the stage and progression of the disease, in: *Estrogen Receptors in Human Breast Cancer* (W. L. McGuire, E. P. Vollmer, and P. P. Carbone, eds.), pp. 157–174, Raven Press, New York (1975).

67. D. M. Barnes, G. G. Ribeiro, and L. G. Skinner, Two methods for measurement of oestradiol-17-beta and progesterone receptors in human breast cancer and correlation with response treatment, *Eur. J. Cancer* **13,** 1133–1143 (1977).

68. T. Ratajczak and R. Hähnel, The protection, stabilization, and reactivation of estradiol receptors in human myometrial cytosol, *Biochim. Biophys. Acta* **338,** 104–107 (1974).

69. H. Braunsberg, Factors influencing the estimation of oestrogen receptors in human malignant breast tumors, *Eur. J. Cancer* **11,** 499–507 (1975).

70. N. E. Good, G. D. Winget, W. Winter, T. N. Connolly, S. Izawa, and R. M. M. Singh, Hydrogen ion buffers for biological research, *Biochemistry* **5,** 467–477 (1966).

71. R. Hähnel, Properties of the estrogen receptor in the soluble fraction of human uterus, *Steroids* **17,** 105–132 (1971).

72. W. L. McGuire, M. de la Garza, and G. C. Chamness, Evaluation of estrogen receptor assays in human breast cancer tissue, *Cancer Res.* **37,** 637–639 (1977).

73. E. V. Jensen, D. J. Hurst, E. R. DeSombre, and P. W. Jungblut, Sulfhydryl groups and estradiol–receptor interaction, *Science* **158,** 385–387 (1967).

74. L. Terenius, SH-groups essential for estrogen uptake and retention in the mouse uterus, *Mol. Pharmacol.* **3,** 423–428 (1967).

75. H. Braunsberg, E. Killen, and S. G. Richardson, The effect of thiols on oestradiol binding by components of human malignant breast tumours, *Biochem. J.* **130,** 38P (1972).

76. W. L. McGuire and M. de la Garza, Improved sensitivity in the measurement of estrogen receptor in human breast cancer, *J. Clin. Endocrinol. Metab.* **37,** 986–989 (1973).

77. R. Hähnel and A. B. Vivian, Estrogen receptors and prognosis in cancer of the breast, in: *Estrogen Receptors in Human Breast Cancer* (W. L. McGuire, E. P. Vollmer, and P. P. Carbone, eds.), pp. 205–235, Raven Press, New York (1975).

78. R. A. Hawkins, A. Hill, B. Freedman, S. M. Gore, M. M. Roberts, and A. P. Forrest, Reproducibility of measurements of oestrogen-receptor concentration in breast cancer, *Br. J. Cancer* **36,** 355–361 (1977).

79. L. P. Pertschuk, E. H. Tobin, D. J. Brigatti, D. S. Kim, N. D. Bloom, E. Gaetjens, P. J. Berman, A. C. Carter, and G. A. Degenschein, Immunofluorescent detection of estrogen receptors in breast cancer, *Cancer* **41**, 907–911 (1978).

80. K. A. Kyser, *The Tissue, Subcellular and Molecular Binding of Estradiol to Dimethylbenzanthracene-Induced Rat Mammary Tumor*, Ph.D. thesis, Department of Physiology, University of Chicago, Chicago (1970).

81. R. A. Hawkins, A. Hill, and B. Freedman, A simple method for the determination of oestrogen receptor concentrations in breast tumors and other tissues, *Clin. Chim. Acta* **64**, 203–210 (1975).

82. J. P. Van Netten, F. T. Algard, G. Montessori, and B. Weare, Electrophoretic assay of specific estrogen receptors: A contribution to methodology, *Clin. Chem.* **23**, 2059–2065 (1977).

83. M. Little, P. Szendro, C. Teran, A. Hughes, and P. W. Jungblut, Biosynthesis and transformation of microsomal and cytosol estradiol receptors, *J. Steroid Biochem.* **6**, 493–500 (1975).

84. R. Hähnel and E. Twaddle, Estradiol binding by human breast carcinoma cytosols: The influence of commonly used reference parameters on the results, *Eur. J. Cancer* **14**, 125–131 (1978).

85. J. R. Masters, R. A. Hawkins, K. Sangster, W. Hawkins, I. I. Smith, A. A. Shivas, M. M. Roberts, and A. P. Forrest, Oestrogen receptors, cellularity, elastosis and menstrual status in human breast cancer, *Eur. J. Cancer* **14**, 303–307 (1978).

86. B. G. Mobbs and I. E. Johnson, *In vitro* estrogen-binding by human breast carcinomas, *Can. Med. Assoc. J.* **114**, 216–219 (1976).

87. K. Burton, A study of the conditions and mechanism of the diphenylamine reaction for the colorimetric estimation of deoxyribonucleic acid, *Biochem. J.* **62**, 315–323 (1956).

88. R. W. Hubbard, W. T. Matthew, and D. A. Dubowik, Factors affecting the determination of DNA with indole, *Anal. Biochem.* **38**, 190–201 (1970).

89. W. J. Waddell, A simple ultraviolet spectrophotometer method for the determination of protein, *J. Lab. Clin. Med.* **48**, 311–314 (1956).

90. O. H. Lowry, N. J. Rosebrough, A. L. Farr, and R. J. Randall, Protein measurement with the Folin phenol reagent, *J. Biol. Chem.* **193**, 265–275 (1951).

91. C. G. Vallejo and R. Lagunas, Interferences by sulfhydryl, disulfide reagents, and potassium ions on protein determination by Lowry's method, *Anal. Biochem.* **36**, 207–212 (1970).

92. P. J. Geiger and S. P. Bessman, Protein determination by Lowry's method in the presence of sulfhydryl reagents, *Anal. Biochem.* **49**, 467–473 (1972).

93. G. Mancini, O. A. Carbonara, and J. F. Heremans, Immunochemical quantitation of antigens by single radial immunodiffusion, *Immunochemistry* **2**, 235–254 (1965).

94. S. Sander, The *in vitro* uptake of estradiol in biopsies from 25 breast cancer patients, *Acta Pathol. Microbiol. Scand.* **74**, 301–302 (1968).

95. H. Maass, B. Engel, H. Hohmeister, F. Lehmann, and G. Trams, Estrogen receptors in human breast cancer tissue, *Am. J. Obstet. Gynecol.* **113**, 377–382 (1972).

96. H. Johansson, L. Terenius, and L. Thoren, The binding of estradiol-17β to human breast cancers and other tissues *in vitro*, *Cancer Res.* **30**, 692–698 (1970).

97. A. F. Hoge, J. M. Hartsuck, G. M. Kollmorgen, and J. A. Schilling, Endocrine and immunologic studies in breast cancer, *Am. J. Surg.* **126**, 722–728 (1973).

98. E. V. Jensen, G. E. Block, S. Smith, and E. R. DeSombre, Hormonal dependency of breast cancer, *Recent Results Cancer Res.* **42**, 55–62 (1973).

99. H. Maass, B. Engel, G. Trams, H. Nowakowski, and G. Stolzenbach, Steroid hormone receptors in human breast cancer and the clinical significance, *J. Steroid Biochem.* **6**, 743–749 (1975).

100. L. Terenius, A. Rimsten, L. Thoren, and A. Lindgren, Estrogen receptors and prognosis in cancer of the breast, in: *Estrogen Receptors in Human Breast Cancer* (W. L. McGuire, E. P. Vollmer, and P. P. Carbone, eds.), pp. 237–245, Raven Press, New York (1975).

101. W. L. McGuire, Estrogen receptors in human breast cancer, *J. Clin. Invest.* **52**, 73–77 (1973).

102. E. S. Boylan and J. L. Wittliff, Specific estrogen binding *in vivo* in the R3230AC mammary adenocarcinoma of the rat, *Cancer Res.* **33**, 2903–2908 (1973).

103. R. G. Martin and B. N. Ames, A method for determining the sedimentation behavior of enzymes: Application to protein mixtures, *J. Biol. Chem.* **236**, 1372–1379 (1961).

104. G. C. Chamness and W. L. McGuire, Estrogen receptor in the rat uterus: Physiological forms and artifacts, *Biochemistry* **11**, 2466–2472 (1972).

105. I. Reti and T. Erdos, On the "native state" of the uterine estradiol "receptor," *Biochimie* **53**, 435–437 (1971).

106. J. L. Wittliff, R. Hilf, W. F. Brooks, Jr., E. D. Savlov, T. C. Hall, and R. A. Orlando, Specific estrogen-binding capacity of the cytoplasmic receptor in normal and neoplastic breast tissues of humans, *Cancer Res.* **32**, 1983–1992 (1972).

107. U. Spaeren, S. Olsnes, I. Brennhovd, J. Efskind, and A. Pihl, Content of estrogen receptors in human breast cancer, *Eur. J. Cancer* **9**, 353–357 (1973).

108. W. L. McGuire, O. H. Pearson, and A. Segaloff, Predicting hormone responsiveness in human breast cancer, in: *Estrogen Receptors in Human Breast Cancer* (W. L. McGuire, E. P. Vollmer, and P. P. Carbone, eds.), pp. 17–30, Raven Press, New York (1975).

109. E. V. Jensen, T. Z. Polley, S. Smith, G. E. Block, D. J. Ferguson, and E. R. DeSombre, Prediction of hormone dependency in human breast cancer, in: *Estrogen Receptors in Human Breast Cancer* (W. L. McGuire, E. P. Vollmer, and P. P. Carbone, eds.), pp. 37–56, Raven Press, New York (1975).

110. E. V. Jensen, S. Smith, and E. R. DeSombre, Hormone dependency in breast cancer, *J. Steroid Biochem.* **7**, 911–917 (1976).

111. E. D. Savlov, J. L. Wittliff, and R. Hilf, Further studies of biochemical predictive tests in breast cancer, *Cancer* **39**, 539–541 (1977).

112. S. L. Schneider and T. L. Dao, Effect of Ca^{2+} and salt on forms of estradiol cytoplasmic receptor in human neoplastic breast tissue, *Cancer Res.* **37**, 382–387 (1977).

113. A. W. Steggles and R. J. B. King, The use of protamine to study 6,7-³H: oestradiol-17β binding in rat uterus, *Biochem. J.* **118**, 695–701 (1970).

114. B. K. Vonderhaar, U. H. Kim, and G. C. Mueller, The heterogeneity of soluble estrogen receptors from rat uteri and their modification by temperature, imidazole compounds and estradiol, *Biochim. Biophys. Acta* **208**, 517–527 (1970).

115. D. Toft, The interaction of uterine receptors with DNA, *J. Steroid Biochem.* **3**, 512–522 (1972).

116. J. M. Sala-Trepat and C. Vallet-Strouve, Binding of the estradiol receptor from calf uterus to the chromatin: Active forms, *Biochim. Biophys. Acta* **371**, 186–202 (1974).

117. D. T. Kiang and B. J. Kennedy, Estrogen receptor assay in the differential diagnosis of adrenocarcinomas, *J. Am. Med. Assoc.* **238**, 32–34 (1977).

118. H. Bojar, J. L. Wittliff, K. Balzer, R. Dreyfürst, F. Boeminghaus, and W. Staib, Properties of specific estrogen-binding components in human kidney and renal carcinoma, *Acta Endocrinol. (Copenhagen) Suppl.* **193**, 51 (1975).

119. O. M. Griffith, Rapid density gradient centrifugation using short column techniques, *Anal. Biochem.* **90**, 435–443 (1978).

120. V. C. Jordan and G. Prestwich, Binding of [³H]tamoxifen in rat uterine cytosols: A comparison of swinging bucket and vertical tube rotor sucrose density gradient analysis, *Mol. Cell. Endocrinol.* **8**, 179–188 (1977).

121. B. Powell, R. E. Garola, G. C. Chamness, and W. L. McGuire, Measurement of progesterone receptor in human breast cancer biopsies, *Cancer Res.* (in press).

122. S. G. Korenman, Radio-ligand binding assay of specific estrogens using a soluble uterine macromolecule, *J. Clin. Endocrinol. Metab.* **28,** 127–130 (1968).

123. S. G. Korenman and B. A. Dukes, Specific estrogen binding by the cytoplasm of human breast carcinoma, *J. Clin. Endocrinol. Metab.* **30,** 639–645 (1970).

124. P. Feherty, G. Farrer-Brown, and A. E. Kellie, Oestradiol receptors in carcinoma and benign disease of the breast: An *in vitro* assay, *Br. J. Cancer* **25,** 697–710 (1971).

125. R. Hähnel and E. Twaddle, Estrogen receptors in human breast cancer. 1. Methodology and characterization of receptors, *Steroids* **18,** 653–680 (1971).

126. C. B. Korsten and J. P. Persijn, Simple assay for estrogen-binding capacity in human mammary tumors, *Z. Klin. Chem. Klin. Biochem.* **10,** 502–508 (1972).

127. G. LeClerq, J. C. Heuson, R. Schoenfeld, W. H. Mattheiem, and H. J. Tagnon, Estrogen receptors in human breast cancer, *Eur. J. Cancer* **9,** 665–673 (1973).

128. B. S. Leung, W. S. Fletcher, T. D. Lindell, D. C. Wood, and W. W. Krippaehne, Predictability of response to endocrine ablation in advanced breast carcinoma, *Arch. Surg.* **106,** 515–519 (1973).

129. Y. Nomura, Estrogen receptor in breast cancer of the Japanese, *Gann* **67,** 703–711 (1976).

130. P. P. Rosen, C. J. Menendez-Botet, J. S. Nisselbaum, J. A. Urban, V. Miké, A. Fracchia, and M. K. Schwartz, Pathological review of breast lesions analyzed for estrogen receptor protein, *Cancer Res.* **35,** 3187–3194 (1975).

131. C. B. Korsten and J. P. Persijn, Evaluation of and additional data on an improved simple charcoal method to determine oestrogen receptors, *J. Clin. Chem. Clin. Biochem.* **15,** 297–301 (1977).

132. E. J. Peck, Jr. and J. H. Clark, Effect of ionic strength on charcoal adsorption assays of receptor–estradiol complexes, *Endocrinology* **101,** 1034–1043 (1977).

133. E. E. Baulieu, A. Alberga, I. Jung, M. C. LeBeau, C. Mercier-Rodbard, E. Milgrom, J. P. Raynaud, C. Raynaud-Jammet, H. Rochefort, H. Truong, and P. Robel, Metabolism and protein binding of sex steroids in target organs: An approach to the mechanism of hormone action, *Recent Prog. Horm. Res.* **27,** 351–419 (1971).

134. E. Milgrom, M. Perrot, M. Atger, and E. E. Baulieu, Progesterone in uterus and plasma: V. An assay of the progesterone cytosol receptor of the guinea pig uterus, *Endocrinology* **90,** 1064–1070 (1972).

135. D. Williams and J. Gorski, Kinetic and equilibrium analysis of estradiol in uterus: A model of binding-site distribution in uterine cells, *Proc. Natl. Acad. Sci. U.S.A.* **69,** 3464–3468 (1972).

136. J. A. Katzenellenbogen, H. J. Johnson, Jr., and K. E. Carlson, Studies on the uterine, cytoplasmic estrogen binding protein. Thermal stability and ligand dissociation rate. An assay of empty and filled sites by exchange, *Biochemistry* **12,** 4092–4099 (1973).

137. V. C. Godefroi and S. C. Brooks, Improved gel-filtration method for analysis of estrogen receptor binding, *Anal. Biochem.* **51,** 335–344 (1973).

138. A. Singhakowinta, H. G. Potter, T. R. Buroker, B. Samal, S. C. Brooks, and V. K. Vaitkevecius, Estrogen receptor and natural course of breast cancer, *Ann. Surg.* **183,** 84–88 (1976).

139. P. W. Jungblut, S. Hughes, A. Hughes, and R. K. Wagner, Evaluation of various methods for the assay of cytoplasmic oestrogen receptors in extracts of calf uteri and human breast cancers, *Acta Endocrinol. (Copenhagen)* **70,** 185–195 (1972).

140. R. E. Gore-Langton, M. J. Ashwood-Smith, F. T. Algard, and J. P. van Netten, A thin-layer gel filtration assay of cytoplasmic oestrogen receptors. A possible screening method for hormone dependent tumours, *Br. J. Cancer* **28,** 310–315 (1973).

141. M. Töpert, I. Zabel, and M. Ziegler, Thin layer gel filtration as a method for routine steroid receptor binding studies, *Anal. Biochem.* **62**, 514–522 (1974).

142. J. F. Kapp, H. Koch, J. Casals-Stenzel, M. Töpert, and E. Gerhards, Untersuchungen zur Pharmakologie von 6α,9-Difluor-11β-hydroxy-16-methyl-21-valeryloxy-1,4-pregnadien-3,20-dion (Diflucortolon valerianat), *Arzneim. Forsch.* **26**, 1463–1475 (1976).

143. C. Cochet, M. Chedin, and E. Chambaz, Characterization of steroid-binding macromolecules in small biological samples by a rapid minigel filtration method, *Anal. Biochem.* **76**, 351–357 (1976).

144. V. Sica, E. Nola, G. A. Puca, and F. Bresciani, Estrogen binding proteins of calf uterus. Inhibition of aggregation and dissociation of receptor by chemical perturbation with NaSCN, *Biochemistry* **15**, 1915–1923 (1976).

145. M. Ginsburg, B. D. Greenstein, N. J. Maclusky, I. D. Morris, and P. J. Thomas, An improved method for the study of high-affinity steroid binding: Oestradiol binding in brain and pituitary, *Steroids* **23**, 773–792 (1974).

146. V. C. Jordan and L. J. Dowse, Tamoxifen as an anti-tumour agent: Effect on oestrogen binding, *J. Endocrinol.* **68**, 297–303 (1976).

147. V. C. Jordan and T. Jaspan, Tamoxifen as an anti-tumour agent: Oestrogen binding as a predictive test for tumour response, *J. Endocrinol.* **68**, 453–460 (1976).

148. R. K. Wagner, Characterization and assay of steroid hormone receptors and steroid-binding serum proteins by agar gel electrophoresis at low temperature, *Hoppe-Seyler's Z. Physiol. Chem.* **353**, 1235–1245 (1972).

149. C. B. Korsten, E. Engelsman, and J. P. Persijn, Clinical value of estrogen receptors in advanced breast cancer, in: *Estrogen Receptors in Human Breast Cancer* (W. L. McGuire, E. P. Vollmer, and P. P. Carbone, eds.), pp. 93–105, Raven Press, New York (1975).

150. R. K. Wagner and P. W. Jungblut, Estradiol and dihydrotestosterone receptors in normal and neoplastic mammary tissue, *Acta Endocrinol. (Copenhagen)* **82**, 105–120 (1976).

151. F. A. G. Teulings, J. Blonk-vanderWijst, H. Portengen, M. S. Herkelman, R. E. Treuerriet, and H. A. vanGilse, Quantitation of estrogen receptors in human breast cancer by agar gel electrophoresis, *Clin. Chim. Acta* **64**, 27–38 (1975).

152. G. Trams and H. Maass, Specific binding of estradiol and dihydrotestosterone in human mammary cancers, *Cancer Res.* **37**, 258–261 (1977).

153. G. Bastert, H. Schmidt-Mattheisen, R. T. Michel, H. P. Fortmeyer, R. Sturm, D. Nord, and R. Gerner, Human mammary cancers in *nu/nu* mice. A model for testing in research and clinic, *Klin. Wochenschr.* **55**, 83–84 (1977).

154. E. R. DeSombre and T. A. Gorell, Purification of estrogen receptors, *Methods Enzymol.* **36A**, 349–365 (1975).

155. P. L. Corvol, A. Chrambach, D. Rodbard, and C. W. Bardin, Physical properties and binding capacity of testosterone–estradiol-binding globulin in human plasma, determined by polyacrylamide gel electrophoresis, *J. Biol. Chem.* **246**, 3435–3443 (1971).

156. M. R. Sherman, F. B. Tuazon, S. C. Diaz, and L. K. Miller, Multiple forms of oviduct progesterone receptors analyzed by ion exchange filtration and gel electrophoresis, *Biochemistry* **15**, 980–989 (1976).

157. M. J. Duffy and G. J. Duffy, Measurement of estradiol receptors in human breast tumors by polyacrylamide gel electroporesis, *Clin. Chim. Acta* **74**, 161–166 (1977).

158. K. S. Korach and T. G. Muldoon, Studies on the nature of the hypothalamic estradiol-concentrating mechanism in the male and female rat, *Endocrinology* **94**, 785–793 (1974).

159. G. C. Chamness, K. Huff, and W. L. McGuire, Protamine-precipitated estrogen receptor: A solid-phase ligand exchange assay, *Steroids* **25**, 627–635 (1975).

160. M. Lippman and K. Huff, A demonstration of androgen and estrogen receptors in a human breast cancer using a new protamine sulfate assay, Cancer 38, 868–874 (1976).

161. K. B. Horwitz, M. E. Costlow, and W. L. McGuire, MCF-7: A human breast cancer cell line with estrogen, androgen, progesterone, and glucocorticoid receptors, Steroids 26, 785–795 (1975).

162. T. Erdos, M. Best-Belpomme, and R. Bessada, A rapid assay for binding estradiol to uterine receptor(s), Anal. Biochem. 37, 244–252 (1970).

163. D. Williams and J. Gorski, Equilibrium binding of estradiol by uterine cell suspensions and whole uteri in vitro, Biochemistry 13, 5537–5542 (1974).

164. E. J. Pavlik and P. B. Coulson, Hydroxylapatite "batch" assay for estrogen receptors: Increased sensitivity over present receptor assays, J. Steroid Biochem. 7, 357–368 (1976).

165. G. C. Chamness, T. W. King, and P. J. Sheridan, Androgen receptor in the rat brain—assays and proterties, Brain Res. 161, 267–276 (1979).

166. R. E. Garola and W. L. McGuire, A hydroxylapatite micro-method for measuring estrogen receptor in human breast cancer, Cancer Res. 38, 2216–2220 (1978).

167. A. I. Coffer and R. J. B. King, Isoelectric focusing of [³H]oestradiol in flat beds of Sephadex, Biochem. Soc. Trans. 2, 1269–1272 (1974).

168. A. I. Coffer and R. J. B. King, Separation of [³H]estradiol-17β binding proteins by electrofocusing in flat beds of Sephadex. Anal. Biochem. 72, 172–183 (1976).

169. O. Wrange, B. Nordenskjöld, C. Silfverswärd, P. O. Granberg, and J. Gustafsson, Isoelectric focusing of estradiol receptor protein from human mammary carcinoma—a comparison to sucrose gradient analysis, Eur. J. Cancer 12, 695–700 (1976).

170. O. Wrange, B. Nordenskjöld, and J. A. Gustafsson, Cytosol estradiol receptor in human mammary carcinoma: An assay based on isoelectric focusing in polyacrylamide gel, Anal. Biochem. 85, 461–475 (1978).

171. D. V. Santi, C. H. Sibley, E. R. Perriand, G. M. Tomkins, and J. D. Baxter, A filter assay for steroid hormone receptors, Biochemistry 12, 2412–2416 (1973).

172. G. Barbanel, J. L. Borgna, J. C. Bonnafous, and J. C. Mani, Development of a microassay for estradiol receptors, Eur. J. Biochem. 80, 411–423 (1977).

173. E. Casteneda and S. Liao, The use of anti-steroid antibodies in the characterization of steroid receptors, J. Biol. Chem. 250, 883–888 (1975).

174. A. Floridi, G. Citro, E. Sega, and P. G. Natal, Quantitation of estradiol receptors employing a sensitive radioimmunoassay, Immunol. Commun. 4, 603–615 (1975).

175. J. Fishman and J. H. Fishman, Competitive binding assay for estradiol receptor using immobilized antibody, J. Clin. Endocrinol. Metab. 39, 603–606 (1974).

176. J. Fishman, J. H. Fishman, J. S. Nisselbaum, C. Menendez-Botet, M. K. Schwartz, C. Martucci, and L. Hellman, Measurement of the estradiol receptor in human breast tissue by the immobilized antibody method, J. Clin. Endocrinol. Metab. 40, 724–727 (1975).

177. I. Nenci, M. D. Beccati, A. Piffanelli, and G. Lanza, Detection and dynamic localization of estradiol–receptor complexes in intact target cells by immunofluorescence technique, J. Steroid Biochem. 7, 505–510 (1976).

178. I. Nenci, A. Piffanelli, M. D. Beccati, and G. Lanza, In vivo and in vitro immunofluorescent approach to the physiopathology of estradiol kinetics in target cells, J. Steroid Biochem. 7, 883–890 (1976).

179. I. Nenci and E. Marchetti, Concerning the localization of steroids in centrioles and basal bodies by immunofluorescence, J. Cell Biol. 76, 255–260 (1978).

180. L. P. Pertschuk, Detection of estrogen binding in human mammary carcinoma by immunofluorescence: A new technique utilizing the binding hormone in a polymerized state, Res. Commun. Chem. Pathol. Pharmacol. 14, 771–774 (1976).

181. W. E. Mercer, C. A. Carlson, T. M. Wahl, and P. O. Teague, Identification of estrogen receptors in mammary cancer cells by immunofluorescence, *Am. J. Clin. Pathol.* **70**, 330 (1978).

182. W. Mercer, T. Wahl, C. Carlson, and P. Teague, Identification of estrogen receptors in breast cancer cells by immunological techniques, *Fed. Proc. Fed. Am. Soc. Exp. Biol.* **37**, 1312 (1978).

183. W. Mercer, Personal communication.

184. L. Ghosh, B. C. Ghosh, and T. K. DasGupta, Immunocytological localization of estrogen in human mammary carcinoma cells by horseradish–anti-horseradish peroxidase complex, *J. Surg. Oncol.* **10**, 221–224 (1978).

185. S. H. Lee, Cytochemical study of estrogen receptor in human mammary cancer, *Am. J. Clin. Pathol.* **70**, 197–203 (1978).

186. G. L. Greene, L. E. Closs, H. Fleming, E. R. DeSombre, and E. V. Jensen, Antibodies to estrogen receptor: Immunochemical similarity of estrophilin from various mammalian species, *Proc. Natl. Acad. Sci. U.S.A.* **74**, 3681–3685 (1977).

187. K. B. Horwitz and W. L. McGuire, Estrogen control of progesterone receptor in human breast cancer. Correlation with nuclear processing of estrogen receptor, *J. Biol. Chem.* **253**, 2223–2228 (1978).

188. J. Anderson, J. H. Clark, and E. J. Peck, Jr., Oestrogen and nuclear binding sites: Determination of specific sites by [^{3}H]oestradiol exchange, *Biochem. J.* **126**, 561–567 (1972).

189. R. E. Garola and W. L. McGuire, Estrogen receptor and proteolytic activity in human breast tumor nuclei, *Cancer Res.* **37**, 3329–3332 (1977).

190. L. Laing, M. G. Smith, K. C. Calman, D. C. Smith, and R. E. Leake, Nuclear oestrogen receptors and treatment of breast cancer, *Lancet* **2**, 168–169 (1977).

191. D. T. Kiang, Nuclear oestrogen receptor and breast cancer, *Lancet* **2**, 714–716 (1977).

192. W. B. Panko and R. M. MacLeod, Uncharged nuclear receptors for estrogen in breast cancer, *Cancer Res.* **38**, 1948–1951 (1978).

193. J. H. Clark and E. J. Peck, Jr., Nuclear retention of receptor–oestrogen complex and nuclear acceptor sites, *Nature* **260**, 635–637 (1976).

194. T. S. Ruh and L. J. Baudendistel, Different nuclear binding sites for antiestrogen and estrogen receptor complexes, *Endocrinology* **100**, 420–426 (1977).

195. A. M. Traish, R. E. Müller, and H. H. Wotiz, Binding of estrogen receptor to uterine nuclei: Salt-extractable versus salt-resistant receptor–estrogen complexes, *J. Biol. Chem.* **252**, 6823–6830 (1977).

196. E. R. Barrack, E. F. Hawkins, S. L. Allen, L. L. Hicks, and D. S. Coffey, Concepts related to salt resistant estradiol receptors in rat uterine nuclei: Nuclear matrix, *Biochem. Biophys. Res. Commun.* **37**, 829–836 (1977).

197. F. Capony and H. Rochefort, *In vivo* effect of antiestrogens on the localization and replenishment of estrogen receptor, *Mol. Cell. Endocrinol.* **3**, 233–251 (1975).

198. D. T. Zava, N. Y. Harrington, and W. L. McGuire, Nuclear estradiol receptor in the adult rat uterus: A new exchange assay, *Biochemistry* **15**, 4292–4297 (1976).

199. R. E. Garola and W. L. McGuire, An improved assay for nuclear estrogen receptor in experimental and human breast cancer, *Cancer Res.* **37**, 3333–3337 (1977).

200. V. D. Hospelhorn, T. Shida, R. E. DeSombre, and E. V. Jensen, Nuclear estrophilin: Estimation by a novel exchange of bound estradiol, *Endocr. Soc. Abstr.* **60**, 335 (1978).

201. W. L. McGuire and K. B. Horwitz, A role for progesterone in breast cancer, *Ann. N.Y. Acad. Sci.* **286**, 90–100 (1977).

202. L. Terenius, Estrogen and progesterone binders in human and rat mammary carcinoma. *Eur. J. Cancer* **9**, 291–294 (1973).

203. M. L. Freifeld, P. D. Feil, and C. W. Bardin, The *in vivo* regulation of the progesterone "receptor" in guinea pig uterus: Dependence on estrogen and progesterone, *Steroids* **23**, 93–103 (1974).

204. J. R. Reel and Y. Shih, Oestrogen-inducible uterine progesterone receptors. Characteristics in the ovariectomized immature and adult hamster, *Acta Endocrinol. (Copenhagen)* **80**, 344–354 (1975).

205. O. Jänne, K. Kontula, T. Luukkainen, and R. Vihko, Oestrogen-induced progesterone receptor in human uterus, *J. Steroid Biochem.* **6**, 501–509 (1975).

206. W. L. McGuire, J. P. Raynaud, and E. E. Baulieu (eds.), *Progesterone Receptors in Normal and Neoplastic Tissues (Progress in Cancer Research and Therapy*, Vol. 4), Raven Press, New York (1977).

207. B. R. Rao and J. S. Meyer, Estrogen and progestin receptors in normal and cancer tissue, in: *Progesterone Receptors in Normal and Neoplastic Tissues (Progress in Cancer Research and Therapy*, Vol. 4) (W. L. McGuire, J. P. Raynaud, and E. E. Baulieu, eds.), pp. 155–169, Raven Press, New York (1977).

208. M. Lippman, K. Huff, G. Bolan, and J. P. Neifeld, Interactions of R5020 with progesterone and glucocorticoid receptors in human breast cancer and peripheral blood lymphocytes *in vitro*, in: *Progesterone Receptors in Normal and Neoplastic Tissues (Progress in Cancer Research and Therapy*, Vol. 4) (W. L. McGuire, J. P. Raynaud, and E. E. Baulieu, eds.), pp. 193–210, Raven Press, New York (1977).

209. R. J. Seematter, P. G. Hoffman, R. W. Kuhn, P. K. Siiteri, and L. C. Lockwood, Comparison of [³H]progesterone and [6,7-³H]-17,21-dimethyl-19-norpregna-4,9-diene-3,20-dione for the measurement of progesterone receptors in human malignant tissue, *Cancer Res.* **38**, 2800–2806 (1978).

210. D. Philibert and J. P. Raynaud, Progesterone binding in the immature mouse and rat uterus, *Steroids* **22**, 89–98 (1973).

211. D. Philibert and J. P. Raynaud, Progesterone binding in the immature rabbit and guinea pig uterus, *Endocrinology* **94**, 627–632 (1974).

212. J. P. Raynaud, R5020, a tag for the progestin receptor, in: *Progesterone Receptors in Normal and Neoplastic Tissues (Progress in Cancer Research and Therapy*, Vol. 4) (W. L. McGuire, J. P. Raynaud, and E. E. Baulieu, eds.), pp. 9–21, Raven Press, New York (1977).

213. K. B. Horwitz and W. L. McGuire, Specific progesterone receptors in human breast cancer, *Steroids* **25**, 497–505 (1975).

214. P. D. Feil, S. R. Glasser, D. O. Toft, and B. W. O'Malley, Progesterone binding in the mouse and rat uterus, *Endocrinology* **91**, 738–746 (1972).

215. P. C. M. Young and R. E. Cleary, Characterization and properties of progesterone-binding components in human endometrium, *J. Clin. Endocrinol. Metab.* **39**, 425–439 (1974).

216. G. LeClerq, J. C. Heuson, M. C. Deboel, N. Legros, E. Longeval, and W. H. Mattheiem, Estrogen and progesterone receptors in human breast cancer, in: *Progesterone Receptors in Normal and Neoplastic Tissues (Progress in Cancer Research and Therapy*, Vol. 4) (W. L. McGuire, J. P. Raynaud, and E. E. Baulieu, eds.), pp. 141–153, Raven Press, New York (1977).

217. J. Levy and S. M. Glick, Estrogen and progesterone receptors and glucose oxidation in mammary tissue, in: *Progesterone Receptors in Normal and Neoplastic Tissues (Progess in Cancer Research and Therapy*, Vol. 4) (W. L. McGuire, J. P. Raynaud, and E. E. Baulieu, eds.), pp. 211–225, Raven Press, New York (1977).

218. F. May-Levin, F. Guerinot, G. Contesso, J. C. Delarue, and C. Bohuon, Estrogen and progestogen cytosol receptors in human breast carcinoma, *Int. J. Cancer* **19**, 789–795 (1977).

219. L. Liskowski, D. P. Rose, T. Dondlinger, and J. S. Olenick, The determination of progesterone receptors in breast cancer and their relationship to estrogen receptors, *Clin. Chim. Acta* **71**, 309–318 (1976).

220. K. B. Horwitz and W. L. McGuire, Estrogen and progesterone: Their relationship in hormone-dependent breast cancer, in: *Progesterone Receptors in Normal and Neoplastic Tissues (Progress in Cancer Research and Therapy, Vol. 4)* (W. L. McGuire, J. P. Raynaud, and E. E. Baulieu, eds.), pp. 103–124, Raven Press, New York (1977).

221. N. Bloom, E. Tobin, and G. A. Degenschein, Clinical correlations of endocrine ablation with estrogen and progesterone receptors in advanced breast cancer, in: *Progesterone Receptors in Normal and Neoplastic Tissues (Progress in Cancer Research and Therapy, Vol. 4)* (W. L. McGuire, J. P. Raynaud, and E. E. Baulieu, eds.), pp. 125–139, Raven Press, New York (1977).

222. K. Pollow, M. Schmidt-Gollwitzer, and J. Nevinney-Stickel, Progesterone receptors in normal human endometrium and endometrial carcinoma, in: *Progesterone Receptors in Normal and Neoplastic Tissues (Progress in Cancer Research and Therapy, Vol. 4)* (W. L. McGuire, J. P. Raynaud, and E. E. Baulieu, eds.), pp. 313–338, Raven Press, New York (1977).

223. J. A. Gustafsson, N. Einhorn, G. Elfström, B. Nordenskjöld, and O. Wrange, Progestin receptor in endometrial carcinoma, in: *Progesterone Receptors in Normal and Neoplastic Tissues (Progress in Cancer Research and Therapy, Vol. 4)* (W. L. McGuire, J. P. Raynaud, and E. E. Baulieu, eds.). pp. 299–312, Raven Press, New York (1977).

224. R. K. Wagner and P. W. Jungblut, Differentiation between steroid hormone receptors CBG and SHBG in human target organ extracts by a single-step assay, *Mol. Cell. Endocrinol.* **4**, 13–24 (1976).

225. D. Philibert and J. P. Raynaud, Cytoplasmic progestin receptors in mouse uterus, in: *Progesterone Receptors in Normal and Neoplastic Tissues (Progress in Cancer Research and Therapy, Vol. 4)* (W. L. McGuire, J. P. Raynaud, and E. E. Baulieu, eds.), pp. 227–243, Raven Press, New York (1977).

226. A. J. W. Hsueh, E. J. Peck, Jr., and J. H. Clark, Receptor progesterone complex in the nuclear fraction of the rat uterus: Demonstration by ^{3}H-progesterone exchange, *Steroids* **24**, 599–611 (1974).

227. M. R. Walters and J. H. Clark, Nuclear and cytoplasmic progesterone receptors in the rat uterus: Effects of R5020 and progesterone on receptor binding and subcellular compartmentalization, in: *Progesterone Receptors in Normal and Neoplastic Tissues (Progress in Cancer Research and Therapy, Vol. 4)* (W. L. McGuire, J. P. Raynaud, and E. E. Baulieu, eds.), pp. 271–285, Raven Press, New York (1977).

228. M. R. Walters and J. H. Clark, Cytosol and nuclear compartmentalization of progesterone receptors of the rat uterus, *Endocrinology* **103**, 601–609 (1978).

229. E. Milgrom, M. T. VuHai, and F. Logeat, Use of [^{3}H]R5020 for the assay of cytosol and nuclear progesterone receptor in the rat uterus, in: *Progesterone Receptors in Normal and Neoplastic Tissues (Progress in Cancer Research and Therapy, Vol. 4)* (W. L. McGuire, J. P. Raynaud, and E. E. Baulieu, eds.), pp. 261–270, Raven Press, New York (1977).

230. L. P. Bullock and C. W. Bardin, Androgen receptors in mouse kidney: A study of male, female and androgen-insensitive (*tfm/y*) mice, *Endocrinology* **94**, 746–756 (1974).

231. E. Mulder, M. J. Peters, J. deVries, and H. J. van der Molen, Characterization of a nuclear receptor for testosterone in seminiferous tubules of mature rat testes, *Mol. Cell. Endocrinol.* **2**, 171–182 (1975).

232. P. Steins, M. Krieg, H. J. Hollmann, and K. D. Voigt, *In vitro* studies of testosterone binding in benign prostatic hypertrophy, *Acta Endocrinol. (Copenhagen)* **75**, 773–784 (1974).

233. R. K. Wagner, L. Görlich, and P. W. Jungblut, Dihydrotestosterone receptor in human mammary cancer, *Acta Endocrinol. (Copenhagen) Suppl.* **173**, 65 (1973).

234. A. Wirtz, M. Wiedemann, L. Raith, and H. J. Kaul, Studies on the estradiol and 5α-dihydrotestosterone receptors in mammary and prostata tissues, *Acta Endocrinol. (Copenhagen) Suppl.* **177**, 8 (1973).

235. J. P. Persijn, C. B. Korsten, and E. Englesman, Oestrogen and androgen receptors in breast cancer and response to endocrine therapy, *Br. Med. J.* **4**, 503 (1975).

236. J. P. Blondeau, C. Corpechot, C. LeGoascogne, E. E. Baulieu, and P. Robel, Androgen receptors in the rat ventral prostate and their hormonal control, *Vitam. Horm. (N.Y.)* **33**, 319–344 (1975).

237. B. G. Mobbs, I. E. Johnson, J. G. Connolly, and A. F. Clark, Androgen receptor assay in human benign and malignant prostatic tumor cytosol using protamine sulphate precipitation, *J. Steroid Biochem.* **9**, 289–301 (1978).

238. P. Davies, P. Thomas, and K. Griffiths, Measurement of free and occupied cytoplasmic and nuclear androgen receptor sites in rat ventral prostate gland, *J. Endocrinol.* **74**, 393–404 (1977).

239. C. Bonne and J. P. Raynaud, Assay of androgen binding sites by exchange with methyltrienolone (R1881), *Steroids* **27**, 497–507 (1976).

240. H. Ochi, T. Hayashi, K. Nakao, E. Yayoi, T. Kawahara, and K. Matsumoto, Estrogen, progesterone, and androgen receptors in breast cancer in the Japanese: Brief communication, *J. Natl. Cancer Inst.* **60**, 291–293 (1978).

241. D. T. Zava, B. Landrum, K. B. Horwitz, and W. L. McGuire, Measurement of androgen receptor with ³H-methyltrienol-one in systems containing both androgen and progesterone receptors, *Clin. Res.* **26**, 315A (1978).

242. A. G. Fazekas and J. K. MacFarlane, Macromolecular binding of glucocorticoids in human mammary carcinoma, *Cancer Res.* **37**, 640–645 (1977).

243. J. D. Baxter and G. M. Tomkins, Specific cytoplasmic glucocorticoid hormone receptors in hepatoma tissue culture cells, *Proc. Natl. Acad. Sci. U.S.A.* **68**, 932–937 (1971).

244. J. C. Allegra, M. E. Lippman, E. B. Thompson, R. Simon, A. Barlock, L. Green, K. Huff, S. Aitken, M. Do, and R. Warren, Steroid hormone receptors in human breast cancer, *Proceedings of the 14th Annual Meeting of the American Society for Clinical Oncology*, Abstract No. C-118 (1978).

245. M. Lippman, G. Bolan, and K. Huff, The effects of glucocorticoids and progesterone on hormone-responsive human breast cancer in long-term tissue culture, *Cancer Res.* **36**, 4602–4609 (1976).

246. F. A. Teulings and H. A. van Gilse, Demonstration of glucocorticoid receptors in human mammary carcinomas, *Horm. Res.* **8**, 107–116 (1977).

247. J. C. Heuson, E. Longeval, W. H. Mattheiem, M. C. Deboel, R. J. Sylvester, and G. LeClerq, Significance of quantitative assessment of estrogen receptors for endocrine therapy in advanced breast cancer, *Cancer* **39**, 1971–1977 (1977).

248. B. A. Stoll, False-positive oestrogen-receptor assay in breast cancer, *Lancet* **2**, 296–297 (letter) (1977).

6

The Role of Hormones in the Development of Human Breast Cancer

MARVIN A. KIRSCHNER

1. Introduction

It has been long suspected that endocrine factors play a promoting or contributory role in the genesis of human breast cancer. Since growth of normal breast tissue is influenced by the hormonal environment, it seemed reasonable to suspect that growth of neoplastic breast tissue could be similarly influenced by the hormonal milieu. Carcinoma of the breast thus represents one of an intriguing class of cancers arising in target tissues which normally respond to hormonal influences. In humans, such hormone-dependent cancers include also those of the prostate, thyroid, endometrium, and possibly kidney.

Epidemiologic surveys, experimental observations, and clinical observations over the past decades have suggested an association between breast cancer and endocrine function.[1-7] Several of the important lines of evidence showing this association of breast cancer with the endocrine system are listed in Table I; they suggest that gross aspects of endocrine function such as presence or absence of ovarian hormones, some aspect(s) of pregnancy, and menstrual function are important in influencing the genesis of human breast cancer. Other epidemiologic data suggest that lifestyle, dietary patterns, and perhaps obesity are additional factors which influence the development of breast cancer, perhaps by affecting hormone production and metabolism.

MARVIN A. KIRSCHNER • New Jersey Medical School, Newark Beth Israel Medical Center, Newark, New Jersey 07112.

Table I
Endocrine Factors Influencing Breast Cancer

1. Epidemiologic
   Women have 100 times greater incidence of breast cancer than men
   Occurrence after puberty
   Longer menstrual life means more breast cancer
   No breast cancer in ovarian dysgenesis
   Decreased breast cancer after castration
   Protection of early pregnancy
   Higher incidence of postmenopausal breast cancer in Western women
   Higher incidence of postmenopausal breast cancer in obese women
2. Experimental
   Estrogens are cocarcinogens in animal model systems
   Estrogen manipulations influence course of breast cancer
3. Clinical
   Endocine ablation   ⎫ Remission of patients
   Endocrine additives ⎬   with breast cancer
   Antiestrogens   ⎭
   Estrogen exacerbation of breast cancer

As a direct extension of our thinking about hormone-responsive neoplasms, we have long searched for evidence that tumor growth may occur in a given woman because the hormonal environment of that individual is different from that of other women. If such were true, we might be able to define these hormonal differences in patients with or destined to develop breast cancer, so that: (1) we could predict more accurately those patients at risk, and, even more importantly, (2) we might be able to modify these hormonal differences, thereby reducing the risk of breast cancer in the given woman.

Over the past decades many attempts have been made to define the hormonal influences on breast cell growth and to determine if differences exist in the hormonal environment of women who develop breast cancer versus those who do not. These studies have been limited to the available methodology of the time. Initially, urinary hormone metabolites were examined; then direct measurement of hormones in plasma became possible. More recently, it has been possible to accurately examine hormone production rates and interconversion rates. Ultimately, it should be possible to accurately define hormonal events at the subcellular level. In the following review, I will consider several aspects of hormonal investigation in women with breast cancer, an area recently referred to as metabolic epidemiology.[8] Most of the findings attempting to relate breast cancer risk with endocrine function are not well understood and do not fit into a cohesive scheme consistent with our current understanding of hormonal influences on the human breast. Nonetheless, several intriguing hypotheses have emerged from these fragmentary attempts to relate breast cancer to endocrine function.

2. Estrogens

As noted in Table I, many epidemiologic and clinical observations have suggested that estrogenic hormones are important in influencing the risk of developing breast cancer and/or in promoting the growth of already established malignant foci. Earlier attempts at measuring estrogen production in women with breast cancer or at high risk were limited to measurement of urinary estrogen metabolites. Most of these early surveys of urinary estrogen metabolites failed to reveal consistent differences in total estrogens or in individual estrogen metabolites.[9-12] Since then, methodologic advances have permitted accurate assessment of urinary metabolites, plasma concentrations, metabolic interconversions, and overall production rates. Assessment of possible hormonal changes at the breast-cell level remains an undefined area.

2.1. Estriol

In 1966, Lemon and associates[13,14] reported that women with breast cancer excreted less estriol (E_3) as compared to estrone (E_1) and estradiol (E_2). Since E_3 had been shown to have much less estrogenic potency in various bioassay systems when compared with E_1 or E_2, these workers postulated that E_3 could normally serve as a modulator of the more potent estrogens in breast growth, and that patients with decreased urinary E_3 could be at increased risk for breast cancer because of the uncontrolled stimulation of breast cells by the more potent estrogens. This hypothesis, of course, was based on the assumption that urinary E_3 mirrored E_3 production rates and E_3 blood levels. Subsequently, it was shown that E_3 binds to the target tissue (breast cell) with similar affinity to the more potent estrogens.[15] This discovery provided the link for the concept that E_3 could act as a competitive inhibitor of estrogen binding to the breast cell, thereby competing and modulating the action of the more potent estrogens, E_1 and E_2. This "impeded-estrogen hypothesis" was greatly strengthened by the findings of MacMahon et al.[16] and Dickinson et al.,[17] who reported relatively higher levels of E_3 in the urine of Japanese women (low risk for breast cancer) and low urinary E_3 ratios in the urine of Caucasian women (high risk for breast cancer). Similar data were obtained in Israel,[18] where women of European and American origin (high risk for breast cancer) had low urinary E_3 ratios, and women of African or Asian origin (low risk for breast cancer) had relatively high urinary E_3 excretion. The "estriol hypothesis" popularized by Cole and MacMahon[2,19] proposed that E_3, a weak estrogen, modulated or opposed the action of E_1 and E_2, as illustrated in Fig. 1. Women with relatively high production rates of E_3 as compared to E_1 and E_2 could be protected against the increased risk of breast stimulation leading to breast cancer.

The estriol hypothesis relating breast cancer risk to a particular hormonal effect has been a most attractive idea; unfortunately, this construct has not withstood the test of time. First, studies of Hellman *et al.*[20] could not confirm low E_3 excretion in women with breast cancer; in fact, this laboratory and other groups found elevated urinary E_3 in women with breast cancer. Tracer studies showed increased peripheral metabolism of E_2 to E_3 in women with breast cancer. Most recently, Fishman and colleagues[21] examined urinary estrogen metabolites in 30 premenopausal women at high risk for breast cancer (increased family history) versus low-risk controls and reported no differences in urinary E_3 in both follicular and luteal phases of the menstrual cycle.

Over the past decade it has become possible to directly measure circulating E_3 levels by radioimmunoassay. Lipsett,[22] Rotti[23] and Fishman[24] have reported that circulating E_3 levels are extremely low as compared to E_1 and E_2, making it quite unlikely that circulating E_3 could effectively compete with E_1 or E_2 for target-cell cytosol receptor. Pratt and Longcope[25] reported no difference in circulating E_3 levels of women with breast cancer versus normals, and Fishman[24] could find no difference in plasma E_3 of high-risk versus low-risk women. Further, the

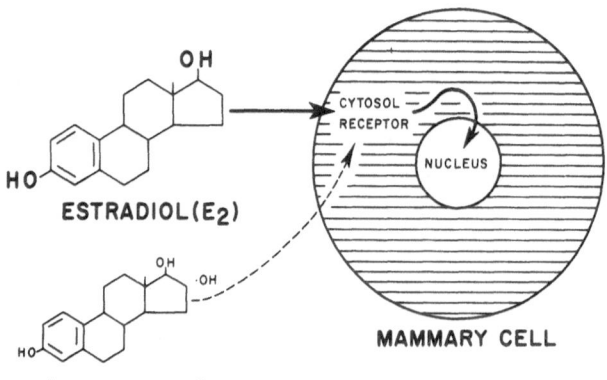

Fig. 1. The "estriol hypothesis" (after Lemon, Cole, *et al.*). Estriol, a weak estrogen, competes for cytosol binding sites, thereby modulating the stimulatory effects of the more potent estrogens (E_2). Reprinted with the permission of *Cancer*.

marked elevations of plasma E_3 during pregnancy are matched by similar increases of other estrogenic steroids, making it difficult to relate the pregnancy effect on breast cancer to a pure E_3 effect.

Recently, Longcope and Pratt[26] measured E_3 blood production rates in normal women with high and low urinary E_3 ratios. No differences were noted between these groups, nor was any relationship observed between E_3 blood production rates and the pattern of urinary estrogen metabolites. Further, Flood[27] examined E_3 production rates of women with breast cancer, and found them to be no different from those of controls. These data, as well as those of Fishman,[21] indicate that urinary E_3 excretory patterns do not reflect differences in E_3 production rates. Finally, the idea that E_3 may serve as a weak "modulating" estrogen has also come under closer scrutiny. Deshpande and colleagues reported that E_3 given orally to breast cancer patients prior to mastectomy did not block tumor uptake of E_2.[28] Noble's group has indicated that E_3 may be as carcinogenic as other estrogens[29] in experimental rodent cancers, and studies by Lippmann showed that E_3 did not antagonize E_2 enhancement of breast cancer growth in a select model system.[30]

These studies conducted over the past decade concerning estrogen blood levels, production rates, and effects on tumor model systems have fairly well disputed the previous hypothesis that the estrogen metabolite E_3 influences the development of breast cancer by modulating breast stimulation by more potent hormones. Nonetheless, the magnificent studies of MacMahon[16] and Dickinson[17] showing differences in urinary estrogen metabolites in Hawaiian subpopulations with differing breast cancer risk cannot be readily dismissed. I propose to examine these data differently,[7] as shown in Fig. 2. Although the circulating estrogen pool may be identical in women with high risk versus low risk for breast cancer, the differing distribution of urinary estrogen metabolites may result from dietary, hepatic, or other metabolic factors which influence the distal metabolism of estrogens. It may well be that one or several of these factors affecting the excretion of individual estrogens may be an important risk factor(s) for breast cancer; and perhaps we have been focusing on the estrogen metabolites rather than on the factors causing the altered estrogen metabolism. One possible shift in estrogen metabolism brought on by external factors may result in formation of 2-hydroxyestrone.[31] This estrogen binds with estrogen receptor proteins and is of potential interest because it has no estrogenic properties of its own and may thus be a competitive inhibitor of the more potent estrogens, as postulated earlier for E_3.[32] Further, formation of this metabolite was shown to be strongly influenced by body weight and/or diet.[31] At this time, however, it would seem that the estriol

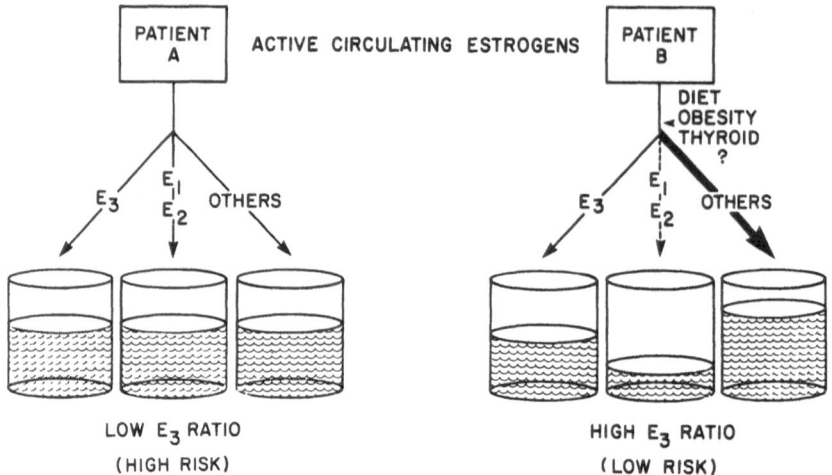

Fig. 2. Reexamination of the estriol hypothesis linking breast cancer risk with patterns of urinary metabolites. In both high-risk and low-risk women, estrogen production and the circulating estrogen pools are identical. However, the distal metabolism and excretory patterns of individual metabolites are different, perhaps influenced by diet, obesity, thyroid status, or other factors. The differing ratios of urinary metabolites thus do not reflect the hormone environment at the level of the breast cell. See text for details.

hypothesis as initially conceived is no longer valid in explaining altered breast cancer risk in certain women or in defined populations.

2.2. Estrone and Estradiol

As discussed above, earlier attempts to quantify "active" estrogen production by measuring urinary E_1 and E_2 metabolites in women with breast cancer or at high risk produced conflicting results, and focused largely on the relationship of urinary E_1 and E_2 versus E_3. It should be pointed out (Fig. 2) that differences in urinary estrogen ratios were caused largely by decreased urinary E_1 and E_2 in women at low risk rather than by differences in E_3 excretion among varying groups. Recently, however, Fishman has reported higher urinary E_1 and E_2 in low-risk women.[21]

Attempts to measure plasma E_1 and E_2 levels in varying groups of women at risk for breast cancer have not produced consistent findings. Hill and colleagues[33] reported that young Japanese and Bantu women (low risk) had significantly higher plasma E_1 and E_2 levels than North American women (high risk) at comparable times of the menstrual cycle. In postmenopausal women, these differences between high-risk and low-risk groups were not seen. Henderson[34] reported that daughters of women with breast cancer (high-risk group) had higher levels of both E_2

and prolactin at comparable times of the menstrual cycle than control populations. These studies are contrasted with those of Fishman,[24] who found no differences in plasma E_1 and E_2 levels in 30 women at high risk compared to an equal number of women at low risk. Thus, there is no consensus at the present time that plasma levels of E_1 or E_2 are altered in women with breast cancer or at high risk for this disease.

Several studies have attempted to define E_1 production rates in women with breast cancer. Poortman and colleagues[35,36] found normal urinary E_1 production rates and my laboratory[37] reported normal E_1 blood production rates in postmenopausal women with established breast cancer. This sensitive assessment of estrogen production needs to be extended to younger women at high and low risk, since changes in hormone production, as with urinary excretion, may become blunted with time and disease, and it would seem possible that differences in E_1 or E_2 production would be most critical during the earlier (induction) years.

2.3. Effect of Diet and Obesity

Much recent interest has focused on the role of diet and/or obesity as potentially important factors associated with both altered breast cancer risk and altered hormone metabolism. The studies of Miller[38] suggest that Canadian women with breast cancer exhibit dietary patterns richer in calories and fats than case-matched controls. Carroll has shown excellent correlation of dietary fat intake and increased breast cancer incidence throughout the world.[39] Hirayama[40] has shown that breast cancer incidence is increasing in postwar affluent Japan. Studies of de Waard showed differing incidence rates of breast cancer in urban versus rural European populations.[41] Further, the changing incidence patterns of breast cancer in Iceland paralleled the shift from rural to urban living in that country.[42] These data seem to support the emerging interest in possible nutritional factors and/or lifestyle as they may influence the incidence and natural history of breast cancer. At present, detailed studies of dietary patterns in Hawaiian and Israeli women are being conducted, since both countries have subpopulations with differing rates of breast cancer incidence.

The relationship of diet to hormone production and metabolism has not been extensively examined. There are some suggestions, however, that dietary alterations may well influence hormone production rates, and, perhaps even more notably, changes in peripheral metabolism of hormones. Spaulding and co-workers[43] reported changes in thyroid hormone metabolism associated with manipulation from high-carbohydrate to low-carbohydrate diets. The effect of fasting on insulin secretion and insulin action is well known.[44] There is further evidence that dietary alterations such as calorie restriction or fasting can influence cortisol,[45,46] androgen metabolism,[47,48] and estrogen production and metabolism, as described above.

The role of obesity as a risk factor for breast cancer was initially reported by de Waard, who subsequently included height and weight as also influencing the incidence of breast cancer.[49] More recently, Miller[50] has confirmed the association of weight, but not height, with increased breast cancer risk. Interest in obesity as a risk factor for breast cancer was heightened by the reports of Grodin,[51] Rizkallah,[52] and Siiteri[53] that obese women have increased peripheral conversion of androstenedione to E_1. Indeed, obese postmenopausal women produce excessive amounts of estrogen from this prehormone pathway.[53,54] Similarly, Schneider et al.[55] have shown that obese men produce excessive amounts of estrogens proportional to the degree of obesity. Again, the prehormone pathway of androgen to estrogens was significantly elevated. Although no systematic study has been performed to explore the origin of estrogens in young, premenopausal women, Edman and MacDonald[56] have reported increased conversion of androstenedione to E_1 in obese young women; in 29 of these women with varying degrees of obesity, the E_1 production rate ranged from 100 to 320 μg/day, as compared to a mean production rate of 60 μg/day in lean women studied at similar times during the menstrual cycle.[57] Similar pilot studies by Longcope[58] and my laboratory[59] found E_1 production rates of 147 to 430 μg/day and elevated blood-to-urine urinary transfer constants ($\rho_{BU}{}^{\Delta E_1}$) of 2.03 to 4.23%. It thus seems likely that obesity does indeed influence both sex hormone production rates and peripheral metabolism (see Table II). At the present time, however, there are no data available

Table II
Effects of Obesity on Sex Hormone Production and Metabolism

Estrogens
1. Increased plasma E_1 and E_2
2. Increased production rate of E_1 and E_2
3. Increased conversion of prehormones to estrogens
   androstenedione to E_1
   testosterone to E_2
4. Increased conversion of E_2 to E_3
5. Decreased conversion of E_2 to 2-hydroxyestrone

Androgens
1. Decreased binding protein (SHBG)
2. Increased metabolic clearance rate of testosterone and androstenedione
3. Decreased plasma testosterone in men and women
4. Normal "free" testosterone

on whether differing diets *per se* can influence steroid hormone production and metabolism, although Hill and Wynder[60] report that a vegetarian diet decreases prolactin levels in young women. Based on available data, it seems legitimate to ask, "Is the obese woman chronically overproducing estrogens from peripheral metabolism of androgens?" and, if so, are the elevated estrogen production rates in the young obese woman causally associated with the increased incidence of breast cancer in the obese postmenopausal woman?

2.4. Exogenous Estrogens

The potential role of exogenous estrogens in the genesis of human breast cancer has come sharply into focus as the result of reports linking diethylstilbestrol usage with vaginal cancer in offspring, and menopausal estrogen usage with increased risk of endometrial cancer.[61–63] Estrogens have been most widely used in several settings: (1) as an abortion preventive in pregnant women, (2) as a component of oral contraceptives, along with a progestin, and (3) for treatment of perimenopausal symptoms.

The potential relationship of oral contraceptive usage to the development of breast cancer has been widely monitored by epidemiologic studies from a variety of sources. To date these studies have presented no convincing clinical evidence to support a significant association between oral contraceptive usage and subsequent breast cancer.[64–69] Indeed, several groups have reported a decreased incidence of benign breast disease in women on the pill.[65,67,68,70] As for menopausal estrogen use and breast cancer risk, available data are limited. Most studies to date show no increased incidence of breast cancer in women receiving this therapy.[65,69,71,72] Hoover *et al.*[73] have suggested, however, that breast cancer incidence rates increase after a latency period in excess of 10 years. Clearly more data are needed in this area. As yet, there are no data on breast cancer incidence in women or daughters of women who received estrogens during pregnancy.

3. Androgens

3.1. Urinary Metabolites

Among the earliest attempts to define hormonal differences in women with breast cancer were those of Bulbrook and collaborators,[74–76] who reported lower levels of individual 17-ketosteroid metabolites in women with breast cancer who responded poorly to endocrine ablative procedures. These differences were best described as the "Bulbrook discriminant," relating excretion of urinary etiocholanolone to that of the 17-hydroxysteroids:

$$D = 80 - 80[17\text{-hydroxycorticoids (mg/24 hr)}] + \text{etiocholanolone } (\mu g/24 \text{ hr})$$

A given woman with a positive discriminant value had a better prognosis and more favorable response to endocrine ablation when compared with a patient exhibiting a negative discriminant. A variety of factors such as age, nutritional state, and stress were shown to influence this value.[48] Subsequently, it was observed that other C-19 urinary androgen metabolites could be substituted into suitable formulae[77,80] which would roughly predict hormonal responsiveness in women with breast cancer. These findings of altered urinary 17-ketosteroids have been confirmed by some[78] and denied by others.[79,80]

More recently, Bulbrook and co-workers have been conducting an ongoing long-term prospective study in Guernsey to determine possible differences in urinary steroid metabolites in women who were destined to develop breast cancer. These workers again reported lower urinary etiocholanolone levels in women who subsequently developed breast cancer, but at a time well before the disease was clinically evident.[81,82]

The significance of decreased levels of urinary 17-ketosteroid metabolites in women with breast cancer or in women who are destined to develop breast cancer remains unknown. In other studies of high-risk and low-risk populations, the association between decreased levels of 17-ketosteroids and breast cancer risk could not be demonstrated. In this regard, Zumoff et al.[83] reported altered patterns of androgen metabolism with decreased excretion of 17-ketosteroids in patients with a variety of nonspecific illnesses, including women with breast cancer. These workers raised the strong possibility that breast cancer patients may excrete lesser amounts of androgen metabolites because of nutritional, thyroidal, or other factors, all nonspecific for breast cancer. This thesis, although readily acceptable in explaining altered steroid metabolism in women with advanced breast cancer, hardly seems an adequate answer for the decreased levels of urinary 17-ketosteroid metabolites observed in young women whose urine was collected many years before the breast cancer developed.

3.2. DHEA and DHEA-SO$_4$

Poortman and colleagues reported decreased production rates and excretion of dehydroepiandrosterone (DHEA) and DHEA sulfate

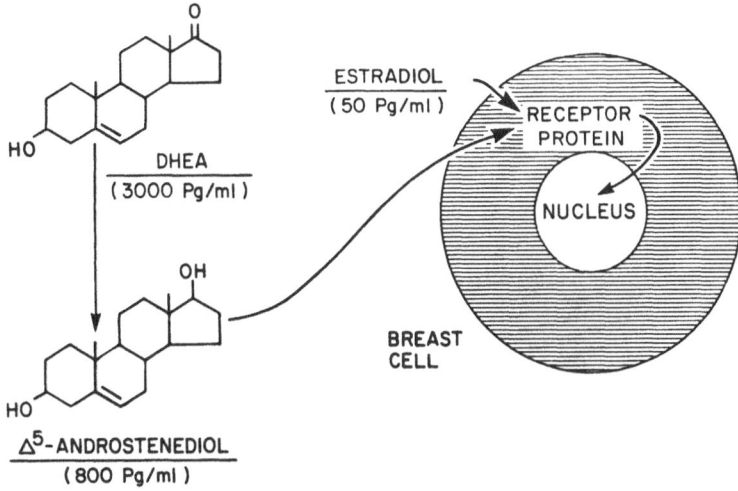

Fig. 3. The potential role of Δ^5-androstenediol as a competitive inhibitor of estrogen binding (after Poortman). Circulating levels of this metabolite are far above those of circulating
estrogens.

(DHEA-SO$_4$) in women with breast cancer.[36,84] In addition, these workers found decreased levels of Δ^5-androstenediol, a metabolite of DHEA,
in women with breast cancer. This metabolite was subsequently shown
to compete for estrogen receptor protein at the target tissue.[84] They
suggest that Δ^5-diol could normally be a modulator of estrogen binding
to its target organ, similar to the role postulated earlier for E$_3$. Lower
levels of Δ^5-diol found in certain instances could lessen the "brake" on
breast cell growth so that estrogen actions might be unopposed, leading
somehow to cancer development. In normal young women, the produc-
tion rate of Δ^5-diol is approximately 500 μg/day, and its circulating level
is 800–1000 pg/ml, making it a more likely competitor for estrogen
cytosol receptor protein at the target cell than E$_3$, whose circulating level
is less than 10 pg/ml (Fig. 3). These data need confirmation, particularly
in young women at high risk for breast cancer.

3.3. Plasma Androgens

Plasma androgen determinations have produced several interesting
and contrasting findings. Plasma testosterone levels seemed to be identical in high-risk American and low-risk Japanese and Bantu women.[33]
In premenopausal women with breast cancer, Malarkey et al.[85] found
elevated plasma testosterone concentrations only in the luteal phase of
the menstrual cycle. In postmenopausal women with breast cancer,
most groups, including my laboratory, found no differences in plasma

testosterone concentrations,[37,85] although McFayden[86] reported minor but significant elevations. Using different methods, both Adami[87] and my laboratory[37] found no differences in the levels of sex-hormone-binding proteins of postmenopausal women with breast cancer.

DHEA and DHEA-SO$_4$ concentrations in plasma have been of interest in view of the potential role of Δ^5 C-19 steroids as competitive inhibitors of estrogen cytosol receptors. Hill[33] reported elevated DHEA levels in normal Bantu women as compared to Japanese and American whites. In this study, Bantu women with established breast cancer had somewhat lower DHEA levels, which were in the same range as those noted in normal American women. No differences were noted in plasma DHEA levels in American women with breast cancer versus controls. The significance of these findings is unclear. As for DHEA-SO$_4$, Wang et al.[88] found decreased circulating levels of this steroid, as well as decreased levels of androsterone sulfate, in breast cancer patients after mastectomy and with advanced disease. These authors reported excellent correlation between plasma DHEA-SO$_4$, androsterone sulfate, and urinary 17-ketosteroid excretion in women with breast cancer. Furthermore, these studies confirm the findings of the Dutch group, referred to above,[36,84] of decreased urinary DHEA-SO$_4$ production rates. The question of whether Δ^5 C-19 steroids are decreased as a nonspecific consequence of disease in general needs further clarification.

3.4. Androstenedione

An androgen of potential importance to the hormonal milieu of women with breast cancer is Δ^4-androstenedione. This C-19 steroid represents the major prehormone of testosterone in women and is excreted in urine as androsterone and etiocholanolone (17-ketosteroids). Perhaps even more important than being a source of 17-ketosteroid metabolites, 1–2% of androstenedione is normally transformed to E$_1$. Androstenedione production rates average 3 mg/day in young women and 1–2 mg/day in postmenopausal women. This androgen is a major prehormone of E$_1$, as noted in Fig. 4. Indeed, in postmenopausal women, androstenedione secreted by both adrenals and ovaries is transformed in its peripheral metabolism to E$_1$, accounting for 80–100% of the total daily E$_1$ production. [51–54] The rate of metabolism of androstenedione to E$_1$ is influenced by aging as well as by obesity. Thus, overnutrition or specific dietary factors might influence the rate of androstenedione metabolism to E$_1$, providing more or less estrogen for breast stimulation. Plasma concentrations of androstenedione were compared in normal premenopausal Bantu versus American women as well as in Bantu and American women with breast cancer. Hill et al.[33] reported that both

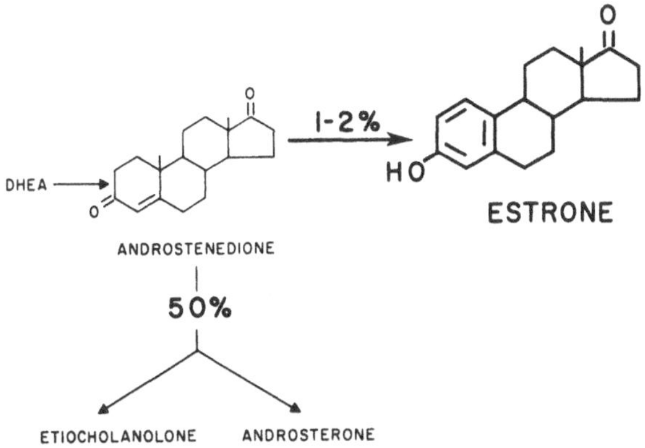

Fig. 4. Schematic diagram of androstenedione metabolism. This androgen serves as a major source of 17-ketosteroid metabolites, as well as being a major prehormone of estrone. In postmenopausal women, androstenedione serves as the chief source of estrogens.

Bantu and American women with breast cancer had higher plasma Δ^4 concentrations as compared to their control groups; however, all values reported for the various groups comprising this study ranged from 280 to 367 ng/dl, considerably higher than Δ^4 values reported by most steroid laboratories, thereby raising questions of technical validation.

In postmenopausal women with breast cancer, Adami[87] reported that Δ^4 values averaged 167 ng/dl, which was significantly higher than the mean of 144 ng/dl noted in age-matched controls, thus supporting the data of Hill's group. By contrast, Thijssen,[89] Longcope,[54] and my laboratory[37] reported no differences in plasma Δ^4 concentrations in breast cancer patients.

Androstenedione production rates have been measured in post-menopausal women with breast cancer, with similar results reported by both Poortman[35,36] and my laboratory.[37] Both laboratories reported that androstenedione production rates were not significantly different in postmenopausal women with breast cancer as compared to age-matched controls. Values noted were in the range of 1.5 to 1.9 mg/day. Further, both laboratories found similar transfer constants (ρ) of Δ to E_1. In the study reported from my laboratory,[37] urinary E_1 production rates averaged 57 μg/day in breast cancer patients, not significantly different from values of 42 and 44 μg/day found in control groups; however, the androstenedione contribution to the total E_1 production rate was decreased in breast cancer patients, as noted in Fig. 5. It thus appears that post-menopausal women with breast cancer have an additional source of E_1, beyond the androstenedione contribution.

A theoretical scheme depicting the potential influences of andro-

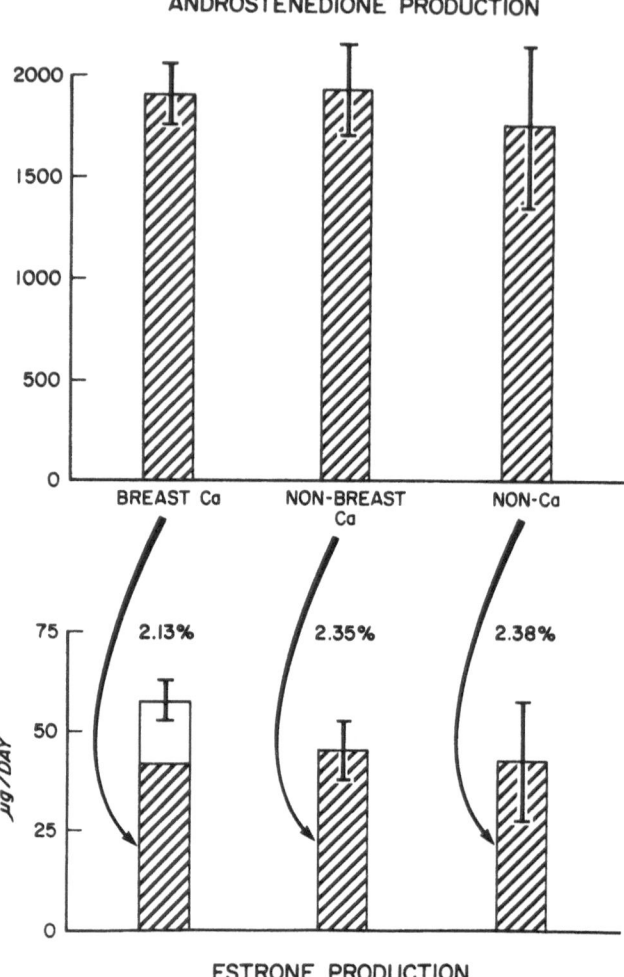

Fig. 5. Androstenedione production rates, conversion to estrone, and estrone production rates in postmenopausal women with breast cancer, non-breast cancer, and non-cancer controls. In women with breast cancer, only 72% of the total estrone production arises from androstenedione metabolism. By contrast, virtually all estrone produced in the control patients comes from androstenedione. Reprinted with the permission of *Cancer Research*.

gens on breast cell growth is presented in Fig. 6. This scheme indicates that androstenedione serves as a prehormone for E_1, and that certain factors might influence this rate of transformation, producing more active estrogen to stimulate cell growth. Androstenediol might also influence the breast cell by serving as a competitive inhibitor of estrogen

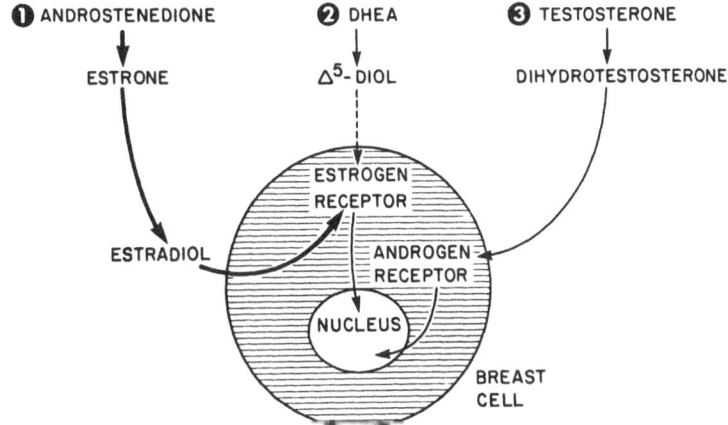

Fig. 6. Schematic representation of potential influences of androgens on the breast cell. See text for details. Reprinted with the permission of *Cancer*.

binding, and thus modulate estrogen action. Finally, studies indicate that breast tissue contains specific androgen receptor sites,[84,90,91] leaving open the possibility that alterations in testosterone and dihydrotestosterone production *per se* could influence breast cell growth. The role of any or all of these potential factors in influencing or promoting breast cancer, however, remains unclear.

4. Progesterone

In normal human breast tissue, progesterone acts to bring about cell growth and alveolar proliferation. Estrogen stimulation is essential for progesterone to be fully effective. In the normal menstruating woman, progesterone is produced almost entirely in the corpus luteum of the ovary. Proper luteinization of the ovarian follicle requires an orderly sequence of pituitary follicle-stimulating hormone (FSH) and luteinizing hormone (LH) secretion, ovarian follicular growth, estrogen production, and ovulation as a prerequisite for normal progesterone secretion.[92,93] In many past studies, normal progesterone production was assumed if women had normal menstrual intervals, mittelschmerz, and prior fertility. Recent studies, however, have shown that these assumptions are frequently incorrect,[92,94,95] and that accurate assessment of corpus luteum function and progesterone production in women requires frequent blood sampling throughout the menstrual cycle.

To date, there have been very few studies of progesterone production in women with breast cancer or at high risk for this disease.

Grattarola,[96] found that young women with a recent history of breast cancer exhibited a higher incidence of anovulatory cycles and a higher incidence of primary and secondary sterility as compared to normal women.

The possible significance of progesterone as an important factor in the development of human breast cancer has been suggested by Sherman and Korenman.[97] These workers surveyed various risk factors associated with breast cancer and called attention to the fact that many of these risk factors are associated with menstrual irregularities and inadequate corpus luteum phase cycles. From their survey, Sherman and Korenman proposed that estrogenic stimulation of breast cell growth in the absence of sufficient cyclic progesterone secretion may provide a setting favorable for the development of breast cancer. Indeed, it has been suggested that the progestogen component of oral contraceptives may be responsible for the decreased incidence of benign breast disease, and possibly breast cancer, in women receiving long-term contraceptives.

In a recent study of integrated 24-hour plasma progesterone concentrations, Malarkey et al.[85] were unable to discern differences in luteal-phase values in premenopausal women with malignant or benign breast disease versus controls, nor in postmenopausal women with breast cancer, benign disease, or no disease. Despite these negative plasma progesterone data, the Sherman–Korenman hypothesis is intriguing and is being pursued by a long-term prospective study of breast cancer incidence in young women with a variety of menstrual patterns.

5. Prolactin

A prominent hormone influencing the growth and function of mammary tissue is prolactin. This pituitary protein hormone acts directly on the stimulated mammary gland, resulting in the initiation and maintenance of lactation. The importance of prolactin as a stimulatory hormone for breast tissue has been reaffirmed by the finding of specific prolactin receptor sites in normal breast tissue[98,99] and in breast cancer tissue.[100,101]

Interest in prolactin as a hormone potentially involved in the genesis of breast cancer has been heightened by several laboratory and clinical observations. In animal model systems and in tissue culture, prolactin stimulates breast tumor growth.[102–105] In the sphere of clinical observations, it was noted that breast cancer incidence is greater in women with hypothyroidism (elevated prolactin levels)[106–109] and that

drugs that decrease prolactin secretion (i.e., L-dopa and ergot derivatives) have been used with limited success in the treatment of disseminated breast cancer.[110–112] Reserpine is a drug that stimulates release of
prolactin; however, earlier reports that reserpine usage was associated
with higher incidence rates of breast cancer[113–115] have not been confirmed.[116–118] Plasma prolactin levels have been examined in several
groups of women at varying risk for breast cancer. Both Kwa[119] and
Henderson[34] reported higher serum prolactin levels in daughters of
women with breast cancer. More recently, however, Pike[120] found in-
significant differences in daytime plasma prolactin values in daughters
of women with breast cancer. Hill et al.[121] reported no significant differences in plasma prolactin levels in young, normal Bantu, Japanese, or
Caucasian women (differing risk groups). These workers, however, reported extraordinarily high serum prolactin levels (155 ng/ml) in
seemingly normal Caucasian women whose first pregnancy occurred
after age 35 (higher risk). Indeed, these data need confirmation since
most investigators would suspect pituitary pathology in women exhibiting such high prolactin levels. Of considerable interest have been the
observations of Hill and Wynder[60] that normal Western women who
switched to vegetarian diets for a month exhibited a 60% decrease in
nocturnal plasma prolactin values. When vegetarian diets were continued for longer periods, the volunteer women exhibited decreased
prolactin levels at several points throughout the day. Further, these
workers reported that menstrual cycles of women on this diet were
shortened by two days. These observations are indeed of considerable
interest in view of the developing evidence that fat content, obesity, or
perhaps other dietary factors (alluded to previously) are associated with
altered breast cancer risk.

In women with established breast cancer, most studies to date have
shown that prolactin levels in blood are within normal limits. Hill and
colleagues[121] were unable to show differences in prolactin levels in
Caucasian, Bantu, and Japanese patients with established breast cancer.
It should be emphasized again that prolactin levels in blood are quite
labile and fluctuate greatly, making single determinations of this hormone of little value. Provocative tests for prolactin release [i.e.,
thyrotropin-releasing hormone, (TRH) stimulation tests] in women with
breast cancer have produced normal prolactin responses.[122] Recently,
Malarkey et al., [123] cognizant of the marked fluctuations in serum prolactin levels, measured prolactin levels on an hourly basis. This group
reported decreased nocturnal prolactin levels in postmenopausal
women with breast cancer, but not at other times of the day. These
workers also observed elevated nocturnal prolactin levels in two of five

premenopausal women with breast cancer. The significance of the seemingly disordered prolactin secretion in women with breast cancer needs expansion.

6. Thyroid Hormones

The association of thyroid hormones with breast cancer is unclear, although the finding that TRH also causes prolactin secretion has provoked new interest in the thyroid gland and its diseases as relating to breast cancer. Several groups have suggested that patients with breast cancer have a higher incidence of hypothyroidism,[106-108,124] and that breast cancer is uncommon in hyperthyroid women.[3,125] A report suggested that Japanese women with Hashimoto's thyroiditis had an increased incidence of breast cancer.[83] These results, however, could not be confirmed in a study of American women.[126,127] A report by Kapdi and Wolfe[109] that women receiving exogenous thyroid hormones had a higher incidence of breast cancer provoked much concern. These data could not be confirmed by Wallace[128] or Adami[87] and, indeed, reinterpretation of the data within given age groups of women failed to show a correlation between thyroid hormone usage and breast cancer.[129] Subsequently, Gorman et al.[130] reviewed the biological and statistical evidence for the role of thyroid hormone usage in the development of breast cancer and could find no such association. Treatment of breast cancer patients with thyroid hormones has not appreciably altered the course of the disease,[131,132] although hypothyroid women with breast cancer seem to have a poorer prognosis.[107,133-135]

In women with established breast cancer, results of thyroid function tests have generally been within normal limits[136,139] Mittra[140] reported normal thyroid function tests and normal prolactin levels in women with breast cancer; in their patients, however, thyroid-stimulating hormone (TSH) was elevated, and there was excessive TSH response to its hypothalamic-releasing hormone (TRH). These authors postulated that women with breast cancer have subnormal levels of thyroid hormone (subclinical hypothyroidism), accounting for the elevated plasma TSH. They further proposed that the subclinical hypothyroid state sensitizes the breast epithelium to hyperrespond to normal levels of prolactin. Adami[87] similarly found elevated TSH levels in 179 breast cancer patients of all ages registered in four Swedish counties. These findings were associated with elevated reverse T_3 and slightly decreased T_3 levels, and were interpreted as being a nonspecific consequence of disease and debility. Malarkey *et al.*[85] could not confirm differences in TSH or T^4 levels in young or postmenopausal women with benign or malignant breast disease.

Thyroid hormones have been shown to significantly alter peripheral metabolism of several hormones, including androgens[141] and estrogens.[31,142] Previous studies by Hellman *et al.*[141] have shown that hypothyroidism is associated with a shift in steroid ring-A reduction in favor of 5β metabolites, such as etiocholanolone. Fishman *et al.* further demonstrated that hyperthyroidism favors 2-hydroxylation versus 16-hydroxylation of estrogens, giving rise to increased production of 2-hydroxyestrone at the expense of E_3.[143] McGuire and Tomkins[144] demonstrated that thyroid function alters metabolism of the 11-oxo adrenocortical steroids. Furthermore, studies have shown that hyperthyroidism is associated with a considerable increase in circulating levels of sex-hormone-binding globulin.[145] Elevations of this binding protein may significantly influence the biological availability of both androgens and estrogens at the cellular level.

At the present time, no unified hypothesis has emerged implicating thyroid function in increased incidence of breast cancer. There are, however, a number of intriguing findings linking abnormalities of thyroid function with alterations in androgen and estrogen metabolism, which may bear more directly as stimulatory agents on growth of mammary cells. The possible link between thyroid status and prolactin secretion has not as yet resulted in new experimental or clinical advances.

7. Other Pituitary Hormones

7.1. Growth Hormone

In women with breast cancer, both Greenwood[146] and Pearson[147] observed normal basal growth hormone (GH) levels and normal responses to insulin-induced hypoglycemia. Interestingly, however, the latter group observed paradoxical elevations of GH following glucose loading. Carter and colleagues[148] observed slight increases in resting GH levels and confirmed Pearson's observations of paradoxical elevations following glucose loading. This group further noted blunting of the lipolytic effect of administered GH in women with breast cancer, which they felt could not be explained by age, nutritional state, or stress. More recently, Malarkey *et al.* reported normal integrated 24-hour plasma GH levels in young and postmenopausal women with benign and cancerous breast lesions.[85] It would seem that abnormalities reported to date are minimal and inconstant and that the GH axis in women with breast cancer is probably normal.

7.2. Gonadotropins

Earlier studies of total urinary gonadotropin excretion in women with breast cancer were inconclusive. Loraine[149] and Boyland[150] reported somewhat higher total urinary gonadotropins in patients who subsequently failed to respond to endocrine therapy, whereas Hayward[108] reported changes in the opposite direction. Beck[79] reported no abnormalities in urinary gonadotropin levels, nor differences in the urine of responders versus nonresponders to endocrine therapy. More recently, both Malarkey[85] and McFayden[86] have reported no differences in serial measurements of plasma FSH or LH in women with breast cancer. The general consensus at present is that the gonadotropin axis is not altered in women with breast cancer.

8. Comments

From the foregoing review of hormone production and metabolism in women with or at high risk for developing breast cancer, it becomes apparent that no clearcut pattern of hormonal abnormalities has been found to date. Although breast tissue represents a target organ for the action of many hormones, and in spite of the fact that many of the epidemiologic variables associated with altered risk for breast cancer are seemingly related to endocrine function, attempts to define these endocrine differences have been elusive. Indeed, "femaleness," the presence or absence of ovarian function, and the presence or absence of pregnancy, are all factors that represent gross influences of endocrine function. Yet, when it comes to measuring parameters of hormonal function in terms of urinary metabolites, circulating blood levels, or hormone production rates, the findings have been confusing, equivocal, and generally not abnormal. Maybe the next level of exploration for hormonal differences in women who develop breast cancer should be at the cellular level. Perhaps target-cell transformation or steroids, as suggested by Adams[151] and Dao and colleagues,[152] needs to be further emphasized. It would seem that attempts to define hormonal events at the breast-cell level by measuring these in breast fluids have thus far been unrewarding.

Differences in excretion of certain androgen and estrogen metabolites noted in women with breast cancer, which aroused much interest and spawned exciting hypotheses, may in fact be secondary factors relating to as yet undefined influences on breast growth and breast cancer induction. For example, the differences in E_3 excretion observed in women with increased risk for breast cancer are probably the result of alterations in steroid disposal secondary to dietary factors, obesity, etc., rather than an indication of altered hormone production leading to the disease. Similarly, the differences observed in urinary androgen metabolites in women with breast cancer or at high risk may be reflective of other, possibly more important, phenomena rather than causative for breast cancer. The suggestion of progesterone insufficiency, leading to unbridled stimulation of the breast, the potential relation between prolactin secretion and breast cancer, and possible associations between thyroid and breast have thus far been unconvincing.

Despite three decades of intensive investigation into the relationships between breast cancer and hormones, and despite the tantalizing associations that have been attempted from inconsistent data, there is as yet no clearcut pattern of abnormal hormone production or abnormal hormone milieu in women at increased risk for breast cancer.

9. References

1. M. B. Lipsett, Hormonal induction of breast cancer, in: *Breast cancer: A Challenging Problem* (M. L. Griem, E. V. Jensen, J. E. Ultman, and R. W. Wissier, eds.), pp. 28–30, Springer-Verlag, New York (1973).
2. B. MacMahon, P. Cole, and J. B. Brown, Etiology of human breast cancer: A review, *J. Natl. Cancer Inst.* **50**, 21–42 (1973).
3. E. L. Wynder, I. J. Bross, and T. Hirayama, A study of the epidemiology of cancer of the breast, *Cancer* **13**, 559–601 (1960).
4. M. Kirschner, Relation of endocrine function to epidemiological characteristics in breast cancer, in: *Report to the Profession, Breast Cancer*, pp. 35–44, Breast Cancer Task Force, National Cancer Institute, U.S. Department of Health, Education, and Welfare, Bethesda, Maryland (September, 1974).
5. B. E. Henderson, V. R. Gerkins, and M. C. Pike, Sexual factors and pregnancy, in: *Persons at High Risk of Cancer: An Approach to Cancer Etiology and Control* (J. F. Fraumeni, ed.), pp. 267–284, Academic Press, New York (1975).
6. H. P. Leis, Hormones in the epidemiology of breast cancer, *Dis. Breast* **2**, 7–13 (1976).
7. M. A. Kirschner, The role of hormones in the etiology of human breast cancer, *Cancer* **39**, 2716–2726 (1977).
8. E. L. Wynder, Point of view: Metabolic epidemiology, *Lancet* **1**, 260 (1978).
9. R. D. Bulbrook, F. C. Greenwood, G. J. Hadfield, and E. F. Scowen, Oophorectomy in breast cancer; an attempt to correlate clinical results with estrogen production, *Br. Med. J.* **2**, 7–11 (1958).
10. R. A. McAllister, A. W. Sim, R. Hobkirk, H. Stewart, D. W. Blair, and A. P. M. Forrest, Urinary oestrogens after endocrine ablation, *Lancet* **1**, 1102–1105 (1960).
11. W. T. Irving, E. H. Aitken, D. F. Rendelman, and P. J. Folca, Urinary oestrogen

measurements after oophorectomy and adrenalectomy for advanced breast cancer, *Lancet* **2**, 791–797 (1961).

12. G. I. M. Sawyer, A. E. Lee, and M. B. Masterton, Oestrogen excretion of patients with breast cancer, *Br. Med. J.* **1**, 617–619 (1961).

13. H. M. Lemon, Endocrine influences on human mammary formation, a critique, *Cancer* **23**, 781–790 (1969).

14. H. M. Lemon, H. H. Wotiz, L. Parsons, and P. J. Mozden, Reduced estriol excretion in patients with breast cancer prior to endocrine therapy, *J. Am. Med. Assoc.* **196**, 112–120 (1966).

15. P. I. Brecher and H. H. Wotiz, Competition between estradiol and estriol for end organ receptor proteins, *Steroids* **9**, 431–437 (1967).

16. B. MacMahon, P. Cole, J. B. Brown, Urine oestrogen profiles of Asian and North American women, *Int. J. Cancer* **14**, 161–167 (1974).

17. L. E. Dickinson, B. MacMahon, P. Cole, and J. B. Brown, Estrogen profiles of Oriental and Caucasian women in Hawaii, *N. Engl. J. Med.* **291**, 1211–1213 (1974).

18. J. Gross, B. Modan, B. Bertini, O. Spira, F. de Waard, J. H. H. Thijssen, and P. Vestergaard, Relationship between steroid excretion patterns and breast cancer incidence in Israeli women of various ethnic origin, *J. Nat. Cancer Inst.* **59**, 7–11 (1977).

19. P. Cole and B. MacMahon, Oestrogen fractions during early reproductive life in the etiology of breast cancer, *Lancet* **1**, 604–606 (1969).

20. L. Hellman, B. Zumoff, J. Fishman, and T. F. Gallagher, Peripheral metabolism of ^{3}H-estradiol and the excretion of endogenous estrone and estriol glucosiduronate in women with breast cancer, *J. Clin. Endocrinol. Metab.* **33**, 138–144 (1971).

21. J. Fishman, D. Fukushima, J. O'Connor, R. S. Rosenfeld, H. T. Lynch, J. F. Lynch, H. Guirgis, and K. Maloney, Plasma hormone profiles of young women at risk for familial breast cancer, *Cancer Res.* **38**, 4006–4011 (1978).

22. M. B. Lipsett, Oestrogen profiles and breast cancer, *Lancet* **2**, 1378 (1971).

23. K. J. Rotti, J. Stevens, D. Watson, and C. Longcope, Estriol concentrations in plasma of normal, non-pregnant women, *Steroids* **25**, 807–812 (1975).

24. J. Fishman, D. Fukushima, J. O'Connor, and R. S. Rosenfeld, Low urinary estrogen glucuronides in women at risk for familial breast cancer, *Science* (in press).

25. J. H. Pratt and C. Longcope, Estriol production rates and breast cancer, *J. Clin. Endocrinol.* **46**, 44–47 (1978).

26. C. Longcope and J. H. Pratt, Blood production rates of estrogens in women with differing ratios of urinary estrogen conjugates, *Steroids* **29**, 483–492 (1977).

27. C. Flood, J. H. Pratt, and C. Longcope, The metabolic clearance and blood production rates of estriol in normal, non-pregnant women, *J. Clin. Endocrinol. Metab.* **42**, 1–8 (1976).

28. N. Deshpande, P. Carson, and J. Horner, Oestriol in human breast tumors, *J. Steroid Biochem.* **7**, 11–14 (1976).

29. R. L. Noble, B. C. Hockachka, and D. King, Spontaneous and estrogen-produced tumors in Nb rats and their behavior after transplantation, *Cancer Res.* **35**, 766–780 (1975).

30. M. Lippman, M. Monaco, and G. Bolan, Effects of estrone, estradiol and estriol on human breast cancer in tissue culture, *Cancer Res.* **37**, 1901–1907 (1977).

31. J. Fishman, R. M. Boyar, and L. Hellman, Influence of body weight on estradiol metabolism in young women, *J. Clin. Endocrinol. Metabl.* **41**, 989–991 (1975).

32. B. Zumoff, J. Fishman, H. L. Bradlow, and L. Hellman, Hormone profiles in hormone-dependent cancers, *Cancer Res.* **35**, 3365–3373 (1975).

33. P. Hill, E. L. Wynder, P. Helman, R. Hickman, and G. Rona, Plasma hormone profiles in populations at different risk for breast cancer, *Cancer Res.* **36**, 1883–1885 (1976).

34. B. E. Henderson, V. Gerkins, I. Rosario, J. Casagrande, and M. Pike, Elevated serum levels of estrogen and prolactin in daughters of patients with breast cancer, N. Engl. J. Med. **293**, 790–795 (1975).

35. J. Poortman, J. H. H. Thijssen, and F. Schwarz, Androgen production and conversion to estrogens in normal post-menopausal women and in selected breast cancer patients, J. Clin. Endocrinol. Metab. **37**, 101–109 (1973).

36. J. Poortman, Geslachtshormonen en mamma-carcinoom, Thesis, University of Utrecht (1974).

37. M. A. Kirschner, F. B. Cohen, and C. Ryan, Androgen–estrogen production rates in post-menopausal women with breast cancer, Cancer Res. **38**, 4029–4035 (1978).

38. A. B. Miller, Role of nutrition in the etiology of breast cancer, Cancer **39**, 2704–2708 (1977).

39. K. K. Carroll, Experimental evidence of dietary factors and hormone-dependent cancers, Cancer Res. **35**, 3374–3383 (1975).

40. T. Hirayama, Socio-economic factors in breast cancer incidence, U.S.–Japan Cooperative Cancer Research Program, Tokyo (May, 1976).

41. F. de Waard, Diet and nutrition as environmental factors in the pathogenesis of breast cancer, in: Report to the Profession, Breast Cancer, pp. 21–30, Breast Cancer Task Force, National Cancer Institute, Department of Health, Education, and Welfare, Bethesda, Maryland (September, 1974).

42. O. Bjarnason, N. Day, G. Snaedal, and H. Tulunius, The effect of year of birth on the breast cancer age incidence curve in Iceland, Int. J. Cancer **13**, 689–696 (1974).

43. S. W. Spaulding, I. J. Chopra, R. S. Sherwin, and S. S. Lyall, Effect of caloric restriction and dietary composition on serum T_3 and reverse T_3 in man, J. Clin. Endocrinol. **42**, 197–200 (1976).

44. J. A. Archer, P. Gorden, and J. Roth, Defect in insulin binding to receptors in obese men: Amelioration with calorie restriction, J. Clin. Invest. **55**, 166–174 (1975).

45. S. H. Schachner, R. G. Wieland, D. E. Maynard, F. A. Kruger, and G. J. Hamwi, Alterations in adrenal cortical function in fasting, obese subjects, Metabolism **14**, 1051 (1965).

46. A. L. Schultz, A. Kerlow, and R. A. Ulstrom, Effect of starvation on adrenal cortical function in obese subjects, J. Clin. Endocrinol. **24**, 1253 (1964).

47. A. Hendriks, W. Heyns, and P. De Moor, Influence on low-calorie diet and fasting on the metabolism of DHEA-SO_4 in adult obese subjects, J. Clin. Endocrinol. **28**, 1525–1533 (1968).

48. M. C. Metcalf, The breast cancer discriminant: Effect of age, obesity, hirsutism, starvation and change in adrenocortical and gonadal activity, J. Endocrinol. **63**, 263–272 (1977).

49. F. W. de Waard, Breast cancer incidence and nutritional status with particular reference to body weight and height, Cancer Res. **35**, 3351–3356 (1975).

50. A. B. Miller, An overview of hormone-associated cancers, Cancer Res. **38**, 3985–3990 (1978).

51. J. M. Grodin, P. K. Siiteri, and P. C. MacDonald, Source of estrogen production in postmenopausal women, J. Clin. Endocrinol. Metabl. **36**, 207–214 (1973).

52. T. H. Rizkallah, H. M. M. Tovell, and W. G. Kelly, Production of estrone and fractional conversion of circulating androstenedione to estrone in women with endometrial carcinoma, J. Clin. Endocrinol. **40**, 1045–1055 (1975).

53. P. K. Siiteri, J. E. Williams, and N. K. Takaki, Steroid abnormalities in endometrial and breast carinoma: A unifying hypothesis, J. Steroid Biochem. **4**, 897–904 (1976).

54. C. Longcope, Steroid production in pre- and post-menopausal women, in: The Menopausal Syndrome (R. B. Greenblatt, V. B. Mahesh, and P. C. MacDonald, eds.), pp. 6–18, Medcom Press, New York (1974).

55. G. Schneider, M. A. Kirschner, R. Berkowitz, and N. H. Ertel, Increased estrogen production in obese men, *J. Clin. Endocrinol.*, April (1979).

56. C. D. Edman and P. C. MacDonald, Effect of obesity on conversion of plasma androstenedione to estrone in ovulatory and anovulatory young women, *Am. J. Obstet. Gynecol.* **130**, 456–462 (1978).

57. C. D. Edman, Personal communication.

58. C. Longcope, Personal communication.

59. M. A. Kirschner, Unpublished observation.

60. P. Hill and E. L. Wynder, Diet and prolactin release, *Lancet* **1**, 806–807 (1976).

61. H. K. Ziel and W. D. Finkle, Increased risk of endometrial carcinoma among users of conjugated estrogens, *N. Engl. J. Med.* **293**, 1167–1170 (1975).

62. Estrogens and endometrial cancer, *FDA (Food Drug Adm.) Drug Bull.* **6**, 18–20 (1976).

63. D. Thomas, Role of exogenous female hormones in altering the risk of benign and malignant neoplasms in humans, *Cancer Res.* **38**, 3991–4000 (1978).

64. F. G. Arthes, P. E. Sartwell, and E. F. Lewison, The pill, estrogens and the breast: Epidemiologic aspects, *Cancer* **28**, 1391–1394 (1971).

65. Boston Collaborative Drug Surveillance Programme, Oral contraceptives and venous thromboembolic disease surgically confirmed, gall bladder disease, and breast tumor, *Lancet* **1**, 1399–1404 (1973).

66. F. G. Arthes, P. E. Sartwell, E. F. Lewison, and J. Tonascia, Breast cancer, estrogens and the pill, *Proceedings of XI International Cancer Congress*, pp. 247–248, Florence, Italy (1974).

67. M. P. Vessey, R. Doll, and K. Jones, Oral contraceptives and breast cancer, *Lancet* **1**, 941–943 (1975).

68. E. Fasal and R. S. Paffenbarger, Oral contraceptives as related to cancer and benign lesions of the breast, *J. Natl. Cancer Inst.* **55**, 767–773 (1975).

69. E. F. Lewison, Role of exogenous estrogens, in: *Risk Factors in Breast Cancer: New Aspects of Breast Cancer* (B. A. Stoll, ed.), pp. 67–70, Wm. Heinemann Medical Books, Ltd., London (1976).

70. H. Ory, P. Cole, B. MacMahon, and R. Hoover, Oral contraceptives and reduced risk of benign breast diseases, *N. Engl. J. Med.* **294**, 419–422 (1976).

71. J. C. Burch, B. F. Byrd, and W. K. Vaughn, The effects of long-term estrogen administration to women following hysterectomy, estrogens in the post-menopause, *Front. Horm. Res.* **3**, 208–214 (1975).

72. S. Wallach and P. H. Henneman, Prolonged estrogen therapy in postmenopausal women, *J. Am. Med. Assoc.* **171**, 1637–1642 (1959).

73. R. Hoover, L. A. Gray, P. Cole, and B. MacMahon, Menopausal estrogens and breast cancer, *N. Engl. J. Med.* **295**, 401–405 (1976).

74. R. D. Bulbrook, F. C. Greenwood, and J. L. Hayward, Selection of breast cancer patients for adrenalectomy or hypophysectomy by determination of 17-hydroxycorticosteroids and aetiocholanolone, *Lancet* **2**, 1154–1157 (1960).

75. R. D. Bulbrook, J. L. Hayward, C. C. Spicer, and B. S. Thomas, A comparison between the urinary steroid excretion of normal women and women with advanced breast cancer, *Lancet* **2**, 1235–1237 (1962).

76. R. D. Bulbrook, J. L. Hayward, C. C. Spicer, and B. S. Thomas, Abnormal excretion of urinary steroids by women with early breast cancer, *Lancet* **2**, 1238–1240 (1962).

77. H. Miller, J. A. Durant, A. G. Jacobs, and J. G. Allison, Alternative discriminating function for determining hormone dependency of breast cancer, *Br. Med. J.* **1**, 147–149 (1967).

78. S. Kumaoka, N. Sakauchi, N. Abe, M. Kusama, and O. Takatini, Urinary 17-ketosteroid excretion of women with advanced breast cancer, *J. Clin. Endocrinol.* **28**, 667–672 (1968).

79. J. C. Beck, A. J. Blair, M. M. Griffiths, M. W. Rosenfeld, and E. E. McGarry, In search of hormonal factors as an aid in predicting the outcome of breast cancer, *Proc. Can. Cancer Res. Conf.* **6**, 3–35 (1966).

80. R. E. Wilson, D. W. Crocker, J. Fairgrieve, A. F. Bartholomay, K. Emerson, and F. D. Moore, Adrenal structure and function in advanced carcinoma of the breast. II. The relation of steroid excretion to adrenal morphology and the outcome of adrenalectomy with description of a new discriminant function, *J. Am. Med. Assoc.* **199**, 474–482 (1967).

81. R. D. Bulbrook and J. L. Hayward, Abnormal urinary steroid excretion and subsequent breast cancer: A prospective study in the Island of Guernsey, *Lancet* **2**, 519–521 (1967).

82. J. L. Hayward, Androgens and corticosteroids—the Guernsey trial in: *Hormones and Human Breast Cancer*, Chapter 9, pp. 121–135, Springer-Verlag, New York (1970).

83. B. Zumoff, H. L. Bradlow, T. F. Gallagher, and L. Hellman, Decreased conversion of androgens to normal 17-ketosteroid metabolites: A non-specific consequence of illness, *J. Clin. Endocrinol. Metab.* **32**, 824–832 (1971).

84. J. Poortman, J. A. C. Prenen, F. Schwarz, and J. H. H. Thijssen, Interaction of Δ^5-androstene-3β, 17β-diol with estradiol and dihydrotestosterone receptors in human myometrium and mammary cancer tissue, *J. Clin. Endocrinol. Metab.* **40**, 373–379 (1975).

85. W. B. Malarkey, L. L. Schroeder, V. C. Stevens, A. G. James, and R. R. Lanese, Twenty-four hour preoperative endocrine profiles in women with benign and malignant breast disease, *Cancer Res.* **37**, 4655–4659 (1977).

86. J. McFayden, R. J. Prescott, G. V. Groom, A. P. M. Forrest, A. Golden, D. R. Fahmy, and K. Griffith, Circulating hormone concentrations in women with breast cancer, *Lancet* **1**, 1100–1102 (1976).

87. H. O. Adami, Epidemiology and endocrinology in breast cancer. Results of case-control study, Centraltryckeriet, A. B. Uppsala, Sweden (1977).

88. D. Y. Wang, J. L. Hayward, and R. D. Bulbrook, Testosterone levels in the plasma of normal women and patients with benign breast disease or with breast cancer, *Eur. J. Cancer* **2**, 373 (1966).

89. J. H. H. Thijssen, J. Poortman, F. Schwartz, and F. de Waard, Post-menopausal estrogen production, with special reference to patients with mammary carcinoma, *Front. Horm. Res.* **3**, 45–62 (1975).

90. R. P. Persijn, C. B. Korsten, and E. Engelsman, Oestrogen and androgen receptors in breast cancer and response to endocrine therapy, *Br. Med. J.* **4**, 503 (1975).

91. R. K. Wagner, L. Gorlick, and P. W. Jungblut, Dihydrotestosterone receptors in human mammary cancer, *Acta. Endocrinol. (Copenhagen) Suppl.* **173**, 65 (1973).

92. G. T. Ross, C. M. Cargills, M. D. Lipsett, P. Rayford, J. R. Marshall, C. A. Strott, and D. Rodbard, Pituitary and gonadal hormones in women during spontaneous and induced ovulatory cycles, *Recent Prog. Horm. Res.* **26**, 1–62 (1970).

93. R. L. Vande Wiele, J. Bogamil, I. Dyrenfurth, M. Ferin, R. Jewelewicz, M. Warren, T. Rizkallah, and G. Mikhail, Mechanisms regulating the menstrual cycle in women, *Recent Prog. Horm. Res.* **26**, 63–103 (1970).

94. B. M. Sherman and S. G. Korenman, Hormonal characteristics of the human menstrual cycle throughout reproductive life, *J. Clin. Invest.* **55**, 699–706 (1975).

95. B. M. Sherman, J. H. West, and S. G. Korenman, The menopausal transition: Analaysis of LH, FSH, estradiol and progesterone concentrations during menstrual cycles of older women, *J. Clin. Endocrinol. Metab.* **42**, 629–636 (1976).

96. R. Grattarola, The premenstrual endometrial pattern of women with breast cancer, *Cancer* **17**, 1119–1122.

97. B. M. Sherman and S. G. Korenman, Inadequate corpus luteum function: A

pathophysiological interpretation of human breast cancer epidemiology, *Cancer* **33**, 1306–1312 (1974).

98. W. L. Frantz, J. H. MacIndoe, and R. W. Turkington, Prolactin receptors. 1. Characteristics of the particulate binding activity, *J. Endocrinol.* **60**, 485–497 (1974).

99. R. W. Turkington, G. C. Majumder, N. Kadohama, J. H. MacIndoe, and W. L. Frantz, Hormonal regulation of gene expression in mammary cells, *Recent Prog. Horm. Res.* **29**, 417–455 (1973).

100. M. E. Costlow, R. A. Buschow, N. J. Richert, and W. L. McGuire, Prolactin and estrogen binding in transplantable hormone-dependent and autonomous rat mammary carcinoma, *Cancer Res.* **35**, 970–794 (1975).

101. R. W. Turkington, Prolactin receptors in mammary carcinoma cells, *Cancer Res.* **34**, 758–763 (1974).

102. O. Mioduszewska, T. Koszarowski, and C. Gorski, The influence of hormones in breast cancer *in vitro* in relation to the clinical course of the disease, in: *Prognostic Factors in Breast Cancer* (A. P. M. Forrest and P. B. Kunkler, eds.), pp. 347–353, E. & S. Livingstone, Edinburgh (1968).

103. O. H. Pearson, A. Molina, A. Butler, L. Lerena, and H. Nasr, Estrogens and prolactin in mammary cancer, in: *Estrogen Target Tissues and Neoplasia* (T. L. Dao, ed.), p. 287, University of Chicago Press, Chicago (1972).

104. S. K. Quadri and J. Meites, Regression of spontaneous mammary tumors in rats by ergot drugs, *Proc. Soc. Exp. Biol. Med.* **138**, 999–1001 (1971).

105. P. K. Talwalker, J. Meites, and H. Mizuno, Mammary tumor induction by estrogen or anterior pituitary hormones in ovariectomized rats given dimethylbenzanthracene, *Proc. Soc. Exp. Biol. Med.* **116**, 531–534 (1962).

106. G. M. Bogardus and J. W. Finley, Breast cancer and thyroid disease, *Surgery* **49**, 461–468 (1961).

107. K. Backwinkel and A. S. Jackson, Some features of breast cancer and thyroid deficiency, *Cancer* **17**, 1174–1176 (1964).

108. J. Hayward, *Hormones and Human Breast Cancer*, Ch. 10, Springer-Verlag, New York (1970).

109. C. C. Kapdi and J. M. Wolfe, Breast cancer. Relationship to thyroid supplements for hypothyroidism, *J. Am. Med. Assoc.* **236**, 1124–1127 (1976).

110. J. P. Minton and R. P. Dickey, Levodopa test to predict response of carcinoma of the breast to surgical ablation of endocrine glands, *Surg. Gynecol. Obstet.* **136**, 1325 (1974).

111. E. E. Cassell, J. Meites, and C. W. Welsch, Effects of ergocornine and ergocryptine on growth of dimethylbenzanthracene-induced mammary tumors in rats, *Cancer Res.* **31**, 1051–1053 (1971).

112. H. Nagasawa and J. Meites, Suppression by ergocornine and iproniazid of carcinogen-induced mammary tumors in rats; effect on serum and pituitary prolactin levels, *Proc. Soc. Exp. Biol. Med.* **135**, 469–472 (1970).

113. B. Armstrong, N. Stevens, and R. Foll, Retrospective study of the association between use of rauwolfia derivatives and breast cancer in English women, *Lancet* **2**, 672–675 (1974).

114. O. P. Heinonen, S. Shapiro, L. Tuominen, and M. I. Turunen, Reserpine use in relation to breast cancer, *Lancet* **2**, 675–677 (1974).

115. H. Jick, D. Slone, S. Shapiro, O. P. Heinonen, and S. C. Hartz, Reserpine and breast cancer, *Lancet* **2**, 669–671 (1974).

116. E. M. Laska, M. Meisner, C. Siegel, S. Fischer, and J. Wanderling, Matched pair study of reserpine use and breast cancer, *Lancet* **2**, 296–300 (1975).

117. T. M. Mack, B. E. Henderson, V. R. Gerkins, J. Baptista, and M. C. Pike, Reserpine and breast cancer in a retirement community, *N. Engl. J. Med.* **292**, 1366–1371 (1975).

118. W. M. O'Fallon, D. P. Labarthe, and G. T. Kurland, Rauwolfia derivatives and breast cancer, *Lancet* **2**, 773–775 (1975).
119. H. G. Kwa, E. Engelsman, M. De Jong-Bakker, and F. J. Cuton, Plasma prolactin in human breast cancer, *Lancet* **1**, 433–435 (1974).
120. M. C. Pike, J. T. Cassagrande, J. B. Brown, V. Gerkins, and B. E. Henderson, Comparison of urinary and plasma hormone levels in daughters of breast cancer patients and controls, *J. Natl. Cancer Inst.* **59**, 1351–1355 (1977).
121. P. Hill, E. L. Wynder, H. Kemar, P. Helman, G. Rorea, and K. Kuno, Prolactin levels in populations at risk for breast cancer, *Cancer Res.* **36**, 4102 (1976).
122. I. Mittra, J. L. Hayward and A. S. McNeilly, Hypothalamic–pituitary–prolactin axis in breast cancer, *Lancet* **1**, 889–891 (1974).
123. W. B. Malarkey, L. L. Schroeder, V. C. Stevens, A. G. James, and R. R. Lanese, Disordered nocturnal prolactin regulation in women with breast cancer, *Cancer Res.* **37**, 4650–4654 (1977).
124. G. A. Edelstyn, A. R. Lyons, and R. B. Welbourn, Thyroid function in patients with mammary cancer, *Lancet* **1**, 670–673 (1958).
125. L. J. Humphrey and M. Swerdlow, The relationship of breast disease to thyroid disease, *Cancer* **17**, 1170 (1964).
126. L. T. Kurland and J. F. Annegers, Breast cancer and Hashimoto's thyroiditis, *Lancet* **1**, 808 (1976).
127. N. Maruchi, J. F. Annegers, and L. T. Kurland, Hashimoto's thyroiditis and breast cancer, *Mayo Clin. Proc.* **51**, 263–265 (1976).
128. R. B. Wallace, B. M. Sherman, J. A. Bean, and J. Leepr, Thyroid human use in patients with breast cancer—absence of an association, *J. Am. Med. Assoc.* **239**, 958 (1978).
129. P. Mustacchi, and F. Greenspan, Thyroid supplementation: An iatrogenic cause of breast cancer? *J. Am. Med. Assoc.* **237**, 1446–1447 (1977).
130. C. A. Gorman, D. V. Becker, and F. S. Greenspan, Breast cancer and thyroid therapy: Statement by the American Thyroid Association, *J. Am. Med. Assoc.* **237**, 1459–1460 (1977).
131. E. W. Emergy and B. Trotter, Triiodothyronine in advanced breast cancer, *Lancet* **1**, 358–359 (1963).
132. A. R. Lyons and G. A. Edelstyn, Thyroid hormone as a prophylactic agent following radical treatment of breast cancer, *Br. J. Cancer* **19**, 116–121 (1965).
133. R. D. Liechty, R. E. Hodges, and J. Burket, Cancer and thyroid function, *J. Am. Med. Assoc.* **183**, 30–32 (1963).
134. A. R. Moossa, D. A. Price Evans, and A. C. Brewer, Thyroid status and breast cancer, *Ann. R. Coll. Surg. Engl.* **53**, 178–188 (1973).
135. A. R. Lyons, Thyroid hormones and breast cancer, in: *Prognostic Factors in Breast Cancer* (A. P. M. Forrest and P. B. Kunkler, eds.), pp. 165–173, Williams & Wilkins, Baltimore (1968).
136. A. C. Carter, E. B. Feldman, and H. L. Schwartz, Level of serum protein-bound iodine in patients with metastatic carcinoma of the breast, *J. Clin. Endocrinol.* **20**, 477–482 (1960).
137. B. A. Stoll, Breast cancer and hypothyroidism, *Cancer* **18**, 1431–1436 (1965).
138. J. Myhill, T. S. Reeve, and I. B. Heald, Thyroid function in breast cancer, *Acta Endocrinol. (Copenhagen)* **51**, 290–300 (1966).
139. K. Sicher and J. A. H. Waterhouse, Thyroid activity in relation to prognosis in mammary cancer, *Br. J. Cancer* **21**, 512–518 (1967).
140. I. Mittra, J. L. Hayward, and A. S. McNeilly, Hypothalamic–pituitary–thyroid axis in breast cancer, *Lancet* **1**, 885–888 (1974).

141. L. Hellman, H. L. Bradlow, B. Zumoff, D. Fukushima, and T. F. Gallagher, Thyroid–androgen interrelationships and the hypercholesteremic effect of androsterone, *J. Clin. Endocrinol. Metab.* **19,** 936–948 (1959).

142. J. Fishman, L. Hellman, B. Zumoff, and T. F. Gallagher, Influence of thyroid hormone on estrogen metabolism in man, *J. Clin. Endocrinol. Metab.* **22,** 389–392 (1962).

143. J. Fishman, L. Hellman, B. Zumoff, and T. F. Gallagher, Effect of thyroid on hydroxylation of estrogen in man, *J. Clin. Endocrinol. Metab.* **25,** 365–368 (1965).

144. J. S. McGuire and G. Tomkins, The effects of thyroxin administration on the enzymatic reduction of Δ^4-3 ketosteroids, *J. Biol. Chem.* **234,** 791–794 (1959).

145. H. M. Ruder, P. Corval, J. A. Mahoudeau, G. T. Rose, and M. B. Lipsett, Effects of induced hyperthyroidism on steroid metabolism in man, *J. Clin. Endocrinol. Metab.* **33,** 382–387 (1971).

146. F. C. Greenwood, V. H. T. James, B. F. Megitt, J. D. Miller, and P. H. Taylor, Pituitary function in breast cancer, in: *Prognostic Factors in Breast Cancer* (A. P. M. Forrest and P. B. Kunkler, eds.), pp. 409–420, Williams & Wilkins, Baltimore (1968).

147. O. H. Pearson, O. Llerena, N. Samaan, and D. Gonzalez, Serum growth hormone and insulin levels in patients with breast cancer, in: *Prognostic Factors in Breast Cancer* (A. P. M. Forrest and P. B. Kunkler, eds.), pp. 421–430, Williams & Wilkins, Baltimore (1968).

148. A. C. Carter, B. W. Lefkon, M. Farlin, and E. B. Feldman, Metabolic parameters in women with metastatic breast cancer, *J. Clin. Endocrinol. Metab.* **40,** 260–265 (1975).

149. J. A. Loraine, The estimation of anterior pituitary hormones in patients with mammary carcinoma, in: *Endocrine Aspects of Breast Cancer* (A. P. Currie, ed.), pp. 158–169, E. & S. Livingstone, Edinburgh (1958).

150. E. Boyland, B. Godsmark, W. P. Greening, P. Rigby-Jones, J. J. Stevenson, and M. A. M. Abdul-fadl, The effect of irradiation of the pituitary on gonadotropin excretion in women with advanced mammary cancer, in: *Endocrine Aspects of Breast Cancer* (A. P. Currie, ed.), pp. 170–183, E. & S. Livingstone, Edinburgh (1958).

151. J. B. Adams, Steroid hormones and human breast cancer. An hypothesis, *Cancer* **40,** 320–333 (1977).

152. T. L. Dao and P. R. Libby, Steroid sulfate formation in human breast tumors and hormone dependency, in: *Estrogen Target Tissues and Neoplasm* (T. L. Dao, ed.), pp. 181–200, University of Chicago Press, Chicago (1972).

7

Risks and Benefits of Mammography

J. BAILAR, III

1. Introduction

In general, screening programs for the early detection of cancer have not been as successful as was once expected. Two areas of success are cervical cytology, which has almost certainly reduced mortality from cervical cancer, and screening for breast cancer, which can be helpful for women past the age of 50. On the other hand, breast cancer screening at younger ages has been of no apparent benefit, there is no demonstrated value in testing for occult blood in the stool to detect colon cancer, screening for cancer of the urinary bladder is of little value because of the limited range of treatment options, several well-designed trials for early diagnosis of lung cancer have not yet been successful in reducing mortality, and there has been no benefit shown for screening of persons at high risk for thyroid cancer.

This chapter considers just one of these problems: the role of X-ray mammography in programs for the early detection of breast cancer, particularly in women under the age of 50. It is based largely on several earlier reviews of the same subject.[1-3] The problem in general is that there is strong evidence of a small risk from radiation and no evidence of any benefit.

Some experts have urged that every woman 35 years of age or older undergo mammography at least once a year. Other experts have noted that a significant radiation hazard is involved in mammography, that

J. BAILAR, III • National Cancer Institute, National Institutes of Health, Bethesda, Maryland 20205.

mammography can be of value with only some breast cancers, and that the long-term health costs will outweigh the long-term health benefits for a large proportion of potential screenees. These matters must be considered very carefully before any recommendations are made for an increase in the use of mammography. A second, and clearly secondary, reason for caution is the extremely high economic cost of the procedure.

I am particularly concerned by overoptimistic expectations of what mammography can accomplish. My interest in this problem was first stimulated not because the risks were being ignored, but because the public seemed to be misinformed about the benefits. Mammographers themselves seem to be particularly susceptible to this optimism; many simply do not have a realistic view of the limitations of their procedure.

2. Definition of "Screening"

To me, the word "screening" implies a search for any medical condition for which there are no signs or symptoms that reasonably suggest that condition. This definition excludes any consideration of "risk factors" in the absence of signs or symptoms. Risk factors may help to determine whether screening should be done, but the presence of one, two, or even more risk factors does not keep an examination from being "screening" if the subject is free of signs and symptoms. In other words, one can screen high-risk persons, but examinations of persons with signs or symptoms of cancer should be considered diagnosis, not screening. (Diagnosis may, of course, include mammography or other procedures also used in screening.) Most women have minor breast complaints from time to time; such women are not considered symptomatic unless there is real suspicion that the symptoms may indicate cancer.

3. Risks of Yearly Screening for Asymptomatic Women under the Age of 50

3.1. Carcinogenic Effects of Radiation

This paper does not reexamine the basic data on radiation carcinogenesis in the human breast. Upton et al. [4] recently considered all available human data suitable for this purpose; no additional data have been reported since then, and I know of no other significant data sources that could add much to our knowledge on this matter within the next few years. Upton concluded that "... the risk may be assumed to approximate 3.5–7.5 cases of breast cancer per million women of ages 35 or older at risk per year per rad to both breasts, from the tenth year after irradiation throughout the remainder of life." I accept that estimate as the best that can be derived today. It implies a strictly additive, linear, nonthreshold dose–response relationship. Those who believe that other models should be used may come to significantly different risk estimates for discussion of these points (see references 5-11). This estimate also implies that the female breast is one of the most sensitive human organs for radiation carcinogenesis.[12] There is some reason to believe that the risk of radiation to the breast is highest before age 20 and declines at older age; Upton's estimate was meant to apply to women in age groups commonly subjected to mammographic screening.

The well-known study of the Health Insurance Plan of Greater New York (H.I.P.)[13] showed, beyond serious question, that annual screening by a combination of modalities (medical history, physical examination, and mammography) can reduce mortality from breast cancer for women over the age of 50. The mortality reduction was almost 40% in that age group, a result of great practical importance. In contrast, no mortality reduction whatever occurred in younger women. These results refer to the effect of the three screening modalities together. The H.I.P. study was not designed to provide reliable assessments of the effect of each modality separately, and the problems involved in attempts to obtain such estimates include length bias, lead-time bias, self-selection, and many other factors.[1-3] Thus we do not know how much mammography contributed to the good results from screening older women. We can conclude, however, that mammography was not beneficial to women 50 years of age and younger, because even the three modalities together did not seem to be helpful.

The H.I.P. study used the radiologic techniques of the early 1960s, and significant technical advances have been made since then. The most modern equipment, properly used, can produce distinctly better images now than then, so that detection of more lesions at earlier stages is possible. However, no data are available to determine by direct means whether this earlier detection is beneficial for women 50 years of age and younger. All of the evidence is indirect, and much of it depends on the assumption that breast cancer in women over 50, essentially all postmenopause, is the same disease in all important biologic respects as is breast cancer in younger women. This assumption may well be false. Whereas breast cancers in these two age groups tend to have the same microscopic appearance, they differ substantially in epidemiologic features, hormonal and biochemical concomitants, response to treatment, and other factors. Thus we cannot ignore the fact that the H.I.P. study, the only reliable source of data on the long-term effects of breast cancer screening, produced entirely negative results for women under 50 years of age. Large-scale studies with modern mammographic equipment are now or soon will be in progress in the Netherlands, Sweden, and perhaps Canada. Their results, when available, may modify present conclusions.

With respect to the radiation risks of mammography, again no direct evidence exists. There are no data on the long-term follow-up of women exposed to ionizing radiation of the same dose level, type of ionizing, and fractionation pattern as that used in breast cancer screening. Most of the arguments have centered on whether the dose-response relationship is linear; that is, whether the likelihood of causing breast cancer is in direct proportion to the total amount of radiation absorbed. I believe that the linear model should be used for doses up to several hundred rads, although some people (including many radiologists) believe that it overstates risks, and many others (including some eminent radiation biologists) believe that it understates risks. The linear model for X-ray carcinogenesis in the breast should be regarded as a "best estimate," not a "conservative" model, for three reasons: (1) it fits all available data very well,[14-17] (2) it has a direct interpretation in terms of present understanding of cellular and molecular events in radiation carcinogenesis, and (3) it avoids the unnecessary "looseness" and complexity of models with larger numbers of fitted parameters. That the survivors of the atomic explosions in Japan have had a distinct elevation in the incidence of breast cancer after exposure to just 17 rads is significant.[16]

Application of the linear model requires some knowledge of the radiation doses used in the practice of mammography. These have varied widely, with occasional reports of extremely high doses.[2,3] Radiation doses in mammography need to be quite high (even with so-called "low-dose" methods) because of the need for good contrast in differentiating among small differences in radiographic density among fat, fibrous and glandular tissue, and masses of malignant cells. In the United States, the average midbreast exposure for a complete examination (2 films/breast) may have been in the range of 3–5 rads at the time of the H.I.P. study. Over time, and with the partial shift from early methods to xeromammography, average doses declined to perhaps 1–2 rads by the summer of 1975. At that time, public and professional awareness of the radiation hazards in mammography increased rapidly. As a result, there was a sharp acceleration in the move toward low-dose methods, and film–screen combinations were more widely used. Also, the degree of caution and control over the use of existing equipment increased. Average midbreast exposures for a complete examination may now be about 0.5 rads in the United States.[18] Further significant reductions are likely as more hospitals and clinics adopt improved techniques. This recent rapid drop in average exposure was due mostly to public pressure and should be regarded as one of several beneficial effects of extensive coverage of the subject by general newspapers, magazines, radio, and television.

Radiation risks are not the only health hazards of breast cancer screening. Other authors have commented on the high frequency of negative biopsies, on surgical morbidity and even mortality, and on other matters (see, for example, references 19 and 20, and reference 20 with following discussion). Some of the research needs on radiation risks have been described by Dethlefsen and others.[22]

As discussed above, data on the risks of mammography are not entirely satisfactory, while no data exist to show benefits in women under 50 years of age. Just these two points provide reason to be cautious in the use of mammography to screen asymptomatic young women from the general population. Two additional problems make the broad-scale, indiscriminate use of mammography before the age of 50 distinctly unwise. These problems are the overdiagnosis of "cancer" and the likelihood of synergism between radiation and other risk factors.

3.2. Overdiagnosis

Overdiagnosis has also received extensive public exposure in the United States, especially during late 1977 and early 1978. A group of 27 large demonstration centers for breast cancer screening had reported a total of 1808 "cancers" found during a series of examinations of about 280,000 women. Five hundred ninety were described as "minimal cancer." A group of eminent pathologists examined slides for 504 of these minimal cancers. Their final conclusion was that 48 were entirely benign, 27 were noninvasive but could not be definitely classified as benign, and 262 were considered noninvasive neoplasms.[23] Thus there was no evidence that 337 lesions, or two-thirds of the "cancers" reviewed by this group, presented any real threat to life and health. This fact is particularly significant because the promoters of mammography have given great emphasis to the "minimal cancers" as evidence that screening can detect cancers at an early stage.

The 48 benign lesions are a serious matter, but more serious is the large group of noninvasive neoplasms (262 of the 504 lesions reviewed). We simply do not know what proportion, if any, of these neoplasms will ever progress to the more usual forms of breast cancer that invade, metastasize, and kill. That some do is likely, but recent work indicates that the proportion may be small. For example, Lattes[24] has reported on a series of 210 patients with lobular noninvasive neoplasms incidentally detected. Seventeen percent had developed invasive cancers after an average of seven to eight years of observation, but half were in the breast contralateral to the lobular lesion. Others[25-28] have also noted a relatively low frequency or rate of incidence of invasive cancer following the detection of noninvasive neoplasms, although results have differed on whether lobular or ductal lesions present a greater long-term hazard. At present we do not know whether and how to treat such conditions. Answers to these questions will depend in part on the development of a better understanding of the biology and multicentric origin of breast cancer neoplasms, particularly the noninvasive lesions found at early stages by screening.[29,30]

3.3. Synergism between Radiation Risk and Other Risk Factors

With respect to the likelihood of synergism between the carcinogenic effects of radiation and the effects of other risk factors, we again have no data. However, the fact that carcinogenic agents are generally synergistic in laboratory animals is widely accepted, and good evidence demonstrates synergy in some human cancers. For example, the relation between lung cancer and cigarette smoking is very much magnified by exposure to either asbestos[31] or radiation.[32] At least two other studies are in progress to determine whether radiation is synergistic with other causes of cancer in the human female breast, but that work is not yet complete.[33,34]

If a significant degree of synergy exists, of course, women at high risk for breast cancer should be actively excluded from general X-ray screening programs. This would be contrary to current practice in the United States and elsewhere, and we may in time come to regret the present emphasis on preferential screening of women who are at especially high risk for developing breast cancer.

It is difficult to assess the meaning and impact of risk factors taken one at a time, even without the complications of synergism. Recent work on the implications of fibrocystic disease has generally suggested a modest elevation in the risk of developing breast cancer.[35,36] Family history is important,[37] but no good evidence supports the idea that cancer incidence is correlated with the size of the breast, which is largely composed of fat and supporting tissues (see, for example, Robertson et al.[38]). Suggestions that fibrocystic disease may be associated with cancers having a favorable prognosis[39] cannot yet be confirmed or denied. Several authors[40-42] have developed models for estimating the effects of two or more risk factors in combination, but those models need much testing and further development before they can be applied with confidence to estimate risks for specific individuals. Kessner[43] has considered some of the broader issues in identifying segments of high-risk populations for special attention in screening programs.

3.4. False-Negative Screening Results

An additional point should be considered in discussions of breast cancer screening for women under the age of 50, although it is a problem in the use of screening results, not in the screening itself. One justification for the periodic examination of young women has been the value of providing reassurance to most screenees that breast cancer is not present. Unfortunately, not all cancers are detectable at screening, and this problem is particularly acute in young women because the denser breast tissue makes radiologic examination more difficult. Several reports (see, for example, reference 44) have shown that mammographic screening of young women has more often led to a significant delay in diagnosis than it has advanced the date of cancer detection. To the extent that screening programs are used to provide reassurance, this problem of false-negative results will continue to be a serious one.

4. Conclusions

In the United States, many radiologists recommend that each woman have one or two so-called "baseline mammography studies" at ages 35–40.[45] Two reasons have been advanced. The first is to have the films on file for comparison with later X-rays, if any should be taken. However, that would be of value only if the use of baseline films really changes the interpretation of later results in a significant proportion of cases. Colleagues who are radiologists tell me that baseline films can provide welcome reassurance that later films have been correctly interpreted, but that they rarely affect the final diagnosis or the management of patients.

The second reason given for baseline mammography is to identify from the appearance of the breast parenchyma a small subgroup of women who are at an especially high risk for breast cancer. This argument is based primarily on the work of John Wolfe,[46,47] who has reported very impressive results. However, other radiologists[48–53] have had limited success in duplicating those results in well-controlled studies. Thus, to recommend baseline mammography seems unwise unless Wolfe's classification can be refined and improved for general application.

There is a large and expanding literature on newer techniques of mammography, or radiation exposure levels with various techniques, and on methods of quality control. That literature will not be reviewed here, except for brief comment on a few recent reports that illustrate important points. Several authors believe that a single view is sufficient for screening mammography (see, for example, references 54 and 55). There is widespread concern as well as some evidence that breast cancer screening often fails to meet minimum quality standards for both radiologic[56,57] and clinical[3] examinations. Much active research is in progress on the development of entirely new imaging systems and on new ways of using present systems.[58,59]

These and many other questions about breast cancer screening have been examined by a long series of committees. Perhaps it should not be surprising that committees composed primarily or exclusively of radiologists have generally advocated vigorous promotion of mammography with loose control and a low age limit for starting periodic examinations. Committees with a broader membership, including surgeons, pathologists, epidemiologists, radiation biologists, and persons from other relevant disciplines, in addition to radiologists, have come to different conclusions. Recently, five such committees[4,23,60-64] have arrived at nearly identical conclusions with respect to the appropriate role of mammography. The most recent report,[63] which drew in part on the others, was summarized by Thier[64] as follows:

> It seems reasonable to screen women over 50 years of age with a combination of physical examination and X-ray mammography. Mammographic equipment should be well calibrated, and the dose of radiation should be less than 1 rad. The patient should ask for and keep a record of her radiation exposure. Women under 50 may continue to be screened by physical examination, but should be screened with X-ray mammography only if they have already had breast cancer or if they are between the ages of 40 and 49 and have a mother or sister who has had cancer of the breast. Though the risk from X-ray mammography may be small, it is finite, and must be balanced against the absence of any demonstrable benefit from screening women below 50 years of age. When screening is done, it should probably be on a yearly basis. Lesions of less than 1 cm should be evaluated by more than two pathologists before any definitive operation is performed, and before a firm diagnosis of cancer is reported to the patient.

For reasons outlined above, I endorse these guidelines. I do have some reservations about them, also outlined above, but basically I believe these guidelines to be both reasonable and defensible. They were recently adopted as official policy in all agencies of the U.S. Government.[65] In one large screening program, approximately 17% of women aged 35–49 years actually attending the screening clinic qualified for mammography under guidelines very similar to these.[66] These guidelines apply only to screening, that is, to the examination of women who do not have signs or symptoms that specifically suggest the possibility of breast cancer. Strax[67] and Lester[68] have summarized the views of persons advocating less restrictive guidelines.

I hope that other groups will examine the matter with equal care before launching breast cancer screening programs that may be either too broad or too narrow.

5. References

1. J. C. Bailar, III, Mammography: A contrary view, *Ann. Int. Med.* **84**, 77–84 (1976).
2. J. C. Bailar, III, Screening for early breast cancer: Pros and cons, *Cancer* **39**, 2783–2795 (1977).
3. J. C. Bailar, III, Mammographic screening: A reappraisal of benefits and risk, *Clin. Obstet. Gynecol.* **21**, 1–14 (1978).
4. A. C. Upton, G. W. Beebe, J. M. Brown, E. H. Quimby, and C. Shellabarger, Report of NCI ad hoc working group on the risks associated with mammography in mass screening for the detection of breast cancer, *J. Natl. Cancer Inst.* **59**, 481–493 (1977).
5. K. Z. Morgan, Radiation-induced health effects, *Science* **195**, 344–348 (1977).
6. M. Brown, Letters, *Science* **195**, 348–349 (1977).
7. J. M. Brown, The shape of the dose–response curve for radiation carcinogenesis. Extrapolation to low-doses, *Rad. Res.* **71**, 34–50 (1977).
8. H. H. Rossi, Symposium on the Radiobiological Response Relationships at Low Doses. The effects of small doses of ionizing radiation. Fundamental biophysical characteristics, *Rad. Res.* **71**, 1–8 (1977).
9. M. M. Elkind, The initial part of the survival curves. Implications for low-dose, low-dose-rate radiation responses, *Rad. Res.* **71**, 9–23 (1977).
10. H. R. Withers, Response of tissues to multiple small dose fractions, *Rad. Res.* **71**, 24–33 (1977).
11. A. C. Upton, Radiobiological effects of low doses. Implications for radiological protection, *Rad. Res.* **71**, 51–74 (1977).
12. R. H. Mole, The sensitivity of the human breast to cancer induction by ionizing radiation, *Br. J. Radiol.* **51**, 401–405 (1978).
13. S. Shapiro, Evidence on screening for breast cancer from a randomized trial, *Cancer* **39**, 2772–2781 (1977).
14. J. D. Boice, Jr. and R. R. Monson, Breast cancer in women after repeated fluoroscopic examinations of the chest, *J. Natl. Cancer Inst.* **59**, 823–832 (1977).
15. R. E. Shore, L. H. Hempelmann, E. Kowaluk, P. S. Mansur, B. S. Pasternack, R. E. Albert, and G. E. Haughie, Breast neoplasms in women treated with X-rays for acute postpartum mastitis, *J. Natl. Cancer Inst.* **59**, 813–822 (1977).
16. D. H. McGregor, C. E. Land, K. Choi, S. Tokuoka, P. I. Liu, T. Wakabayashi, and G. W. Beebe, Breast cancer incidence among atomic bomb survivors, Hiroshima and Nagasaki, 1950–69, *J. Natl. Cancer Inst.* **59**, 799–811 (1977).
17. E. Baral, L. Larsson, and B. Mattsson, Breast cancer following irradiation of the breast, *Cancer* **40**, 2905–2910 (1977).
18. R. Jans, Personal communication (1978).
19. M. R. Coates, Y. H. Pilch, and J. R. Benfield, Changing concepts in establishing the diagnosis of breast masses, *Am. J. Surg.* **134**, 77–79 (1977).
20. M. A. Schneiderman and L. M. Axtell, "Surgical deaths" among female breast cancer patients treated by surgery only, *Surg. Gynecol. Obstet.* **148**, (Feb.), 193 (1979).

21. J. D. Lewis, J. R. Milbrath, K. A. Shaffer, J. C. Darin, and J. J. DeCosse, Which breast to biopsy: An expanding dilemma, *Ann. Surg.* **184**, 253–256 (1976).

22. L. A. Dethlefsen, J. M. Brown, A. V. Carrano, and S. Nandi, Report of the BCTF Ad Hoc Committee on X-Ray Mammographic Screening for Human Breast Cancer: Can animals and *in vitro* studies give new, relevant answers? Unpublished report (1977).

23. O. H. Beahrs, Report, Supplemental Report, and Concluding Report of the Working Group to Review the National Cancer Institute–American Cancer Society Breast Cancer Detection Demonstration Projects, *J. Natl. Cancer Inst.* **62**, 639–709 (1979).

24. C. D. Haagensen, N. Lane, R. Lattes, and C. Bodian, Lobular neoplasia (so-called lobular carcinoma *in situ*) of the breast, *Cancer* **42**, 737–769 (1978).

25. E. R. Fisher and B. Fisher, Lobular carcinoma of the breast: An overview, *Ann. Surg.* **185**, 377–385 (1977).

26. D. L. Page, R. Vander Zwaag, L. W. Rogers, L. T. Williams, W. E. Walker, and W. H. Hartmann, Relation between component parts of fibrocystic disease complex and breast cancer, *J. Natl. Cancer Inst.* **61**, 1055–1063 (1978).

27. C. Toker and J. D. Goldberg, The small cell lesion of mammary ducts and lobules, *Pathobiol. Annu. (Part 1)* **12**, 217–249 (1977).

28. W. L. Betsell, Jr., P. P. Rosen, P. H. Lieberman, and G. F. Robbins, Intraductal carcinoma: Long term follow-up after "treatment" by biopsy alone, *Lab. Invest.* **38**, 4 (1978).

29. M. D. Lagios, Multicentricity of breast carcinoma demonstrated by routine correlated serial subgross and radiographic examination, *Cancer* **40**, 1726–1734 (1977).

30. A. S. Patchefsky, G. S. Shaber, G. F. Schwartz, S. A. Feig, and R. E. Nerlinger, The pathology of breast cancer detected by mass population screening, *Cancer* **40**, 1639–1670 (1977).

31. I. J. Selikoff, E. C. Hammond, and J. Churg, Asbestos exposure, *J. Am. Med. Assoc.* **204**, 106–112 (1968).

32. F. E. Lundin, Jr., J. W. Lloyd, E. M. Smith, V. E. Archer, and D. A. Holaday, Mortality of uranium miners in relation to radiation exposure, hard-rock mining and cigarette smoking—1950 through September 1967, *Health Phys.* **16**, 571–578 (1969).

33. J. D. Boice and B. J. Stone, Interaction between radiation and other breast cancer risk factors, in: *Late Biological Effects of Ionizing Radiation*, Vol. 1, pp. 231–249, International Atomic Energy Agency, Vienna, Austria (1978).

34. A. Miller, Personal communication (1977).

35. R. R. Monson, S. Yen, B. MacMahon, and S. Warren, Chronic mastitis and carcinoma of the breast, *Lancet* **2**, 224–226 (1976).

36. A. Nomura, G. W. Comstock, and J. A. Tonascia, Epidemiologic characteristics of benign breast disease, *Am. J. Epidemiol.* **105**, 505–511 (1977).

37. D. E. Anderson, Genetic study of breast cancer: Identification of a high risk group, *Cancer* **34**, 1090–1097 (1974).

38. A. J. Robertson, J. Clark, A. W. Hall, J. S. Beck, and A. Cushieri, Breast size and cancer, *Br. Med. J.* **1**, 1283 (1977).

39. T. C Bernstein, What are my chances of getting breast cancer? *J. Am. Med. Assoc.* **238**, 345–346 (1977).

40. V. T. Farewell, B. Math, and M. Math, The combined effect of breast cancer risk factors, *Cancer* **40**, 931–936 (1977).

41. D. F. Davies, A. Torng, E. B. Morris, and J. Sebes, Estimates of the composite risk factors for death from breast cancer, *J. Natl. Cancer Inst.* **61**, 41–48 (1978).

42. F. van der Linde, Definition der Bevölkerungsgruppen mit hohem Risiko beim Mammakazinom, *Schweiz. Med. Wochenschr.* **107**, 962–968 (1977).

43. D. M. Kessner, Screening high-risk populations: A challenge to primary medical care, *J. Commun. Health* **1**, 216–225 (1976).
44. G. J. Lesnick, Detection of breast cancer in young women, *J. Am. Med. Assoc.* **237**, 967–969 (1977).
45. American College of Radiology, Board approves mammography policy, *Bull. Am. Coll. Radiol.* **32**,(8), 1 (August 1976).
46. J. N. Wolfe, Risk for breast cancer development determined by mammographic parenchymal pattern, *Cancer* **37**, 2486–2492 (1976).
47. J. N. Wolfe, Breast parenchymal patterns and their changes with age, *Radiology* **121**, 545–552 (1976).
48. R. G. Peyster, L. Kalisher, and P. Cole, Mammographic parenchymal patterns and the prevalence of breast cancer, *Radiology* **125**, 387–391 (1977).
49. R. L. Egan and R. C. Mosteller, Breast cancer mammography patterns, *Cancer* **40**, 2087–2090 (1977).
50. L. Mendell, M. Rosenbloom, and A. Naimark, Are breast patterns a risk index for breast cancer? A reappraisal, *Am. J. Roentgenol.* **128**, 547 (1977).
51. E. Wilkinson, C. Clopton, J. Gordonson, R. Green, A. Hill, and M. C. Pike, Mammographic parenchymal pattern and the risk of breast cancer, *J. Natl. Cancer Inst.* **59**, 1397–1400 (1977).
52. M. Moskowitz, S. Pemmaraja, P. Russell, L. Gardella, P. Gartside, and I. DeGroot, Observations on the natural history of carcinoma of the breast, its precursors, and mammographic counterparts. Part 2. Mammographic patterns, *Breast* **3**, 37–41 (1977).
53. D. F. Rideout and P. Y. Poon, Patterns of breast parenchyma on mammography, *J. Can. Assoc. Radiol.* **28**, 257–258 (1977).
54. B. Lundgren and S. Jakobsson, Single view mammography. A simple and efficient approach to breast cancer screening, *Cancer* **38**, 1124–1129 (1976).
55. B. B. Lundgren, The oblique view at mammography, *Br. J. Radiol.* **50**, 626–628 (1977).
56. J. R. Huppe and H.-J. Schneider, Qualitatsprobleme der Mammographie. Vermeidbare Fehler bei Anfertigung und Betrachtung von Mammogrammen, *Radiologie* **17**, 197–202 (1977).
57. P. L. Pressman, Mammography in surgical practice, *Am. J. Surg.* **133**, 702–704 (1977).
58. K. T. Smith, S. L. Wagner, R. B. Guenther, and D. C. Solomon, The diagnosis of breast cancer in mammograms by the evaluation of density patterns, *Radiology* **125**, 383–386 (1977).
59. W. W. Logan, ed., *Breast Carcinoma. The Radiologist's Expanded Role*, John Wiley & Sons, New York (1978).
60. L. Breslow, L. B. Thomas, and A. C. Upton, Final reports of National Cancer Institute ad hoc Working Groups on Mammography in Screening for Breast Cancer and a summary report of their joint findings and recommendations, *J. Natl. Cancer Inst.* **59**, 467–541 (1977).
61. L. Breslow, B. Henderson, F. Massey, Jr., M. Pike, and W. Winkelstein, Jr., Report of NCI ad hoc Working Group on the Gross and Net Benefits of Mammography in Mass Screening for the Detection of Breast Cancer, *J. Natl. Cancer Inst.* **59**, 473–478 (1977).
62. L. B. Thomas, L. V. Ackerman, R. W. McDivitt, T. A. S. Hanson, B. F. Hankey, and P. C. Prorok, Report of NCI ad hoc Pathology Working Group to Review the Gross and Microscopic Findings of Breast Cancer Cases in the HIP Study (Health Insurance Plan of Greater New York), *J. Natl. Cancer Inst.* **59**, 495–510 (1977).
63. Panel on Breast Cancer Meeting (Samuel O. Thier, chairman), NIH/NCI Consensus Development Meeting on Breast Cancer Screening Issues and Recommendations, Bethesda, Maryland, September 14–16, 1977, *Yale J. Biol. Med.* **51**, 3–7 (1978).

64. S. O. Thier, Breast-cancer screening: A view from outside the controversy, *N. Engl. J. Med.* **297,** 1063–1065 (1977).
65. *Fed. Regist.* **43,** 4377 (1978).
66. D. J. Fink, Personal communication (1977).
67. P. Strax, Consensus meeting, National Institutes of Health, September 14–16 (1977).
68. R. G. Lester, Consensus meeting, National Institutes of Health, September 14–16 (1977).

8

Male Breast Cancer

RICHARD B. EVERSON AND MARC E. LIPPMAN

1. Introduction

About 1 of every 100 cases of human breast cancer occurs in a male, resulting in a disease both similar and dissimilar to breast cancer in females. The disorder accounts for about 0.2% of malignant neoplasia in men.[1] Although the basic clinical characteristics of male breast cancer (MBC) had been well characterized even before Wainwright's classic description in 1927,[2] the relative rarity of the disorder and the consequent reporting of numerous small series have led to frequent disagreement in the literature and insufficient firm data concerning its less prominent features.

This review will attempt to focus on a critical evaluation of several controversial aspects of literature data and on more recent investigations of the disease. Four especially notable recent reviews of MBC deserve special citation: a review of the large (198-patient) series at Memorial Hospital by Holleb et al.[3–5]; a thorough compilation of the 20th-century literature by Crichlow[6]; a series of articles exhaustively describing 265 Danish cases by Scheike and others[7–14]; and a recent review by Meyskens and colleagues.[15]

RICHARD B. EVERSON AND MARC E. LIPPMAN • National Cancer Institute, National Institutes of Health, Bethesda, Maryland 20014.

2. Incidence and Geographic Distribution

The average annual age-adjusted breast cancer incidence rates for cases reported by the United States Third National Cancer Survey were 0.7 per 100,000 males and 73.8 per 100,000 females of all races, roughly a 100-fold difference.[1] That series, including 194 MBC cases diagnosed or treated during 1969–1971 in several large United States metropolitan areas and two states, was population based and should avoid selection factors frequently encountered in hospital series. The average age at diagnosis was higher for men (64.6 years) than for women (59.8 years). Cases of MBC have been reported at ages as young as 5 and as old as 93 years,[6] but rarely before age 35.[1]

Figure 1 displays incidence data by age from the Third National Cancer Survey report: Only one MBC case occurred per 170 female breast cancer cases in patients less than 65 years old, whereas after age 65 one case of MBC occurred per 87 female breast cancer cases. The same relationship can be seen in other reports of incidence[11,16] and mortality.[17] Thus, the ratio of male to female cases seems to be age

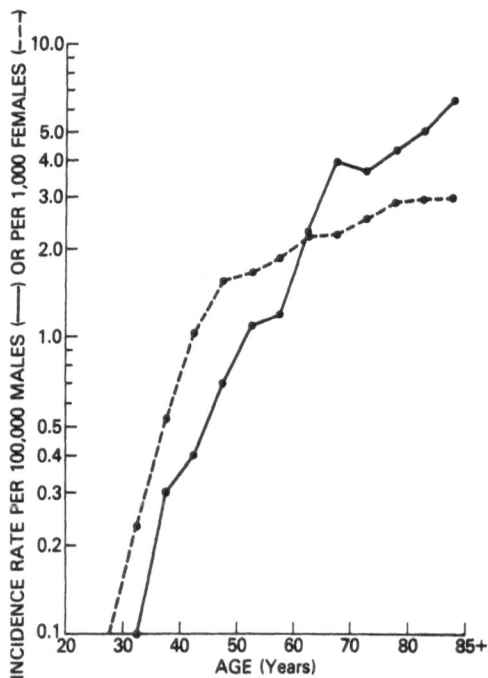

Fig. 1. Average annual age-specific breast cancer incidence rates per 100,000, U.S. population of all races.[1] Note two log differences in scales between male and female rates.

dependent, with a larger fraction of cases among males with increasing age, perhaps accounting for some of the variability in literature reports.[18] Also, as shown in Fig. 1, the log-scale slope for females seems to consist of two components, with a more rapid premenopausal and a slower postmenopausal rise, while the slope for males appears to continue with a more exponential rise. Similar relationships were noted by Schottenfeld and Lilienfeld for mortality in the United States.[17] However, Brunet *et al.*, surveying world incidence data for MBC, have recently reported a bimodal distribution consisting of two normal-distribution curves with means at 47 and 66.5 years.[19]

The United States geographic distribution of breast cancer deaths for 1950–1969 is shown by state economic area for males in Fig. 2 and by county for females in Fig. 3.[20] Although thorough analysis of such geographic clustering is complex, roughly similar clustering of cases in the urban Northeast is noted for both sexes. Data by race for this relatively rare disease are sparse; in one report, mortality rates in the United States were shown to be higher for nonwhites than whites.[17]

Worldwide, the reported annual incidence of MBC ranges more than 10-fold from a high of 1 case per 100,000 in West Germany and Connecticut to 0.1 case per 100,000 in Yugoslavia, Uganda, and Singapore. Finland and Japan, countries with relatively low rates for female breast cancer, also tend to have low MBC rates.[16]

Several authors reported a high incidence of MBC in areas of Africa

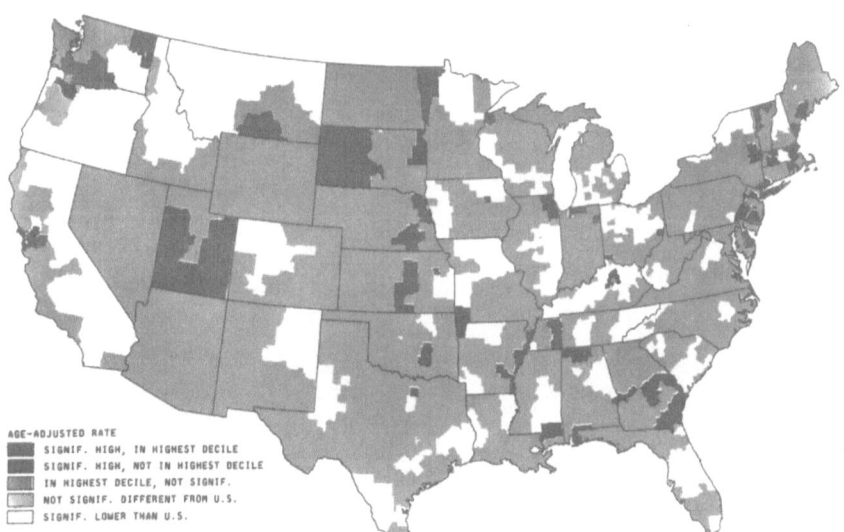

AGE–ADJUSTED RATE
◼ SIGNIF. HIGH, IN HIGHEST DECILE
◼ SIGNIF. HIGH, NOT IN HIGHEST DECILE
◼ IN HIGHEST DECILE, NOT SIGNIF.
◻ NOT SIGNIF. DIFFERENT FROM U.S.
◻ SIGNIF. LOWER THAN U.S.

Fig. 2. Age-adjusted rates for breast cancer mortality among white males, 1950–1969, by U.S. state economic area.

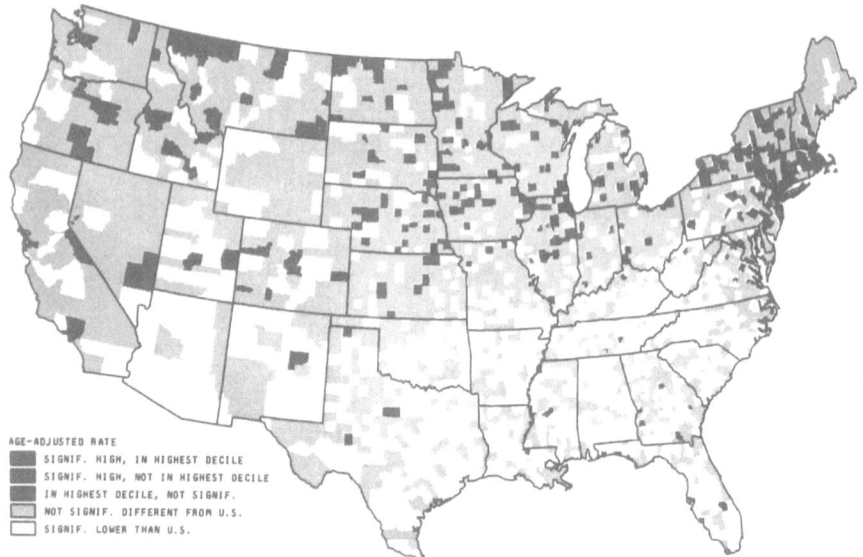

AGE-ADJUSTED RATE
- ■ SIGNIF. HIGH, IN HIGHEST DECILE
- ▨ SIGNIF. HIGH, NOT IN HIGHEST DECILE
- ▨ IN HIGHEST DECILE, NOT SIGNIF.
- ▨ NOT SIGNIF. DIFFERENT FROM U.S.
- ☐ SIGNIF. LOWER THAN U.S.

Fig. 3. Age-adjusted rates for breast cancer mortality among white females, 1950–1969, by U.S. county.

and related this to chronic liver disease from malnutrition.[21,22] Two areas have reported more recently that MBC accounted for a high proportion of total breast cancer cases: 6% of all cases in Egypt[23] and 15% in Zambia.[24] In both these series, the age of onset was unusually young, with a mean of 41 years for the Egyptian series and between 40 and 55 years for 77% of Zambian cases. Even considering the difference in age distribution of the general population between these countries and the United States, this early age of onset suggests an effect of different or more intense etiologic influences. The high male-to-female ratio for breast cancer in Egypt was felt by El-Gazayerli and Abdel-Aziz[23] to be associated with hyperestrogenism resulting from bilharzial hepatic fibrosis but biochemical studies supporting this suggestion have not appeared.

3. Etiology

Possible risk factors for MBC are presented in Table I. While it is possible that the study of MBC etiology could provide important clues to the pathogenesis of female breast cancer, as we will demonstrate, such rewards are not yet firmly apparent; furthermore, several of the few proposed risk factors for MBC are imperfectly established.

Table I
Proposed Risk Factors for Male Breast Cancer

Exogenous estrogen exposure
Atypical endogenous steroid metabolism and excretion
Klinefelter's syndrome
Familial clustering
Radiation
Gynecomastia
Other (orchitis, trauma)

3.1. Epidemiologic Field Studies

Schottenfeld et al.[25] reviewed hospital charts of 120 MBC patients and interviewed 53 of these patients, comparing them with age-matched patients with gynecomastia or colon cancer. No differences in religious distribution or marital status were observed. Although numbers were small and differences not statistically significant, MBC patients had more frequent histories of infectious orchitis, X-ray exposure, gynecomastia, and breast cancer among male family members. Keller, in a case-control study based on clinical records of 181 MBC patients at United States Veterans Administration Hospitals, found no differences between MBC patients and those with urinary cancer or random controls in marital status, religion, race, or geographical origin; liver, endocrine, or other organ disease; and tobacco use. Two MBC patients, but no controls, had Klinefelter's syndrome.[26]

3.2. Exogenous Estrogens

Lacassagne[27] produced mammary carcinoma in male mice by administering an estrogen. Several mouse strains were shown to be susceptible, although large doses were generally required.[28,29] One study reported that castration and ovarian grafts increased the incidence of 3-methylcholanthrene-induced MBC in rats.[30] In 1942, Scarff and Smith reported a proliferative mastitis in two male stilbestrol workers which exhibited a "dangerous" degree of epithelial proliferation.[31] Several case reports of patients developing MBC while on estrogen therapy for prostatic carcinoma appeared subsequently, implicating estrogens in the etiology of this tumor.[32] A questionnaire survey of 150 urologists by the American Medical Association, however, suggested that the risk was probably low: Only 2 of 17,000 patients with prostatic cancer treated by estrogen were reported to have developed MBC,[3] and only 1 of more than 3000 similarly treated patients developed MBC in another report.[33]

Reviews by Campbell and Cummins[34] and Benson[35] suggested that many cases of carcinoma in the breast following treatment for prostatic cancer represented metastases from the prostatic primaries rather than induced MBC. In any case, the number of reported primary and metastatic breast neoplasms in patients with prostatic carcinoma was small: In 1976, Wilson and Hutchinson could find 19 cases in the English literature, 6 of which they accepted as primary breast cancer and 10 as metastatic prostatic lesions, and in 3 the origin was unclear.[32] Two autopsy studies, however, suggested that occult metastases from prostatic carcinoma are common: Malignant deposits interpreted as being of prostatic origin were found in about 5% of autopsies of men with metastatic prostatic carcinoma.[36,37] Also, an autopsy study of breasts from 500 men found 1 primary MBC but 10 metastases to the breast from extramammary tumors.[38] Crichlow, on reviewing the literature, found only 2 reports of previous estrogen therapy among 457 MBC cases.[6]

In summary, although estrogen therapy for prostatic cancer cannot be excluded as a risk factor for MBC, few cases have been reported and the risk appears low.

More convincing evidence for a role of estrogen in the etiology of MBC was presented by Symmers[39] in a case report describing two 30-year-old British transsexuals, both of whom died from metastatic breast carcinoma five years after surgical castration, mammoplasty, and continuous apparently massive estrogen use. The dosage used, young age, and lack of gonads are consistent with typical requirements for estrogen induction of breast cancer in male experimental animals.[30] Indeed, their youth makes an etiologic association likely. Using available United States data, death rates for MBC in males aged 30–34 were 0.3 per million[20]; two deaths would thus be an impressive number for a transsexual population estimated at 3000 to 10,000 in the United States. Orentreich and Durr[40] noted two additional cases of MBC in men treated with estrogen, one in a 59-year-old man treated for ulcer disease and another in a 45-year-old man treated for myocardial infarction; their ages make association by chance more likely than in the transsexual cases.

3.3. Endogenous Hormonal Metabolism

Most studies suggest some alteration in the endocrine physiology of MBC patients. In 1966, Zumoff and associates reported that six men with breast cancer produced less estrone, 2-hydroxyestrone, and 2-methoxyestrone, but more estriol, than controls following a tracer dose of estradiol.[41] They suggested that MBC patients have increased 16α-hydroxylase, leading to a greater production of estriol. Five of these men had recurrent disease and the presence of tumor may have affected the results, as some human mammary tumors can synthesize estrogens from androgens.[42] The relative contributions of different pathways of estrogen metabolism are of critical importance in that estriol is a biologically active estrogen whereas the cathechol metabolites are probably antiestrogenic.

Using chromatographic techniques, Lazarev et al.[43] and Komurdjaev and Rogoznaya[44] reported by 1969 that MBC patients excreted more estrone, estradiol, and estriol than controls. Using gas chromatography, Dao and colleagues[45] reported in 1973 that seven MBC patients excreted significantly more estrone, estradiol, and estriol than controls. Three of their patients were clinically free of disease. In 1974, De Giuli and De Giuli[46] reported that 24 of 29 MBC patients excreted more total estrogens than controls, and Calabresi et al. [47] subsequently showed by radioimmunoassay that 17 MBC patients (10 free of disease) had plasma levels of estrone, estradiol, and estriol higher than those of controls but similar concentrations of androstenedione and testosterone.

The androgens androstenedione and testosterone are direct precursors of estrone and estradiol, respectively. The fact that estrogen levels are higher while androgen precursor levels are unchanged suggests a direct effect on either aromatization or estrogen clearance. Sadoff and Davidson[48] observed elevated estrogen excretion in men with lung, renal pelvis, colon, and pancreas malignancies, as well as three additional cases of MBC; they state that these elevations may represent "a non-specific response to stress" or may "be involved in the actual pathogenesis." Data conflicting with all of these studies, however, were presented by Scheike and colleagues.[8] Their studies used a chemical extraction and fluorimetry technique developed by Brown et al.[49] for estrogens and modifications of techniques by Brown and Giard for metabolism of labeled estradiol. They showed no difference between 19 men with MBC (14 disease free) and age-matched controls for the excretion of total estrogens and for the excretory pattern of administered labeled estradiol as estrone, estradiol, estriol, and 2-methoxyestrone.[49] They suggest that cardiac disease and/or advanced malignant disease in the series of Zumoff et al. may account for the difference in results. They reported, however, increased levels of urinary gonadotropins.[8] Everson et al. observed that two of three healthy, unaffected members of families with multiple cases of MBC excreted elevated levels of estrone, estradiol, estriol, and total estrogens, as measured by radioimmunoassay.[50] Since tumor was not present, this observation supports an association between estrogen excretion and pathogenesis.

Thus, most endocrine-metabolic studies of MBC patients suggest that the disorder is linked to abnormal estrogen metabolism and excretion. The reason for contradictory findings by Scheike and colleagues[8] is unclear, but may relate to patient selection or analytic methodology employed. Several observations hint that these endocrine abnormalities are linked to pathogenesis, but the origin of the elevated amounts of estrogen, whether in glandular secretion or peripheral biotransformation, is unclear.

Some difficulties in interpretation of differences between normal males and MBC patients may reflect problems in obtaining a suitable control population. Aside from matching for age and cardiovascular, renal, and hepatic function, other parameters may be important. For example, since fat is capable of aromatizing androgen precursors such as Δ^4-androstenedione to estrone, differences in body habitus between normal males and MBC patients may be important. In females, excess body fat is a risk factor for both disease occurrence and disease recurrence following primary therapy. These factors should be considered in future studies.

3.4. Klinefelter's Syndrome

Klinefelter's syndrome is typically characterized by a 47,XXY (or mosaic) karyotype, sex-chromatin positivity, a male phenotype with poor development of male secondary sex characteristics including a female escutcheon and gynecomastia, small testes with hyalinized testicular tubules, oligo- or azospermia, Leydig-cell proliferation, and high levels of gonadotropins.[9,51] Breast development can include formation of acini and true lobules typically seen only in females.[38] Association of this syndrome with MBC was reported in a case report by Bauer and Erickson in 1955[52] and in 3 of 21 patients observed by Jackson et al.[51] Further case reports and the screening of MBC cases for sex chromatin have confirmed these findings. This association was reviewed by Scheike et al.[9] By combining case series, they calculated the risk of breast cancer for patients with Klinefelter's syndrome to be roughly one-fifth of the female and 20 times the normal male risk. Of interest in this association was a statistically significant right-sided predominance of the breast primaries[9] and several cases of either bilateral MBC primary tumors or primaries in addition to MBC. These included a case with prostatic and adrenal primaries,[52] bilateral "comedo" MBCs,[53] an interstitial-cell tumor,[54] and an extraordinary case with bilateral Paget's disease of the breast, a sacral chordoma, a temporoparietal spongioblastoma polare, papillary thyroid carcinoma, and multiple bulky lipomas.[55,56] Since Scheike et al.[9] recorded only 14 cases of an association of MBC with Klinefelter's syndrome, it seems likely that these cases have a propensity for developing bilateral disease and, notably, unusual additional second primaries. The physiologic link between Klinefelter's syndrome and MBC is unclear. Since patients with Klinefelter's syndrome are characterized by hormonal differences from normal males (including elevated gonadotropin levels and lower excretion of neutral 17-ketosteroids, pregnanediol, pregnanetriol, estrone, and estradiol[57]) in addition to their chromosomal defect, the association may relate to endocrine or genetic factors.

3.5. Familial Male Breast Cancer

Multiple instances of familial MBC have been reported, among brothers in at least six instances[13,25,50,58–60] and also among other relations.[46,61,62] The rarity of MBC makes these associations seem unlikely on a chance basis, but the extent of familial MBC risk is difficult to assess. In one study, MBC occurred in three brothers in one family, and in a man, his father, and his paternal uncle in another.[50] Male offspring of the latter family were treated by prophylactic subcutaneous mastectomies, with pathologic specimens suggesting mild dysplasia to some consultant pathologists. One of these individuals and the son of another familial case had urinary estrogen measurements exceeding the range of a group of healthy controls, suggesting that hormonal factors may be of etiologic significance in familial MBC cases. An unpublished survey of other family members by one of the authors (R.B.E.) seemed to confirm this finding. Due to the rarity of MBC, recording the risk of breast cancer in female first-degree relatives has been suggested as a means of exploring the extent and sex specificity of familial risk.[59] Currently available data suggest that familial risk is not sex specific[50]; confirmation of these data would suggest the need for investigating mechanisms that are not sex specific in the study of the etiology of male and female breast cancer.

3.6. Gynecomastia

Gynecomastia, or hyperplasia of epithelial or fibrous elements of male breast tissue, has been noted in case series of MBC and an association between the disorders proposed. Evidence cited to favor a relationship with the pathogenesis of MBC includes: (1) the frequent observation of gynecomastia among MBC patients reported by some authors, including 7 of 40 cases in one series,[33] (2) the association of gynecomastia with epithelial atypia in some cases, (3) the association of gynecomastia with Klinefelter's syndrome, and (4) the high frequency of gynecomastia in regions (notably Egypt) where MBC accounts for a relatively high proportion of all breast cancer.[10,63]

Many studies, however, have noted gynecomastia infrequently

among MBC patients: Crichlow[6] could find only 17 reports of gynecomastia among 625 MBC cases in literature series of MBC where gynecomastia was recorded. In addition, gynecomastia has been reported in a high proportion of the general population: Thirty-nine percent of adolescents in one survey had evidence of gynecomastia on physical exam[64] and 40% of an unselected large autopsy series were reported to show histologic gynecomastia, although gross breast enlargement was only noted in 1% of this series.[65] Histologic criteria appear to vary, however, and gynecomastia was reported in only 3% of another autopsy series.[38] Such variations would require that similar diagnostic criteria be applied to both MBC patients and controls if a relationship is to be established. We are not aware of studies with this refinement. In addition, no clear instance of transition from gynecomastia to MBC has been observed in pathologic studies,[66] although the association of other benign and malignant conditions has been substantiated in the absence of such a finding.

In summary, it appears that variable diagnostic criteria and the high frequency of gynecomastia in the general population make both its association with MBC and its role in the etiology of MBC unclear.[10]

3.7. Radiation

MacKenzie implicated radiation exposure from fluoroscopy required for procedures used to treat tuberculosis in the etiology of female breast cancer.[67] The association between radiation exposure and development of breast cancer was confirmed in studies of survivors of atomic bomb explosions.[68,69] Crichlow[6] located five instances in which MBC followed radiation exposure, including cases in which radiation was used for mediastinal lymphoma, eczema, gynecomastia, and other benign breast disease. One of these cases and a review of MBC etiology was presented by Lowell and colleagues.[70] In addition, Deutsch and associates reported MBC in an 18-year-old who had been exposed to an estimated 449 rads of radiation during neonatal treatments for an enlarged thymus.[71]

3.8. Other Proposed Etiologic Factors

Trauma has been cited, especially in the older literature, as potentially predisposing to MBC.[72,73] Crichlow could find only 30 of 532 more recent literature cases reporting trauma preceding MBC,[6] and most evidence suggests that it is coincidental or calls attention to a preexistent malignant lesion.

In addition to a history of orchitis in 4 of 53 cases in the epidemiologic survey noted in Section 3.1,[25] Nicolis and associates[74] reported MBC developing 30 years after severe mumps orchitis in one individual. These findings, plus the association of MBC with Klinefelter's syndrome and the note by Treves[75] that testicular "atrophy" was present in orchiectomy specimens from 24 of 40 men with MBC, suggest, but do not prove, a role for testicular disorders in the etiology of MBC.

4. Diagnosis

4.1. Presenting Symptoms

A painless breast lump first noted by the patient is by far the most common presenting symptom of MBC, accounting for 71% of cases in a Danish series of 257 patients[11] and 87% of another series derived from literature reports of 205 cases.[6] The other presenting signs and symptoms in the Danish series included 8% of patients with pain and breast tenderness and 4% with each of the following: skin ulceration, nipple retraction, and bloody or other discharges. Distant metastases accounted for less than 1% of cases and only 2% were initially discovered by physicians during routine physical examinations.[11] Presentation because of nipple discharge without an underlying mass has led to MBC diagnosis at an apparently early stage in rare cases.[76,77] In one series of patients with breast masses and nipple discharge, a bloody discharge was present in 75% of MBC patients as compared to 45% of patients with benign disease.[76]

Duration of symptoms before presentation averaged 6 months in one recent series.[11] In a review of the literature, an 18-month duration of symptoms was noted for 1228 cases reported since 1900, with a somewhat improved 10-month delay observed for cases diagnosed since 1951.[6] This delay in seeking medical attention is reported to be longer than that for women[78] despite the paucity of other tissue which might obscure the diagnosis in the male breast. This is possibly due to poor awareness of the possibility of MBC in the population[5] or concerns over sexuality.

4.2. Findings at Presentation

A subareolar mass is almost invariably present. Crichlow could identify only two cases of occult MBC in literature reports, both presenting with regional nodes,[6] and Cain[77] described a single case presenting with a completely normal exam but a history of bloody nipple discharge. A mass, however, is infrequently the only clinical finding. In several series, nipple ulceration was present in about 25% of cases and nipple retraction in 33% (Table II).[5,6,11] Nipple discharge was noted at hospital admission in only 2% of Scheike's patients with MBC[11]; but 14% of malignant and 2% of benign lesions reported by Treves et al.[76] had nipple discharge. As shown in Table II, at least 52% of MBC cases with known laterality were left sided and about 1.5% bilateral.[6,11]

Palpable homolateral nodes were present in about 50% of cases in a literature review. About 9% had a malignant disease other than MBC (Table II).[6,11] Although this is not necessarily more than would be expected by chance in a group of this age, Langlands and associates[79] reported significantly more second malignancies in men than women with breast cancer ($p < 0.01$). Their study did not match for age or control for the higher incidence of malignant disease in the general male population, and is therefore also inconclusive; however, a disproportionately high (41%) percentage of cases noted in the literature were large-bowel or rectal primaries.[79] Panettiere felt that the pattern of primary malignancies at other sites were similar for men and women with breast cancer and cited studies indicating an increased risk of primaries at other sites in women with breast cancer.[18]

Scheike reported that tumor size in his series ranged from 1 cm to 28 × 16 cm, with 51% of MBC primaries less than 3 cm. He noted a significant positive correlation between tumor size and both symptom duration and frequency of ulceration.[11]

Table II
Clinical Findings in Male Breast Cancer

	Percentage of cases		
	Holleb[5]	Crichlow[6]	Schieke[11]
At presentation			
Breast mass	91		97
Nipple retraction	33		33
Ulceration	23	28	16
Discharge	16		2
Skin fixation	22		44
Palpable homolateral nodes	50	54	42
Left-sided primaries	57	52	53
At presentation or developing during follow-up			
Bilateral primaries	2	1.4	0.7
Second primaries other than breast	7.5	9	10

5. Differential Diagnosis

MBC must be differentiated from metastatic cancer, gynecomastia, and, in some cases, inflammatory lesions. Holleb[5] estimated that 65% of breast lesions in older males are gynecomastias, 25% MBC, and 10% other benign breast lesions. In one series of male breast lesions, 15 cases of MBC as compared to 114 of gynecomastia were diagnosed during a 16-year period.[80] Youth and bilaterality favor gynecomastia; a firm discoid, subareolar, probably tender mass in an adolescent can be considered a normal accompaniment of puberty and is likely to disappear within one or two years.[64] A hard, poorly defined, irregular mass in an elderly man should be investigated before skin thickening, nipple retraction and ulceration, adherence to the pectoral muscles, and axillary node

Table III

Features Helpful in Differentiating Typical Gynecomastia from Male Breast Cancer[6,81–90]

Male breast cancer	Gynecomastia
Increased incidence with age	Broad age distribution over most of adult life, especially puberty and senescence
Painless (unless ulcerated)	Tender
Unilateral	Significant minority bilateral
Eccentric	Central
Hard	Firm
Poorly defined mass	Well-defined mass
Adheres to pectoral muscles	Can adhere to areola
Associated with	Associated with
Nipple discharge, especially sanguineous	Drug use, including estrogens, androgens, corticosteroids, spironolactone, cimetidine, ergotamine, thyroid extract, reserpine diethylpropion, phenothiazines, marijuana, reserpine, thiazides, digitalis, isoniazid
Enlarged axillary nodes	Medical conditions, including chronic liver disease, central nervous system disease, renal dialysis, thoracic disease, cardiovascular disease, refeeding after starvation
Ulceration	Endocrine disorders, including testicular atrophy secondary to infection, trauma, or hydrocele; eunuchism; male pseudohermaphroditism
	Neoplasms, including testicular, adrenal, pituitary, malignant lymphoma; carcinoma of the lung, colon, or prostate
	Infections, including malaria, tuberculosis, leprosy, bilharziasis
	or Idiopathic

involvement make the diagnosis obvious and the prognosis grave. Nipple discharge, especially sanguineous, should be viewed with similar suspicion. Diagnosis of benign disease frequently does not require biopsy.[61] Nevertheless, especially considering the frequency of gynecomastia associated with senescence or drugs, differentiating MBC from gynecomastia can be difficult. Table III describes features that may be of some utility in making the distinction.[81-90] The frequency of conditions associated with gynecomastia varies in different reports. In a series of 126 cases of gynecomastia, it was associated with cardiovascular disorders in 23 cases (17 on digitalis), Klinefelter's syndrome in 8, chronic liver disease in 6, central nervous system disease in 5, chronic lung disease in 15, use of other various drugs in 9, testicular and adrenocortical tumors in 1 each, miscellaneous disorders in 10, adolescent gynecomastia in 26, and no other disease in 22.[91]

The distinction between primary MBC and deposits of metastatic prostatic carcinoma in the breast is also often difficult but important. As noted by Lome and Austen[92] and Wilson and Hutchinson,[32] metastatic deposits in the breast generally require no treatment but imply a poor survival averaging four months, whereas MBC warrants full surgical treatment and is potentially curable. Thus, the apparently rare case of true MBC, even in the presence of localized prostate cancer, deserves recognition. Histochemical analysis for acid phosphatase can be useful but may require fresh frozen tissue and probably is not definitive.[29,32,36,93]

6. Mammography

Mammography has been employed principally to distinguish gynecomastia from MBC. Radiographically, gynecomastia is characteristically smooth, fans backward from the nipple, and tends to form a symmetric cone. MBC is more likely to be eccentric, is typically dense with irregular margins with or without calcifications, and may have associated skin thickening and nipple retraction. The differential is not absolute, however, and both disorders may coexist.[87,90,94] Mammography should supplement, not replace, physical examination and biopsy.

7. Extent of Disease at Diagnosis

In the series compiled by Scheike,[11] of 396 male patients staged according to the UICC TNM classification scheme as employed for women, 34% presented as Stage I, 14% as Stage II, 40% as Stage III, and

12% as Stage IV. The high frequency of Stage III cases is largely due to patients with skin fixation. The End Results Group of the National Cancer Institute, a large cooperative group including two state cancer registries and other hospitals, numbering among them 393 white MBC patients, reported that between 1950–1954 and 1970–1973 the proportion of cases with localized disease at diagnosis increased from 38% to 58%.[95] In this report the stage at diagnosis was similar for men and women with breast cancer.

In a manner analogous to staging of female breast cancer, staging of MBC should be accomplished before definitive surgery so as to aid in the planning of that surgery. A bone scan and liver function tests are the most useful tests to perform preoperatively. The finding of metastatic disease could spare a portion of the often elderly MBC patients the rigors of radical surgery.

8. Pathology

Except for the absence of *in situ* cases in men, reports of male and female breast pathology are similar. Table IV presents a comparison of histologic subtypes for the sexes. It was adapted from Giffler and Kay's summary table including 684 MBC cases, compared with a series for females reported by the Armed Forces Institute of Pathology.[96] Major

Table IV
Comparative Histology of Male and Female Breast Cancer[a]

Carcinoma	Male (%)	Female (%)
Infiltrating ductal, not otherwise specified	73	78.1
Nonspecified adenocarcinoma	7	
Intraductal	5	
Papillary	5	1.2
Medullary	4	4.3
Mucinous	2	2.6
Squamous	< 1	
Lobular invasive	< 1	8.7
Paget's disease	< 1	
Sarcoma	< 1	
Adenocystic	≪ 1	
Basal-cell	≪ 1	
Lymphoma	≪ 1	
Tubular	≪ 1	
Other (including comedo)	< 1	4.6

[a]Percentages based on cases compiled from Giffler and Kay.[96]

differences include the relative absence of lobular invasive carcinomas and fewer comedo carcinomas in men. Lobules are normally absent from the male breast, and whether true male lobular carcinoma exists remains subject to interpretation. Giffler and Kay reported two cases and cited literature cases which they felt represented male lobular invasive carcinoma, but stated that the *in situ* form (which in women is more common than lobular invasive carcinoma and tends to present bilaterally) has still not been described in men.[96] Yogore and Sahgal reported an additional case of lobular invasive carcinoma.[97]

In a careful review of mastectomy specimens from 187 Danish MBC cases, Visfeldt and Scheike,[7] using the WHO classification and grading scheme, reported a direct and striking relationship between grading and five-year survival: 13% of Grade I, 54% of Grade II, and 94% of Grade III cases not dying from other causes died within five years of developing breast cancer. Haagensen reported MBC to be well differentiated more often than breast cancer in women.[61]

Paget's disease of the male breast has been the subject of several recent reviews.[98–100] Patients typically present because of nipple bleeding, discharge, or ulceration rather than detection of a mass: Only 2 of 13 patients in one series noted a lump, although a mass could usually be detected on physical examination.[98] A poorer prognosis than that for typical MBC has been suggested, with only 4 of 16 five-year survivors and only 1 known 10-year survivor.[100] Otherwise, too few cases have been reported to reliably differentiate clinical or other features of Paget's disease from those of typical MBC or to suggest treatment differing from that for typical MBC.

Inflammatory carcinoma of the male breast has been reported in as many as 2% of cases in some series.[101] Papillary carcinomas have been associated with a good prognosis.[5] Reports of unusual cell types have included cystosarcoma phyllodes,[102] adenoid cystic carcinoma,[103] tubular carcinoma,[104] and granular-cell tumor.[105] Most of these had a more benign course than typical MBC and the latter two lesions are of special import because their low malignant potential may indicate less radical surgical treatment. Local excision only was employed for the two cases of granular-cell tumor in men aged 35 and 36 reported by Hart and Sisely.[105] An ultrastructural study of MBC has been made by Sirsat and colleagues.[106]

9. Steroid Receptors

These have been reviewed recently by Everson and associates, who reported estrogen receptor status in tumor specimens from 34 cases of

MBC and literature reports of 30 cases.[107] Estrogen receptor was present in 84% of samples from MBC patients and progesterone receptor in 73% (Table V). Although these percentages are high, it will be shown shortly that a large proportion (about two-thirds) of MBC patients will respond to endocrine maneuvers. Thus, the proportion of receptor-positive tumors may not be unexpectedly high. However, the presence or absence of estrogen receptor would fail to provide clinically useful discriminants in many MBC cases, so relationships were also viewed quantitatively. The concentration of estrogen receptor appeared to decrease with increasing age but tended to correlate directly with progesterone receptor levels and disease-free interval. Data on therapeutic response to orchiectomy were available for only 13 cases: Although low levels tended to correspond with poor response durations, no statistically significant relationship was established. It was felt that currently available data do not justify therapy for metastatic MBC dictated on the basis of estrogen receptor analysis. This same report noted a low frequency of positive estrogen receptor levels in gynecomastia specimens. Although 9 of 36 specimens (25%) were positive, at least 3 had only a 4 S species of receptor. It has been suggested that female patients whose tumors have the 4 S component of receptor respond to endocrine therapy very infrequently. This finding was similar to the low frequency of estrogen receptor in benign disorders of the female breast and emphasizes the relationship of measurable estrogen receptor to breast malignancy. In a study of steroid receptors and MBC, estrogen and progesterone receptor levels were found to correlate positively with the degree of differentiation of the tumor,[108] but another study reported no relationship.[109] Investigations of dissociation constants and binding specificity as determined by competition studies for MBC tumor specimens gave results similar to those described for breast carcinoma specimens from women.[109–111]

Table V
Steroid Receptors in Male Breast Cancer[a]

	Estrogen receptor[b]	Progesterone receptor[b]	Androgen receptor[b]	Glucocorticoid receptor[b]
Positive	54 (84)	16 (73)	2 (22)	4 (67)
Borderline	2 (3)	1 (4)	1 (11)	0
Negative	8 (13)	5 (23)	6 (67)	2 (33)
TOTALS	64	22	9	6

[a]Compiled from Everson et al.[107]
[b]Number (percentage) of specimens positive, borderline, or negative.

10. Primary Therapy

Literature reports completed by Crichlow[6] concerning 495 men with MBC revealed that 19% were considered inoperable, 13% were treated by simple mastectomy, and 68% were treated by radical mastectomy. Both simple[14,112] and radical[5,18,66,113,114] mastectomy have been advocated; no comparative trials have been attempted and selection factors employed in electing different treatments are such that the dispute cannot be resolved by analysis of available data.[6,12,115] Skin grafting is frequently required and permits wider margins.[5] Postoperative radiation therapy has frequently been employed, but its efficacy has not been subjected to critical review or randomized trial, and patient-selection factors make extrapolation from literature reports of limited value. In at least one series, results were not improved by postoperative radiotherapy.[12] In nonrandomized trials it is possible, but it cannot be assumed, that radiotherapy-treated patients are selected for this therapy because of more advanced disease.

In the absence of data specific for MBC, knowledge of the effect of adjuvant chemotherapy on breast cancer in women provides the only basis for suggesting its value in men. Since the gonads are still functional in most MBC patients, even in instances of advanced age, and since favorable response generally follows castration, it seems most reasonable to equate MBC with premenopausal disease. Although these observations could favor the use of adjuvant chemotherapy for MBC, advanced age of many patients might weigh against this, as might the suggestion that estrogen-receptor-positive disease responds poorly to chemotherapy.[116] Analysis of the response of recurrent MBC to cytotoxic therapy could help resolve these issues.

Unless prospective trials are undertaken (which seems unlikely in view of the rarity of this disorder), the decision to use adjuvant chemotherapy or hormonal manipulation for MBC must be individualized. The high rate of recurrence for node-positive disease may justify the use of adjuvant therapy in many instances.

11. Treatment of Metastatic Disease

Available evidence suggests a similar pattern of metastases for male and female breast cancer.[73,112,117] Indications for systemic treatment are also similar in the advanced-disease setting. Local or isolated recurrence can be managed by excision or radiotherapy, although systemic therapy has recently been advocated for female cases.[118]

11.1. Endocrine Ablation

Reported response rates to endocrine ablation are higher for MBC than for female breast cancer. Table VI compiles statistics from those presented by Meyskens *et al.* in a review of the literature in which a three-month disappearance of all lesions recorded by the author was required for response; due to the nature of data in some reports, this may have been less than total remission.[15] Using that criterion, response was reported in two-thirds of cases treated by orchiectomy and in three-quarters treated by adrenalectomy. Other reviewers cited a three times longer (45-month) duration of orchiectomy responses than ovariectomy response in breast cancer.[119]

Adrenalectomy was used either after a response to orchiectomy (11 patients, 91% adrenalectomy responders with a 32-month median duration), after no response to orchiectomy (8 patients, 50% responders with a 16-month median duration), combined with orchiectomy (3 patients, all responders), or as primary treatment (3 patients, 2 responders). Hypophysectomy was also successful: A total of 10 of 17 patients responded. Responses were observed when hypophysectomy was either primary treatment (2 of 3 patients) or used after response to orchiectomy (3 of 4 patients). No responses to hypophysectomy were noted among 3 orchiectomy failures. Responders to any of these therapies tended to live longer than nonresponders. Data were too sparse to determine whether response rates differed by metastatic site of involvement, although response in osseous, visceral, and soft tissue were noted.[15] As in any study based on case series, it is possible that response rates were inflated by selection of favorable outcomes for publication.[120]

In investigations of the endocrine bases for orchiectomy response, Calabresi and associates[47] showed that this procedure greatly reduced plasma testosterone and estradiol levels and reduced androstenedione, estrone, and estriol levels to a lesser extent. Hellman and Fishman[121]

Table VI
Response of Male Breast Cancer to Endocrine Ablation[a]

	Number of patients	Number of responders (%)	Median response duration (months)
Orchiectomy	70	47 (67)	22
Adrenalectomy	25	19 (76)	26
Hypophysectomy	17	10 (59)	20

[a]Compiled from Meyskens *et al.*[15]

demonstrated a marked decrease in estradiol production following orchiectomy.

11.2. Additive Endocrine Therapy

In his review, Crichlow[6] could find reference to only a few reports
of documented responses to estrogens and Holleb[5] reported no long-
term remissions following estrogen use, despite its application to all
cases with "uncontrolled breast cancer" in his series. Further details
were not given, but Treves, in an earlier review of the series from this
same center, reported that only 2 of 14 patients responded to estrogens,
although the duration of some trials was short and response criteria
poorly defined.[75] Kennedy and Kiang observed a patient who initially
seemed to respond to diethylstilbesterol (DES) but later experienced
rapid growth during two trials with this same agent, with regression
when the drug was discontinued. They felt that the role of estrogen
therapy in the treatment of advanced MBC was not yet defined.[122]

Estrogen therapy, however, was favored in reports from European
centers.[123] Scheike reported a "palliative effect" for more than 6
months in 20 of 63 patients treated with lower doses (generally 1 mg
three times a day of DES) but response criteria and disease sites were
unrecorded. Orchiectomy was not used in his large series.[12] Walach
and Hochman reported that 9 of 14 (60%) of their series were "improved" by DES, but details were not provided.[124] A retrospective survey by Ribeiro of 58 British patients treated with oral DES (5 mg three
times a day) is summarized in Table VII.[125] Using British Breast Group
criteria,[126] objective and partial responses were frequent for soft-tissue
disease and were of long duration: 7 years for objective and 1 year for
partial responders. Four patients included in this report had lung metastases that responded to DES; bone metastases in 2 of them progressed,
however. It is of interest to note that the 2 DES responders in Treves'
series were among the 5 patients he reported with soft-tissue disease.[75]

Table VII
Response of Male Breast Cancer to Diethylstilbestrol[a]

Disease site	Number of patients	Number of responders (%)	Median response duration (months)
Soft tissue	33	21 (64)	60
Multiple sites	14	0 (0)	—
Bone	8	0 (0)	—

[a]Compiled from Ribeiro.[125]

No other sites responded in either study. Few side effects were noted except for intractable nausea in 2 patients, causing them to discontinue the drug after 1 week, and severe gynecomastia with prolonged use in 2 others. Ribeiro's report provides strong support for the use of DES in treatment of MBC with metastases limited to soft tissue.

We are aware of two responses of MBC to androgens (fluoxymesterone[127] and dimethyltestosterone,[128] two to calusterone,[129] and at least two to progestins.[130-132] Androgens are frequently said to stimulate MBC growth but reported evidence for this effect is meager.[127] Corticosteroids have provided short-term palliation for a minority of patients in some series,[12] although Holleb[5] and Crichlow[6] felt their usefulness to be related primarily to subjective effects. Kennedy and Kiang suggested using massive doses of corticosteroids as adrenal ablation in high-surgical risk cases but reported no cases treated with this technique.[122] No reports were located giving response to newer agents such as aminoglutethimide or antiestrogens.

11.3. Chemotherapy

Few observations of the effects of chemotherapy on MBC have been reported. Favorable response to 5-fluorouracil, cytoxan, and combinations of methotrexate and thio-TEPA, and cytoxan, adriamycin, and 5-fluorouracil have been noted.[15,122,133] The high response rates of MBC to endocrine ablations, however, make them the initial treatment of choice. Whether steroid receptor status (see Section 9) will enable selection of appropriate treatment, as it appears to for female breast cancer,[116] is as yet undetermined.

12. Prognosis

Many authors state that breast cancer prognosis is poorer in males than in females.[6,63,134] Norris and Taylor suggested that this might be attributed to the central location of most breast lesions in males, leading to a high incidence of internal mammary node metastases.[63] Several authors, however, developed a strong case for attributing much of the reported difference to higher mortality in males from unrelated causes.[3,12,127] Support for this contention may be taken from reports of the End Results Group (Table VIII), where adjusting for relative survival can be seen to improve male survival rates more than female. Deriving a close approximation of the average rate by averaging the rates for the three reported intervals showed male and female survival to be equivalent (64% and 63.3%, respectively).[95] (This conclusion differs from that of another study using End Results Group data[66] because a broader time period was considered here.)

Other studies of breast cancer that included the experience of comparable groups from both sexes also reported similar male and female relative survival rates (Table VIII).[78,135,136] In addition, when Langlands *et al.* matched male and female breast cancer cases for stage, he found equivalent age-corrected survival rates for both sexes, although overall survival favored women.[79] Ribeiro, however, reported better survival for women with advanced disease in a study matching age and stage.[137] Thus, sex differences in survival may favor women, but only slightly and probably without statistical assurity.

In Scheike's series, relative survival of 246 patients was 46% at five years and 29% at ten years.[12] He reported that clinically positive axillary nodes, tumor ulceration, and fixation to underlying tissues, as well as increasing stage, tumor size, and worsening histologic grade all correlated with worsening prognosis. Prognosis improved during the period 1943–1957 and 1958–1971 in his series; no effect on relative survival was attributable to age at onset, duration of symptoms, or treatment employed. Norris and Taylor stated that microscopic axillary involvement, tumor size greater than 1.9 cm, and skin ulceration unfavorably affect prognosis, but several histologic types including intraductal, papillary, or well differentiated had a more favorable prognosis.[63] Corwin *et al.*,

Table VIII
Cases and Five-Year Survival Rates[a]

	Number of cases	Observed survival (%)	Relative survival (%)
Male			
ERG 1950–1959	113	57	74
ERG 1960–1966	135	40	52
ERG 1967–1973	145	51	66
Brunet *et al.*	293	39	49
MacKay and Sellers	91	36	44
Mausner *et al.*	72	47	60
Female			
ERG 1950–1959	18,220	53	61
ERG 1960–1966	16,403	56	64
ERG 1967–1973	18,216	58	65
Brunet *et al.*	14,008	38	45
MacKay and Sellers	9,742	45	50
Mausner *et al.*	830	57	63

[a]Percentage five-year survival for white breast cancer patients reported by the End Results Group (ERG), Biometry Branch, National Cancer Institute,[95] and patients reported by Brunet *et al.*,[136] MacKay and Sellers,[135] and Mausner *et al.*[78]

Table IX
Correlation of Axillary Node Status and Survival
of Male Breast Cancer Patients Following Radical
Mastectomy[a]

	Node status	
	Negative	Positive
Five-year survivors (Crichlow only)	58 (79)	85 (28)
Ten-year survivors (both authors)	45 (58)	52 (6)

[a]Total number of patients at risk (percentage survivors) among literature cases from reports compiled by Crichlow[6] and Satiani and Powell,[138] with duplication deleted.

in a series of only 15 patients, felt that patient delay in seeking treatment was the most important factor influencing prognosis.[80]

Crichlow[6] and Satiani and Powell[138] observed a striking relationship between axillary node status and crude survival (Table IX). In addition, Ribeiro[137] noted recurrences in 19 of 76 (25%) of Stage I and 27 of 38 (71%) of Stage II patients in a British series of 200 cases. Most recurrences were seen by two years after mastectomy. As noted in Section 8, papillary MBC appeared to have a better and Paget's disease a worse prognosis than typical MBC.

In view of the relatively long delay in seeking therapy, described previously (10 months, according to Crichlow[6]), it may be anticipated that an increasing awareness of physicians and the public as to the need for early detection and treatment of MBC may improve results.

13. References

1. S. J. Cutler and J. L. Young, Jr., eds., Third National Cancer Survey: Incidence Data, *Natl. Cancer Inst. Monogr.* **41**, DHEW Publication No. (NIH) 75-787, U.S. Department of Health, Education, and Welfare (1975) (Tables 5, 7, and 19).
2. J. M. Wainwright, Carcinoma of the male breast: Clinical and pathologic study, *Arch. Surg.* **14**, 836–859 (1927).
3. A. I. Holleb, H. P. Freeman, and J. H. Farrow, Cancer of male breast, Part I, *N.Y. State J. Med.* **68**, 544–553 (1968).
4. A. I. Holleb, H. P. Freeman, and J. H. Farrow, Cancer of male breast, Part II, *N.Y. State J. Med.* **68**, 656–663 (1968).
5. A. I. Holleb, Cancer of the male breast, in: *Breast Cancer: Early and Late*, pp. 245–262, Year Book Medical Publishers, Chicago (1970).

6. R. W. Crichlow, Carcinoma of the male breast, *Surg. Gynecol. Obstet.* **134**, 1011–1019 (1972).

7. J. Visfeldt and O. Scheike, Male breast cancer. I. Histologic typing and grading of 187 Danish cases, *Cancer* **32**, 985–990 (1973).

8. O. Scheike, B. Svenstrup, and V. A. Frandsen, Male breast cancer. II. Metabolism of oestradiol-17β in men with breast cancer, *J. Steroid Biochem.* **4**, 489–501 (1973).

9. O. Scheike, J. Visfeldt, and B. Petersen, Male breast cancer. 3. Breast carcinoma in association with the Klinefelter syndrome, *Acta Pathol. Microbiol. Scand. Sect. A* **81**(3), 352–358 (1973).

10. O. Scheike and J. Visfeldt, Male breast cancer. 4. Gynecomastia in patients with breast cancer, *Acta Pathol. Microbiol. Scand. Sect. A* **81**(3), 359–365 (1973).

11. O. Scheike, Male breast cancer. 5. Clinical manifestations in 257 cases in Denmark, *Br. J. Cancer* **28**, 552–561 (1973).

12. O. Scheike, Male breast cancer. 6. Factors influencing prognosis, *Br. J. Cancer* **30**, 261–271 (1974).

13. O. Scheike, Male breast cancer, *Acta Pathol. Microbiol. Scand. Sect. A*, Supplement **251**, 13–35 (1975).

14. O. Scheike, Factors provoking male breast cancer, in: *Risk Factors in Breast Cancer* (B. A. Stoll, ed.), pp. 173–192, Year Book Medical Publishers, Chicago (1976).

15. F. L. Meyskens, Jr., D. C. Tormey, and J. P. Neifeld, Male breast cancer: A review, *Cancer Treat. Rev.* **3**, 83–93 (1976).

16. B. Modan, U. Mintz, and J. Finkelman, Male breast cancer in Israel. Selected epidemiological and clinical aspects, *J. Chronic Dis.* **23**, 55–60 (1970).

17. D. Schottenfeld and A. M. Lilienfeld, Some epidemiological features of breast cancer among males, *J. Chronic Dis.* **16**, 71–81 (1963).

18. F. J. Panettiere, Cancer in the male breast, *Cancer* **34**, 1324–1327 (1974).

19. M. Brunet, M. Hucher, F. Boutros, and J. Berlie, Is there any bimodality of the age distribution of male mammary cancer? *Rev. Epidémiol. Méd. Soc. Santé Publique* **24**, 405–413 (1976).

20. T. J. Mason, F. W. McKay, R. Hoover, W. J. Blot, and J. F. Fraumeni, Jr., *Atlas of Cancer Mortality for U.S. Counties: 1950–1969*, DHEW Publication No. (NIH) 75-780, U.S. Department of Health, Education, and Welfare.

21. J. N. P. Davies, Sex hormone upset in Africans, *Br. Med. J.* **2**, 676–679 (1949).

22. W. Sinner, Karzinome der männlichen Brüstdruse. Beobachtungen an 27 fällen. Zürcher erfahrungen 1919 bis 1960, *Strahlentherapie* **115**, 522–547 (1961).

23. M. M. El-Gazayerli and A. S. Abdel-Aziz, On bilharziasis and male breast cancer in Egypt: A preliminary report and review of the literature, *Br. J. Cancer* **17**, 566–571 (1963).

24. S. B. Bhagwandeen, Carcinoma of the male breast in Zambia, *East Afr. Med. J.* **49**, 89–93 (1972).

25. D. Schottenfeld, A. M. Lilienfeld, and H. Diamond, Some observations on the epidemiology of breast cancer among males, *Am. J. Public Health* **53**, 890–897 (1963).

26. A. Z. Keller, Demographic, clinical and survivorship characteristics of males with primary cancer of the breast, *Am. J. Epidemiol.* **85**, 183–199 (1967).

27. A. Lacassagne, Hormonal pathogenesis of adenocarcinoma of the breast, *Am. J. Cancer* **27**, 217–228 (1936).

28. W. U. Gardner, Estrogens in carcinogenesis, *Arch. Pathol.* **27**, 138–170 (1939).

29. W. A. Pribe and E. A. Ockuly, Prostatic metastasis to the breast and the role of estrogens: Case report and review, *J. Am. Geriatr. Soc.* **11**, 891–901 (1963).

30. T. L. Dao and M. J. Greiner, Mammary carcinogenesis by 3-methylcholanthrene. III. Induction of mammary carcinoma and milk secretion in male rats bearing ovarian grafts, *J. Natl. Cancer Inst.* **27**, 333–343 (1961).

31. R. W. Scarff and C. P. Smith, Proliferative and other lesions of the male breast with notes on 2 cases of proliferative mastitis in stilboestrol workers, *Br. J. Surg.* **29**, 393–396 (1942).

32. S. E. Wilson and W. B. Hutchinson, Breast masses in males with carcinoma of the prostate, *J. Surg. Oncol.* **8**, 105–112 (1976).

33. R. D. Liechty, J. Davis, and J. Gleysteen, Cancer of the male breast, *Cancer* **20**, 1617–1624 (1967).

34. J. H. Campbell and S. D. Cummins, Metastases, simulating mammary cancer, in prostatic carcinoma under estrogenic therapy, *Cancer* **4**, 303–311 (1951).

35. W. R. Benson, Carcinoma of the prostate with metastases to breasts and testis, *Cancer* **10**, 1235–1245 (1957).

36. T. Berge, Metastases to the male breast, *Acta Pathol. Microbiol. Scand. Sect. A* **79**, 491–496 (1971).

37. W. R. Salyer and D. C. Salyer, Metastases of prostatic carcinoma to the breast, *J. Urol.* **109**, 671–675 (1973).

38. A. T. Sandison, An autopsy study of the adult human breast, *Natl. Cancer Inst. Monogr.* **8**, 75–90 (1962).

39. W. St. C. Symmers, Carcinoma of breast in trans-sexual individuals after surgical and hormonal interference with the primary and secondary sex characteristics, *Br. Med. J.* **2**, 83–85 (1968).

40. N. Orentreich and N. P. Durr, Mammogenesis in transsexuals, *J. Invest. Dermatol.* **63**, 142–146 (1974).

41. B. Zumoff, J. Fishman, J. Cassouto, L. Hellman, and T. F. Gallagher, Estradiol transformation in men with breast cancer, *J. Clin. Endocrinol. Metab.* **26**, 960–966 (1966).

42. W. R. Miller and A. P. M. Forrest, Oestradiol synthesis by a human breast carcinoma, *Lancet* **2**, 866–868 (1974).

43. N. I. Lazarev, K. S. Shasoukhova, N. I. Muravieva, K. D. Smirnova, M. G. Goncharova, and N. P. Makarenko, Peculiarities specific to hormonal metabolism in males with gynecomastia and mammary carcinoma, *Vestn. Akad. Med. Nauk SSSR*, **24**, 28–35 (1969).

44. H. A. Komurdjaev and A. V. Rogoznaya, Mammary gland cancer in males, *Vopr. Onkol.* **1**, 87–93 (1964).

45. T. L. Dao, C. Morreal, and T. Nemoto, Urinary estrogen excretion in men with breast cancer, *N. Engl. J. Med.* **289**, 138–140 (1973).

46. G. De Giuli and S. De Giuli, Urinary excretion of 17-KS, 17-OHCS and phenolsteroids in males with breast cancer, in: *Characterization of Human Tumours* (W. Davis and C. Maltoni, eds.), Vol. 1, pp. 213–217, American Elsevier Publishing Co., New York (1974).

47. E. Calabresi, G. De Giuli, A. Becciolini, P. Giannotti, G. Lombardi, and M. Serio, Plasma estrogens and androgens in male breast cancer, *J. Steroid Biochem.* **7**, 605–609 (1976).

48. L. Sadoff and W. Davidson, Urinary estrogen excretion in men with advanced cancer, *N. Engl. J. Med.* **289**, 863–864 (1973).

49. J. B. Brown, S. C. MacLeod, C. Macnaughtan, M. A. Smith, and B. Smyth, A rapid method for estimating oestrogens in urine using a semiautomatic extractor, *J. Endocrinol.* **42**, 5–15 (1968).

50. R. B. Everson, F. P. Li, J. F. Fraumeni, Jr., J. Fishman, R. E. Wilson, D. Stout, and H. J. Norris, Familial male breast cancer, *Lancet* **1**, 9–12 (1976).

51. A. W. Jackson, S. Muldal, C. H. Ockey, and P. J. O'Connor, Carcinoma of male breast in association with the Klinefelter syndrome, *Br. Med. J.* **1**, 223–225 (1965).

52. D. DeF. Bauer and R. L. Erickson, Male breast cancer. Klinefelter syndrome with prostatic, adrenal and mammary tumors, *Northwest Med.* **54,** 472–476 (1955).
53. M. C. Robson, Q. Santiago, and T. W. Huang, Bilateral carcinoma of the breast in a patient with Klinefelter's syndrome, *J. Clin. Endocrinol.* **28,** 897–902 (1968).
54. O. G. Dodge, A. W. Jackson, and S. Muldal, Breast cancer and interstitial-cell tumor in a patient with Klinefelter's syndrome, *Cancer* **24,** 1027–1032 (1969).
55. G. M. Coley, R. D. Otis, and W. E. Clark II, Multiple primary tumors including bilateral breast cancers in a man with Klinefelter's syndrome, *Cancer* **27,** 1476–1481 (1971).
56. G. M. Coley and P. G. Kuehn, Paget's disease of the male breast, *Am. J. Surg.* **123,** 444–450 (1972).
57. E. P. Giorgi and I. F. Sommerville, Hormone assays in Klinefelter's syndrome, *J. Clin. Endocrinol.* **23,** 197–202 (1963).
58. G. Schmitt and J. Scheffler, Das Karzinom der männlichen Brustdrüse, *Dtsch. Med. Wochenschr.* **96,** 931–937 (1971).
59. D. Marger, N. Urdaneta, and J. J. Fischer, Breast cancer in brothers, *Cancer* **36,** 458–461 (1975).
60. C. Teasdale, J. F. Forbes, and M. Baum, Familial male breast cancer, *Lancet* **1,** 360–361 (1976).
61. C. D. Haagensen, *Diseases of the Breast,* pp. 354–379, 779–792, W. B. Saunders Co., Philadelphia (1971).
62. W. R. Williams, Cancer of the male breast, based on the records of one hundred cases; with remarks, *Lancet* **2,** 261–263, 310–313 (1889).
63. H. J. Norris and H. B. Taylor, Carcinoma of the male breast, *Cancer* **23,** 1428–1435 (1969).
64. M. Nydick, J. Bustos, J. H. Dale, Jr., and R. W. Rawson, Gynecomastia in adolescent boys, *J. Am. Med. Assoc.* **178,** 449–454 (1961).
65. M. J. Williams, Gynecomastia, *Am. J. Med.* **34,** 103–112 (1963).
66. N. H. Moss, Cancer of the male breast, *Ann. N.Y. Acad. Sci.* **114,** 937–950 (1964).
67. I. MacKenzie, Breast cancer following multiple fluoroscopies, *Br. J. Cancer* **19,** 1–8 (1965).
68. C. K. Wanebo, K. G. Johnson, K. Sato, and T. W. Thorslund, Breast cancer after exposure to the atomic bombings of Hiroshima and Nagasaki, *N. Engl. J. Med.* **279,** 667–671 (1968).
69. B. MacMahon, P. Cole, and J. Brown, Etiology of human breast cancer: A review, *J. Natl. Cancer Inst.* **50,** 21–42 (1973).
70. D. M. Lowell, R. G. Martineau, and S. B. Luria, Carcinoma of the male breast following radiation, *Cancer* **22,** 581–586 (1968).
71. M. Deutsch, F. J. Altomare, Jr., A. S. Mastrian, and J. P. Chervenak, Carcinoma of the male breast following thymic irradiation, *Radiology* **116,** 413–414 (1975).
72. J. B. Gilbert, Carcinoma of the male breast, *Surg. Gynecol. Obstet.* **57,** 451–466 (1933).
73. M. D. Sachs, Carcinoma of the male breast, *Radiology* **37,** 458–467 (1941).
74. G. L. Nicolis, R. Sabetghadam, C. C. S. Hsu, A. R. Sohval, and J. L. Gabrilove, Breast cancer after mumps orchitis, *J. Am. Med. Assoc.* **223,** 1032–1033 (1973).
75. N. Treves, The treatment of cancer, especially inoperable cancer of the male breast by ablative surgery (orchiectomy, adrenalectomy, and hypophysectomy) and hormone therapy (estrogens and corticosteroids), *Cancer* **12,** 820–832 (1959).
76. N. Treves, G. F. Robbins, and W. L. Amoroso, Serous and serosanguineous discharge from the male nipple, *A.M.A. Arch. Surg.* **73,** 319–329 (1956).
77. A. S. Cain, Cancer of the male breast: Case report, *Mil. Med.* **142,** 892–893 (1977).
78. J. S. Mausner, M. B. Shimkin, N. H. Moss, and G. P. Rosemond, Cancer of the breast in Philadelphia hospitals 1951–1964, *Cancer* **23,** 260–274 (1969).

79. A. O. Langlands, N. Maclean, and G. R. Kerr, Carcinoma of the male breast: Report of a series of 88 cases, *Clin. Radiol.* **27**, 21–25 (1976).
80. J. H. Corwin, E. F. Ferguson, Jr., T. Moseley, and E. N. Willey, Carcinoma of the male breast, *South. Med. J.* **60**, 777–780 (1967).
81. H. T. Karsner, Gynecomastia, *Am. J. Pathol.* **22**, 235–315 (1946).
82. C. Sirtori and U. Veronesi, Gynecomastia: A Review of 218 cases, *Cancer* **10**, 645–654 (1957).
83. M. Cutler, *Tumors of the Breast*, pp. 426–453, J. B. Lippincott Co., Philadelphia (1962).
84. G. L. Nicolis, R. S. Modlinger, and J. L. Gabrilove, A study of the histopathology of human gynecomastia, *J. Clin. Endocrinol.* **32**, 173–178 (1971).
85. G. A. Bannayan and S. I. Hajdu, Gynecomastia: Clinicopathologic study of 351 cases, *Am. J. Clin. Pathol.* **57**, 431–437 (1972).
86. J. F. Bridgman and J. M. H. Buckler, Drug-induced gynaecomastia, *Br. Med. J.* **3**, 520–521 (1974).
87. L. Kalisher and R. G. Peyster, Xerographic manifestations of male breast disease, *Am. J. Roentgenol.* **125**, 656–661 (1975).
88. W. H. Hall, Breast changes in males on cimetidine, *N. Engl. J. Med.* **295**, 841–842 (1976).
89. R. Marcus and S. G. Korenman, Estrogens and the human male, *Annu. Rev. Med.* **27**, 357–371 (1976).
90. L. G. Michels, R. H. Gold, and R. D. Arndt, Radiography of gynecomastia and other disorders of the male breast, *Radiology* **122**, 117–122 (1977).
91. N. Keddie and P. J. Morris, Male breast tumors, *Surg. Gynecol. Obstet.* **124**, 332–336 (1967).
92. L. G. Lome and G. Austen, Metastatic breast carcinoma of prostatic origin, *Am. J. Surg.* **120**, 113–115 (1970).
93. W. D. Seipel and M. Malament, Carcinoma of the prostate with bilateral breast metastases, *J. Am. Geriatr. Soc.* **20**, 510–513 (1972).
94. M. Forman, Roentgenography of the male breast, *Am. J. Roentgenol.* **88**, 1126–1134 (1962).
95. L. M. Axtell, A. J. Asire, and M. H. Myers, eds., *Cancer Patient Survival: Report Number 5*, pp. 157–163, DHEW Publication No. (NIH) 77-992, U.S. Department of Health, Education, and Welfare (1976).
96. R. F. Giffler and S. Kay, Small-cell carcinoma of the male mammary gland, *Am. J. Clin. Pathol.* **66**, 715–722 (1976).
97. M. G. Yogore III and S. Sahgal, Small cell carcinoma of the male breast, *Cancer* **39**, 1748–1751 (1977).
98. R. W. Crichlow and B. Czernobilsky, Paget's disease of the male breast, *Cancer* **24**, 1033–1040 (1969).
99. A. E. Nehme, Paget's disease of the male breast: A collective review and case report, *Am. Surg.* **42**, 289–295 (1976).
100. B. Satiani, R. W. Powell, and W. H. Mathews, Paget disease of the male breast, *Arch. Surg.* **112**, 587–592 (1977).
101. N. Treves, Inflammatory carcinoma of the breast in the male patient, *Surgery* **34**, 810–820 (1953).
102. I. M. Reingold and G. S. Ascher, Cystosarcoma phyllodes in a man with gynecomastia, *Am. J. Clin. Pathol.* **53**, 852–856 (1970).
103. A. Ferlito and L. Dibonito, Adenoid cystic carcinoma of the male breast: Report of a case, *Am. Surg.* **40**, 72–76 (1974).
104. J. B. Taxy, Tubular carcinoma of the male breast: Report of a case, *Cancer* **36**, 462–465 (1975).

105. S. Hart and L. Sisely, Granular cell tumour in a male breast, *Med. J. Aust.* **2**, 1010–1011 (1973).
106. S. M. Sirsat, A. F. Choksey, and D. J. Jussawalla, Ultrastructural study of mammary cancer in the human male, *Indian J. Cancer* **13**, 201–214 (1976).
107. R. B. Everson, M. E. Lippman, E. B. Thompson, W. L. McGuire, E. R. DeSombre, J. L. Wittliff, A. Singhakowinta, and J. P. Neifeld, Steroid receptors in male breast cancer (submitted for publication).
108. G. Contesso, J.-C. Delarue, F. Guerinot, F. May-Levin, and C. Bohuon, Récepteurs aux estrogènes et aux progestogènes en pathologie mammaire chez l'homme, *Nouv. Presse Méd.* **6**, 1951–1953 (1977).
109. P. P. Rosen, C. J. Menendez-Botet, J. S. Nisselbaum, M. K. Schwartz, and J. A. Urban, Estrogen receptor protein in lesions of the male breast. A preliminary report, *Cancer* **37**, 1866–1868 (1976).
110. E. B. Thompson, E. Perlin, and D. Tormey, Steroid-binding proteins in carcinoma of the human male breast, *Am. J. Clin. Pathol.* **65**, 360–363 (1976).
111. G. Leclercq, A. Verhest, M. C. Deboel, F. Van Schoubroeck, W. H. Mattheiem, and J. C. Heuson, Oestrogen receptors in male breast cancer, *Biomedicine* **25**, 327–330 (1976).
112. W. P. Greening and P. M. Aichroth, Cancer of the male breast, *Br. J. Cancer* **19**, 92–100 (1965).
113. P. Peltokallio and T. V. Kalima, Malignant tumours of the male breast in Finland. A report of 51 cases, *Br. J. Cancer* **23**, 480–487 (1969).
114. R. W. Crichlow, E. L. Kaplan, and W. H. Kearney, Male mammary cancer: An analysis of 32 cases, *Ann. Surg.* **175**, 489–494 (1972).
115. R. W. Crichlow, Management of male breast cancer, in: *Breast Cancer Management—Early and Late* (B. A. Stoll, ed.), pp. 167–173, Year Book Medical Publishers, Chicago (1977).
116. M. E. Lippman, J. C. Allegra, E. B. Thompson, R. Simon, A. Barlock, L. Green, K. K. Huff, H. M. T. Do, S. C. Aitken, and R. Warren, The relation between estrogen receptors and response rate to cytotoxic chemotherapy in metastatic breast cancer, *N. Engl. J. Med.* **298**, 1223–1228 (1978).
117. C. Huggins, Jr. and G. W. Taylor, Carcinoma of male breast, *A.M.A. Arch. Surg.* **70**, 303–308 (1955).
118. C. K. Tashima, A. U. Buzdar, G. R. Blumenschein, and J. U. Gutterman, Adjuvant chemoimmunotherapy of stage IV (NED) breast cancer—an update, *Proc. Am. Soc. Clin. Oncol.* **19**, 332, Abstract No. C-103 (1968).
119. J. P. Neifeld, F. Meyskens, D. C. Tormey, and N. Javadpour, The role of orchiectomy in the management of advanced male breast cancer, *Cancer* **37**, 992–995 (1976).
120. R. L. Stephens and F. M. Muggia, Breast cancer in men, *Am. J. Med.* **57**, 679–682 (1974).
121. L. Hellman and J. Fishman, Oestradiol production rates in man before and after orchiectomy for cancer, *J. Endocrinol.* **46**, 113–114 (1970).
122. B. J. Kennedy and D. T. Kiang, Hypophysectomy in the treatment of advanced cancer of the male breast, *Cancer* **29**, 1606–1612 (1972).
123. P. Juret, Endocrine surgery in male breast cancer (translated by R. Chakravorty and E. Greenberg), in: *Endocrine Surgery in Human Cancers*, pp. 253–256, Charles C. Thomas, Springfield, Illinois (1966).
124. N. Walach and A. Hochman, Male breast cancer, *Oncology* **29**, 181–189 (1974).
125. G. G. Ribeiro, The results of diethylstilboestrol therapy for recurrent and metastatic carcinoma of the male breast, *Br. J. Cancer* **33**, 465–467 (1976).
126. British Breast Group, Assessment of response to treatment in advanced breast cancer, *Lancet* **2**, 38–39 (1974).

127. W. L. Donegan and C. M. Perez-Mesa, Carcinoma of the male breast. A 30-year review of 28 cases, *Arch. Surg.* **106**, 273–279 (1973).
128. T. Battelli, M. Bonsignori, P. Manocchi, and A. Perilli, Progressi in terapia, *Minerva Med.* **68**, 1663–1666 (1977).
129. Y. Horn and B. Roof, Male breast cancer: Two cases with objective regressions from calusterone ($7\alpha,17\beta$-dimethyltestosterone) after failure of orchiectomy, *Oncology* **33**, 188–191 (1976).
130. J. Geller, H. Volk, and M. Lewin, Objective remission of metastatic breast carcinoma in a male who received 17-alpha hydroxy progesterone caproate (Delalutin), *Cancer Chemother. Rep.* **14**, 77–81 (1961).
131. F. M. Muggia, Hormonal management of breast cancer, *Br. Med. J.* **2**, 179 (1969).
132. F. J. Ansfield, H. L. Davis, Jr., G. Ramirez, T. E. Davis, E. C. Borden, R. O. Johnson, and G. T. Bryan, Further clinical studies with megestrol acetate in advanced breast cancer, *Cancer* **38**, 53–55 (1976).
133. M. C. Li, D. E. Janelli, E. J. Kelly, H. Kashiwabara, and R. H. Kim, Metastatic carcinoma of the male breast treated with bilateral adrenalectomy and chemotherapy, *Cancer* **25**, 678–681 (1970).
134. N. Treves and A. I. Holleb, Cancer of the male breast. A report of 146 cases, *Cancer* **8**, 1239–1249 (1955).
135. E. N. MacKay and A. H. Sellers, Breast cancer at the Ontario cancer clinics, 1938–1956: A statistical review, *Can. Med. Assoc. J.* **92**, 647–651 (1965).
136. M. Brunet, M. L. Janin, and J. Berlie, Carcinoma of the breast in man, *Nouv. Presse Méd.* **6**, 721–724 (1977).
137. G. G. Ribeiro, Carcinoma of the male breast: A review of 200 cases, *Br. J. Surg.* **64**, 381–383 (1977).
138. B. Satiani and R. W. Powell, Cancer of the male breast: A thirty-year experience, *Am. Surg.* **44**, 86–93 (1978).

Index